Morrice McCrae has been House Physician and House Surgeon at the Glasgow Royal Infirmary, Hall Fellow at Glasgow University and Consultant Physician at the Royal Hospital for Sick Children, Edinburgh. He is a Fellow of the Royal Colleges of Physicians of Edinburgh and of Glasgow, and College Historian of the Royal College of Physicians of Edinburgh. He is the author of *The National Health Service in Scotland: Origins and Ideals* (2003), *The New Club: A History* (2004) and *Physicians and Society* (2008).

SIMPSON

The Turbulent Life of a Medical Pioneer

Morrice McCrae

BIRLINN

This edition published in 2011 by
Birlinn Ltd
West Newington House
10 Newington Road
Edinburgh
EH9 1QS

www.birlinn.co.uk

First published in 2010 by
John Donald, Edinburgh

ISBN 978 1 78027 025 8
eBook ISBN 978 0 85790 062 3

British Library Cataloguing-in-Publication Data
A catalogue record for this book is available on request
from the British Library

Typeset in Garamond by
Koinonia, Manchester
Printed and bound in Britain by
CPI Cox & Wyman

Contents

Introduction and Acknowledgements   vii
A Note on Sources   x
List of Illustrations   xi

 1 The Ambition to Rise   1
 2 A Sense of Exclusion   13
 3 Revival   30
 4 Professor of Midwifery   43
 5 Physician to the Queen   56
 6 Experimental Medicine: Galvanism and Gynaecology   69
 7 Library Medicine: Evolution of Disease   78
 8 Library Medicine: On Cholera   89
 9 Ether   105
10 Chloroform   117
11 Fortune, Family and Fame   138
12 Homoeopathy, Mesmerism and Blackmail   150
13 Influence and Power   167
14 Private Practice, Archaeology and Semmelweis   187
15 Acupressure and Hospitalism   202
16 Triumph and Decline   218
    Epilogue   234

Appendix I: The Last Illness of Sir James Y. Simpson   237
Appendix II: Publications by James Young Simpson   247

Notes   253
Bibliography   270
Index   275

Introduction and Acknowledgements

Some men are born great, some achieve greatness,
some have greatness thrust upon them.

Shakespeare

On 4 November 1847, James Young Simpson raised a tumbler containing liquid chloroform to his nose, took a deep breath and immediately became unconscious. When he recovered a few minutes later he knew that he had found the general anaesthetic that he had been searching for. Other anaesthetics had been tried but none was so instantly effective, so pleasant to inhale or so convenient to administer. The discovery of chloroform was one of the great moments in the history of medicine. It was cheap and easy to produce. It could be made immediately available everywhere and patients everywhere could be relieved of the appalling agonies of surgery. Surgery itself was transformed, no longer restricted to operative procedures that could be completed within the brief limits of the patient's ability to withstand pain.

Chloroform was the most famous, and is now the best remembered, of Simpson's many great achievements. He was an outstanding clinician but he devoted the greater part of his career to the advance of medicine and medical science. When he graduated there in 1832, Edinburgh University was the most prestigious and most advanced medical school in Britain. Yet even at Edinburgh, candidates for the degree of Doctor of Medicine, the degree that gave them licence to practise, were still examined on the works of Hippocrates and Galen, the authorities of Greek and Roman times. As students, they had been schooled in the ancient concept that good health required that the four body fluids or 'humours' – blood, phlegm, yellow bile and black bile – should be in perfect balance. When ill, the balance of a patient's humours could, in theory, be restored by opening a vein or applying leaches to 'bleed' him; by administering a course of 'clysters' (enemata); or by prescribing substances to make him vomit or to increase the volume of his sputum. To decide on which of these measures was appropriate, it was necessary only to listen carefully to the patient's account of his symptoms, to examine his appearance and his behaviour, to feel his pulse and to inspect his excreta. Even the most successful physicians could not cure their patients; they could only encourage and support them and make their illnesses more bearable by the administration of opium, quinine or digitalis, the only efficacious drugs then available. And, when the illness passed, they could advise their patients on the regime of diet and exercise that would best aid their recovery. For the best part of two centuries discoveries in anatomy, physiology and pathology had been slowly undermining the ancient Hippocratic concept of disease but no new comprehensive model had yet been put in its place. And the advances in anatomy, physiology and pathology had brought little change in the treatment of the sick.

Simpson's earliest ambition was to make his mark in the reform and advancement of medical practice. But to have the necessary authority and influence he saw it as essential that he should first achieve the status of a professorship at Edinburgh University, and that presented him with great difficulties. When he graduated from Edinburgh at the age of twenty-one, the long years of war with Revolutionary France were over but the principles that had inspired that revolution in 1789 were still alive and fears that the same revolutionary movement might spread to Britain still lingered on. The government in Westminster, and the corrupt establishment that it had created to secure the loyalty of every major institution and the holder of every public office in Britain during the dangerous and disturbed years of the war, still saw every movement for change as a threat to the peace and stability of the nation. In 1832, that reactionary and uneasily defensive establishment still held office in Britain's universities and was in very firm control at Edinburgh University. As a student Simpson had taken no active part in politics, but he had associated freely with known radicals and had been open in his sympathy with the principles that had motivated revolution in France. From the beginning of his career it was clear to Simpson that his ambitions could never be achieved without opposition, struggle and conflict.

This biography of Simpson is first the story of the part played by one man in leading medicine and surgery into the modern world. It is also the story of a boy who became a medical student at the age of fifteen and, without family or political influence, became a professor of medicine at the age of twenty-nine and the most celebrated physician in the western world before he was forty.

This account of his life is based largely on works written by Simpson, or written to him or about him by his contemporaries. These many texts are to be found in the collections held in the libraries of the Royal College of Physicians of Edinburgh, the Royal College of Surgeons of Edinburgh, the University of Edinburgh and the West Lothian Local History Library. I am therefore especially grateful for the encouragement and cheerfully efficient assistance that I have received over many months at these libraries from Iain Milne, Estella Dukan, Marianne Smith, Arnott Wilson and Sibyl Cavanagh. Malcolm Nicolson, Chris Short and Jennifer McCrae have very kindly read the text and have provided me with much very helpful and constructive criticism. Alexander Fenton, Iain Donaldson, Gordon Thomson, Tom Smith, Hilary Pearson, Robert Simpson and Michael Barfoot have all responded readily to appeals for their expert advice and assistance on points of particular difficulty. I offer my special thanks to Iain Milne who has marshalled, edited and presented the illustrations. I also wish to thank the Scottish Society of the History of Medicine for its support. To all those who have helped in the writing and production of this biography I am deeply grateful.

A Note on Sources

The source of James Young Simpson's correspondence, as referred to throughout the text, is either J. Duns, *Memoir of Sir James Young Simpson, Bart.,* which he wrote in 1873 (the original correspondence he used is no longer to be found), or the archive of the Royal College of Surgeons of Edinburgh. All of his many pamphlets are in the archive of the Royal College of Physicians of Edinburgh.

List of Illustrations

Plate section 1

Simpson, Fellow of the Royal College of Physicians of Edinburgh at the early age of 25. (Royal College of Physicians of Edinburgh)

The Lawnmarket in 1825 as it was when Simpson arrived in Edinburgh as a student. (Royal College of Physicians of Edinburgh)

Robert Knox (1779–1862), a distinguished comparative anatomist and medical scientist destroyed by his inadvertent involvement in the affair of Burke and Hare in 1829. (Royal College of Surgeons of Edinburgh)

Park House in which Professor James Hamilton established Edinburgh's Lying-in Hospital in 1793. When the building was sold by his heirs in 1842 Simpson transferred the hospital to Queensberry House. (Royal College of Physicians of Edinburgh)

John Thomson (1765–1856), Professor of Military Surgery and later of General Pathology. A prominent Whig, he was Simpson's first professional patron. (Royal College of Surgeons of Edinburgh)

Edinburgh University: the new college building (now Old College) designed by Robert Adam and completed after his death by William Playfair in 1827. (Royal College of Physicians of Edinburgh)

The Royal College of Physicians of Edinburgh: the New Hall designed by Thomas Hamilton in 1844 and, after extensions, completed in 1868. (Royal College of Physicians of Edinburgh)

Simpson's house at 52 Queen Street, enlarged to accommodate his growing practice by the still clearly visible addition of a top floor. (Royal College of Physicians of Edinburgh)

Alexander Simpson, Simpson's brother, born in 1797, a banker and active proprietor of the family bakery and distilling businesses. (Royal College of Physicians of Edinburgh)

Miss Jessie Grindlay of Toxteth in Liverpool, Simpson's second cousin, soon to become his wife. (Royal College of Physicians of Edinburgh)

James Y. Simpson, newly elected Professor of Midwifery and the Diseases of Women and Children, in 1840. (Royal College of Physicians of Edinburgh)

'Class Ticket' for Simpson's lecture course. (Royal College of Physicians of Edinburgh)

Professor Robert Christison (1797–1882), physician and toxicologist: the most influential member of Medical Faculty when Simpson was appointed to his chair at Edinburgh. (Royal College of Physicians of Edinburgh)

Queen Street, Edinburgh: The Royal College of Physicians at no. 9. (Royal College of Physicians of Edinburgh)

The discovery of chloroform. An artist's impression of Simpson, James Matthews Duncan and George Keith intoxicated by their first inhalations of its vapour. (Wellcome Library, London)

Plate section 2 (colour)

Henry Dundas (Viscount Melville), Lord Advocate, in 1775. Later War Secretary, First Lord of the Admiralty and manager of government business in Scotland during his friend William Pitt's years as Prime Minister. (Scottish National Portrait Gallery)

William Hare, body-snatcher, released after giving evidence against William Burke. (Royal College of Physicians of Edinburgh)

William Burke, body-snatcher, executed on 28 January 1829. (Royal College of Physicians of Edinburgh)

Surgeons' Hall when Simpson became a licentiate of the Royal College of Surgeons in 1830. (Royal College of Surgeons of Edinburgh)

Princes Street in the 1840s when Simpson was establishing his fashionable medical practice in Edinburgh's New Town. (The New Club)

James Syme (1799–1870), Professor of Clinical Surgery at Edinburgh and Simpson's long-standing adversary. (Royal College of Surgeons of Edinburgh)

Robert Liston (1794–1847), Simpson's extra-mural tutor on surgery in Edinburgh before becoming Professor of Surgery at the new University of London. One of the first surgeons in Britain to use ether as a general anaesthetic. (Royal College of Surgeons of Edinburgh)

James Miller (1812–1864), Professor of Surgery at Edinburgh Royal Infirmary, who assisted Simpson by making the initial clinical trials of chloroform anaesthesia. (Royal College of Surgeons of Edinburgh)

Rev. Thomas Chalmers. Evangelical and leader in the creation of the Free Church of Scotland in 1843. (Scottish National Portrait Gallery)

Sir James Y. Simpson, Bart., in 1866. (Royal College of Physicians of Edinburgh)

Simpson's Pill Box. (Royal College of Physicians of Edinburgh)

The Coat of Arms of James Y. Simpson, mysteriously matriculated some weeks before he was created a baronet. (Office of the Court of the Lord Lyon)

St Columba's Cell (c.AD 567) discovered by Simpson among the ruins of the ancient abbey on Inchcolm in the Firth of Forth in 1857. (Royal College of Physicians of Edinburgh)

Plate section 3

Simpson's announcement and account of his discovery of chloroform to the general public of Britain and North America. (Royal College of Physicians of Edinburgh)

James Y. Simpson, elected President of the College of Physicians of Edinburgh in 1850. (Royal College of Physicians of Edinburgh)

The apparatus designed by John Snow, London's first anaesthetist, for the administration of chloroform. (Linda Stratman)

An inhaler designed for the recreational use of choloroform. (Linda Stratman)

Newhaven Fishwives who for centuries sold their wares on the streets of Edinburgh. Simpson studied the social conditions in which they lived in their home village near his house, Viewbank, at Trinity. (Royal College of Physicians of Edinburgh)

The first use of chloroform in midwifery recorded in the Edinburgh Royal Maternity Hospital Case Book. (Royal College of Physicians of Edinburgh)

Simpson's *Answer* to the expected religious objections to the use of anaesthesia in childbirth, widely distributed to the general public in Britain and North America. (Royal College of Physicians of Edinburgh)

Lady Simpson. (Royal College of Surgeons of Edinburgh)

Florence Nightingale (1820–1910), who took nurses to serve in the war in the Crimea; Simpson sent surgeons. (Royal College of Physicians of Edinburgh)

Sophia Jex-Blake (1840–1912), founder of the Edinburgh School of Medicine for Women, in 1887. (Royal College of Physicians of Edinburgh)

Joseph Lister (1827–1912), Professor of Surgery at Glasgow from 1860, at Edinburgh from 1869 and at London from 1877: a pioneer of antiseptic surgery. (Royal College of Physicians of Edinburgh)

Sir James in his later years wearing his famous seal-skin coat. (Royal College of Physicians of Edinburgh)

The new Royal Infirmary, completed in 1879. Built as interconnected but distinct pavilions, it shows the influence of Simpson's ideas on the control of hospital infection. (Royal College of Physicians of Edinburgh)

Edinburgh from Warriston Cemetery where Simpson was buried in 1870. (Royal College of Physicians of Edinburgh)

ONE

The Ambition to Rise

*The love of independence, the disdain of being patronised,
the desire to accumulate and the ambition to rise.*

William Cobbett

In 1870, Sir James Y. Simpson died full of honours.[1] Queen Victoria mourned the loss of so great a man. For over twenty years he had been famous in Britain, Europe, North America and elsewhere as the greatest obstetrician of his time. And people everywhere had come to revere him as the man whose chloroform had rescued them from the dread and agonies of surgery and childbirth. His ideas and his methods had been unconventional and had attracted bitter opposition. But he had flourished, even in Edinburgh where medical life was riven by professional enmities and personal polemics to a degree unknown elsewhere in civilised society.[2] At the end of his life he had already been acclaimed as a 'Prometheus among physicians'[3] and he has become the subject of legend.

The legend had it that he had been born and bred in rural poverty. But the story of his life was even more remarkable than the legend, and the key to an understanding of the man is a true understanding of his origins. For generations, his forebears had been subsistence farmers in Linlithgowshire.[4] But he was born in 1811 into the new middle class that had recently emerged and had just begun to make its mark.

His grandfather, Alexander Simpson, was born in 1725, when Scotland was a poor country wasted by centuries of wars and internal strife and still enjoying little of the promised benefit from its recent union with England. The greater part of Scotland's landscape was occupied by hill, moor and low lying marsh. Land fit for cultivation and accessible for the great clumsy old wooden Scots plough was confined mainly to the lower slopes of the hills. On the higher slopes, what fertile soil existed was often little more than a skin over bone. The patches of land where it had been possible to establish farms were oases in a bleak open landscape with few trees and no hedges or boundary walls, drab and colourless except for the yellow of the whins.

Linlithgowshire was fortunate. It offered more land suitable for farming than most other counties in Scotland. The flat land was almost free of bogs and marshes, and the slopes of the low hills could be worked by the plough or provide good pasturage for livestock. But, as elsewhere in Scotland, the system of farming still continued much as it had for centuries. Each farm was let to as many as a dozen tenants housed in cottages grouped together in a 'ferm-toun'. The best land near the cottages of the ferm-toun, (the 'in-field') was routinely manured and ploughed in long ridges ('rigs') up to twenty or more feet wide and separated by deep furrows that, filled with briars and stones, served as a primitive system of drainage; the rigs produced, in a set annual rotation, crops of oats, bere,[5] and barley. The farm's more distant rough land (the 'out-field') offered grazing for livestock and space for occasional crops of grey oats. Each of the farm's many tenants raised his crops on his allotted spaces among the rigs and grazed his due number of beasts on the communal out-field. For many of the tasks on the farm, from cutting peat to the building of houses, the men, women and children of the ferm-toun pooled their labour; and the total produce of the farm, even when harvests were at their most abundant, was consumed locally by the landlord's household[6] and the families of the ferm-toun.[7] But harvests were seldom abundant. The soil of the rigs, tired and often sodden, produced scanty crops and the rank out-field could nourish only thin and scraggy livestock. The rural population was never far from starvation.

At the end of the seventeenth century Scotland's ancient system of agriculture failed utterly. Every year from 1696 until the end of the century, cold, sunless and drenching summers followed by bitter early frosts and deep snow in the autumns had blighted the crops. By January 1697 the people of Scotland were starving. Sir Robert Sibbald, president of Edinburgh's Royal College of Physicians, wrote of seeing 'death in the faces of the poor that abound everywhere; their ghostly looks, their feebleness, their agues and their fluxes threaten them with sudden death. Some die by the wayside, some drop down in the streets, the poor sucking babes are starving from want of milk which the empty breasts of their mothers cannot furnish. Crowds of men and women are forced to prowl and fight for food like beasts.'[8] On the farms, sheep and cattle died in their thousands. The great famine continued until 1700. When it ended, up to a third of the rural population had been lost through death by starvation and disease, by migration to the towns to beg or by emigration to Ireland. Villages and ferm-touns were sadly reduced in size and some had disappeared into ruins. On the farms that remained, little livestock had survived and what would normally have been kept as grain seed had been eaten. Recovery was barely possible as harvests failed again and again until the second half of the century.

Alexander Simpson's parents were tenants on the farm at Winchburgh, in the parish of Kirkliston. Eleven miles from Edinburgh on the coach road to Falkirk, Winchburgh was a settlement of eight cottages, distinguished from other ferm-touns only by its posting-inn, its stables and its smithy. The family had survived the famines and the even longer periods of poor harvests by finding additional employment. As a boy, Alexander Simpson had been apprenticed at the local smithy and had later become a busy journeyman blacksmith and farrier, maintaining the implements of the farm and shoeing the horses at Winchburgh's stables. The farrier was then still looked to as the proper source of advice on animal medicine.[9] Alexander Simpson became well known in the surrounding parishes for his unusual skill in the management of the ailments of farm livestock. He had learned traditional cures during his apprenticeship and many of his animal nostrums were derived from witchcraft. To give a farm lasting protection from disease, he advised that a corner of the farm should be fenced off as the 'Guidman's Croft' and left as an offering to the devil. When a herd was feared to be at risk during an outbreak of 'marain' (cattle plague) he advised that one of the healthy cows should be sacrificed by being buried alive.

Traditionally in Scotland, blacksmiths were also expected to be skilled in the treatment of the broken bones of human patients.[10] Alexander not only treated fractures, he also built up a more general practice as a healer. Bloodletting was part of his answer to almost every human illness and he also made use of some of the ancient folk remedies of rural Scotland; to relieve the pains of childbirth, for example, he recommended the application of white onions in oil to the mother's abdomen.[11] However, as his letters indicate, Alexander Simpson had received some formal education. It is probable that, like parish ministers and the other educated men and women in rural Scotland who, in the absence of trained medical men, were looked to for advice on the care of the sick, he relied for guidance on Buchan's *Domestic Medicine*.[12]

As was the practice for craftsmen serving Scotland's ferm-touns, Alexander took his share in the working of Winchburgh's communal farm, and it was as a resourceful farmer, as well as an educated and enterprising man, that he attracted the attention of his landlord, the Earl of Hopetoun. During the harvest failures that recurred in 1707–8, 1724–5 and 1740–1 many of Lord Hopetoun's tenant farmers had lost everything, including their seed corn and their livestock. Unable to pay their rents, many had been forced to give up their tenancies. By the 1750s, Lord Hopetoun was having difficulty in finding tenants who could afford to rent, seed, equip and stock his farms. To encourage his surviving tenants to continue, he allowed them a stay of their rents for a year; thereafter, he selected for special attention those who had shown willingness to accept new ideas and the ability and drive to make the best of a very difficult situation. For these chosen tenants, of whom Alexander Simpson was one, he did everything possible to inspire them and give them 'the strength and spirit to carry on the work'.[13] The work he had in mind was the introduction of more efficient modern farming methods.

These new farming methods, first developed in the Netherlands, had already been put into practice in some parts of England. In 1723, Thomas Hope of Rankeillor and Robert Maxwell of Arkland had founded the Honourable Society of Improvers to promote these more efficient and more productive farming methods among landowners in Scotland. However, those most eager to make the most of their land were the lairds and lesser aristocracy who depended entirely on the land for their living, and they lacked the capital necessary for modernisation. Some of the most adventurous, notably John Cockburn of Ormiston, invested what they had in improving their properties, but with insufficient capital and no ready access to lucrative markets for their produce, they came almost to bankruptcy; in 1736 Cockburn was obliged to dispose of his estate to Lord Hopetoun.

Then in the middle years of the eighteenth century there came a dramatic change. Scottish merchant adventurers had made their way into the markets of what had once been England's, but were now Britain's, colonies in America and had come to dominate the immensely lucrative trade in tobacco. Thereafter Scotland's transatlantic trade had expanded, and the new banks – Ship Bank, Glasgow Arms Bank, Thistle Bank – that had been established for the capitalisation of the overseas trade had money to invest in agricultural improvement at home. Scotland's landowners were now able to enjoy a bonanza.

The lesser landlords could now find the money for the investment that their properties so urgently needed. When their ventures proved to be highly profitable, the great aristocratic landowners quickly became aware that their estates need not be kept at great expense only as a display of their wealth and place in society, but could be developed as a commercial enterprise and a source of even greater wealth.

Gradually, in estates in almost every part of Scotland, groups of two or three traditional runrig farms were brought together and 'consolidated' as single farms of 300 or more acres, and leased to single tenants. The open runrigs that had occupied the fertile land were replaced by fields enclosed within stone walls. Thousands upon thousands of trees were planted to shelter the crops, the beasts and the new farm buildings. The fields were effectively drained, limed and fertilised; new crop rotations were devised; wheat and potatoes were introduced into the rotations; and better wintering and feeding were provided for livestock.

As more and more runrig farms were consolidated and more efficient farming methods were introduced, ever fewer men were needed to work on the land. Touring Scotland with Boswell in 1773, Dr Johnson wrote of an 'epidemical fury of emigration'.[14] In Linlithgowshire almost all those displaced from the farms were not forced to move overseas but were able to find work in the growing industrial towns of central Scotland. It was said that, in one part of the county, the number of men still working on the land was only one sixth of the number that had once made that their living. The great majority of those who remained were no longer independent small farmers, subtenants or cottars but were members of a new proletariat of paid farm servants. The few who remained as the sole tenants of the new large 'commercial' farms now took no part in common everyday tasks in the fields but had become managers, masters of all the techniques and skill of modern agriculture.

Lord Hopetoun had been one of the founding members of the Honourable Society of Improvers and he was among the first Scottish landowners to take advantage of the new opportunities to invest in commercial farming. Alexander Simpson had not only shown that he was a competent farmer and an enterprising man, but from his work as a blacksmith and his practice as a 'healer' he also had the financial resources to equip and stock a modern farm. In 1764, Lord Hopetoun[15] offered him the tenancy of Slackend, a farm nine miles from Winchburgh in the parish of Torphichen. At the age of thirty-nine, Alexander Simpson was no longer a landless cottar and blacksmith but, as the tenant of a thriving farm of some 300 acres, he had become one of a new farming elite.[16]

When he moved to Slackend, Alexander Simpson and his wife Isabella Grindlay already had a family of one daughter and five sons. The first two sons, Alexander[17] and John,[18] were then just old enough to begin work on the farm. In the years that followed, they helped their father to expand and develop it into a very successful family business. For both farmers and landowners in Scotland, the second half of the eighteenth century was a time of unprecedented prosperity. Investment in extensive and costly programmes of improvement was well rewarded. Grain yields first doubled and later trebled, and the number of slaughtered animals rose six-fold. A rapid increase in Scotland's total population[19] and the growth of its towns created new markets. After years of stagnation, grain and livestock prices increased. In the new commercial farming, rents were no longer paid in kind but in cash. Landowners became cash rich. Some of the largest became extravagantly wealthy and commissioned Robert Adam or Robert Mylne to build great country houses (Inveraray for the Duke of Argyll, Culzean for the Earl of Cassillis). Lesser gentry, who for generations had shared the drudgery and discomfort of their tenants, found themselves rich enough to build and furnish fashionable neo-classical houses, leaving their former homes to serve as barns or shelter for the livestock.

The farm servants also gained. Before the consolidations and enclosures small farmers and cottars had lived in houses that were part of a row of low farm buildings that included the byres for the cattle. They had little furniture apart from bedding, a table, a few stools or chairs and a kist or two. They wore clothes of home-produced wool or flax spun and woven at home and made up into garments by a local tailor. Only the 'guidman' habitually wore boots made by the local cobbler; the women and children normally went barefoot. The staple foodstuff was oats in some form: as porridge made with water, or as 'bread' (oat bannocks), baked on a bake stone set alongside the fire. The bannocks were eaten with milk, livened on special occasions by the addition of a dram of whisky. 'Loaf bread' (bread made with wheat) was a rarity. Meat in any form was an occasional luxury.

By the 1790s, this had all changed. The contributor reporting on a parish in Lithlithgowshire for Sir John Sinclair's *Statistical Account of Scotland* wrote: 'A great alteration in the manner of living has taken place in this parish within the last 40 years. About 1750 there were not above 10 families who used tea and now there is not above twice that number who do not use it. Butchers meat was then not used more than tea; scarcely any cattle or sheep were killed except at Martinmas when families used to salt a whole or part of an ox or cow to serve for winter provision; but now there is a regular flesh market twice a week and almost every family, who can afford it, eats flesh constantly. A much greater quantity of wheaten bread is now consumed in the parish in a month than was in a twelvemonth forty years ago. The alteration in dress is also remarkable. When the good man and his sons went to kirk, market, wedding or burial they were clothed in a suit of friezed cloth or homespun kelt[20] with a blue or brown bonnet; and the good wife and her daughters were dressed in gowns and petticoats of their own spinning with a cloth cloak and hood of the same or a tartan or red plaid. But now the former, when they go abroad, wear suits of English cloth and good hats; and the latter the finest printed cottons and sometimes silk gowns, silk caps and bonnets of different shapes, sizes and colours, white stockings and cloth shoes.'

For the few who, like Alexander Simpson, had been cottars but were now tenant farmers, the change was even more dramatic. Passing through that part of Linlithgowshire in 1787, Robert Burns commented in his diary on the elegant luxury now enjoyed by the local farmers.[21] Alexander Simpson had been particularly successful, and after only a few years his family business ventured into distilling. In the first half of the eighteenth century almost every communal runrig farm had its whisky still. Since the Union with England the excise laws had applied in Scotland, but the owners of these small stills were left undisturbed unless they 'played' their stills on a Sunday. But as the new consolidated and improved farms began to produce barley in commercial quantities whisky distilling became a profitable, legitimate business enterprise. While Alexander Simpson, with his oldest sons, Alexander and John, continued to develop and expand the family farm, he set up Thomas, his third son,[22] as a distiller at Kirkliston; Thomas was later able to buy a small estate some two miles from Slackend and become the Laird of Gormyre. Alexander Simpson's only surviving daughter, Margaret,[23] married William Kay, a prosperous distiller in Torphichen.[24]

Only his youngest sons, David[25] and George,[26] declined at first to join the family business. In 1785, they ran off to make their fortunes in London. They travelled on foot, supporting themselves by casual employment as they went. In London, they had still failed to find any congenial gainful occupation when, in February 1790, a Spanish fleet seized a number of British ships off the north-east coast of the Pacific and made claim to the British trading post at Nootka Sound on Vancouver Island. To counter these 'outrages', the government in London ordered the navy 'to fit out forty ships of the line and to recruit the necessary sailors by press-gang if necessary'.[27] When David and George reported to their father that they had had several narrow escapes from the press-gangs he wrote in reply: 'To run off to London to be made soldiers either by land or sea is what I never thought you or any belonging to me ever intended. The war is about to break out. If you had a mind to shun it you would come home and look like your father's sons.'[28]

Both young men returned to Scotland. George did not immediately report to his father. For two years he made a living as a smuggler on the west coast, but eventually he joined his brother Thomas as a distiller in Kirkliston. David returned home, but not to the family farm. A little over a mile from Slackend was Balbardie, the biggest estate in the parish of Bathgate. It had been inherited in 1766 by Alexander Marjoribanks, an enthusiastic improving landlord and successful entrepreneur. In 1783, he had founded the Glenmavis distillery on his property, leasing it to a succession of tenants. In 1790, Alexander Simpson bought the lease for his son David. As a distiller, David made a very comfortable living and, in January 1792, he married Mary Jarvey, the daughter of the prosperous farmer of Balbardie Mains.

David and Mary Simpson lived at Glenmavis for eight years and had seven children there. For three of these years they lived very well, but in the summer of 1795 poor harvests led to food shortages. Since it was feared these shortages might exacerbate the social and political unrest that was already troubling Scotland,[29] the government prohibited distilling for some months in the winter of 1795–6 in order to ensure an adequate supply of grain for food. There were further short periods of prohibition following the poor harvests that recurred during the next few years. In 1798 and again in 1800, Parliamentary inquiries into the distilling industry resulted in increases in excise duties on whisky.[30] It became increasingly difficult for distillers to make a profit and many of the smaller distilleries went out of business. Then, in 1808, because of wartime shortages of grain, distilling from grain was again prohibited, this time for over a year.[31] David Simpson first tried to make a better living as a brewer; he then tried to make sugar of lead (lead acetate, then used as a sugar substitute or a fixative for dyes) but with disastrous results. In 1810, with the little ready money he still possessed, he moved with his family to set up in a new business in Bathgate.

Bathgate was then a rapidly growing town, eighteen miles from Edinburgh on the main road to Glasgow. In the 1750s Bathgate had only 1,590 inhabitants and almost every one of its families made some part of its living from weaving. But as farming in the surrounding parishes and counties became more commercial, more market driven and more productive, Bathgate grew into a busy and prosperous town. From 1792, a new turnpike road built to link Edinburgh and Glasgow passed through Bathgate, making the town the major agricultural centre in the area with a cattle market second in size only to Scotland's principal market at Falkirk.

The merchants, specialist craftsmen, bankers, lawyers and the other professional men who were needed to service the expanding commercial farming community in Linlithgowshire made Bathgate their centre. By the end of the century the population of the town had risen to 2,300; there was a bank; there were three lawyers where there had been one ('and he had less business than any one of the three now has'); there were two ministers and four surgeons. There were seven shopkeepers but still no bakery, although local farms had begun to grow wheat in addition to the traditional oats and barley and a flour mill had already been built on the Bathgate Water on the outskirts of the town. David Simpson had had some experience of the bakery business during his early travels in England. It seemed to him that there was now an excellent opportunity for him to become the only baker in Bathgate.

In 1810, with his wife and children he moved into a stone cottage on Bathgate's cobbled Main Street; one of its four rooms was made to serve as bedroom, kitchen, bake house and shop. It was over twenty years since David Simpson had had any experience of the bakery business and even then he had not served a full apprenticeship; in addition to his lack of experience and training he did not have the drive and business acumen of his father, his uncles or his brothers. And soon after moving to Bathgate his wife, now aged forty, became pregnant for the eighth time and was unable to provide him with the help and guidance on which he had come to depend. Almost at once his business began to decline and, when his last child, James,[32] was born in May 1811, he was almost bankrupt.

However, within days of her confinement, his wife, Mary Jarvey, took charge of both family businesses. Within months the bakery was flourishing and Mary was able to move her family into larger and more comfortable quarters in a two-storey house on the other side of the Main Street. And when the Treaty of Fontainebleau ended the war with France in 1814, the Glenmavis distillery recovered and again began to show a profit.

James Simpson (not yet James Y. Simpson) was born into a quietly affluent, secure and loving extended family. His father was an amiable man, popular among the people of Bathgate and always welcome as a drinking companion in the local inns. But he was somewhat feckless. He was a fond father, but those who knew him well thought his relationship with his sons peculiar; even when they were still very young they treated him as a companion and friend rather than as a parent. He introduced James to all the legends, the folk tales and the stories of magic and witchcraft that he had learned from his own father. But it was his wife who was the real parent to their children. And it was Mary Jarvey who inspired her youngest son and fired his ambition to become a great man.

On her father's side, Mary Jarvey was descended from a Huguenot family (Gervais) who had fled to Scotland in the 1680s. They had settled first in Stirlingshire but had lived and farmed in Linlithgowshire for the best part of a century. Her mother, Mary Cleland, was the daughter of Cleland of Auchinlea whose ancestors had held land in Lanarkshire since the thirteenth century; one had campaigned with his cousin Sir William Wallace, another had fought alongside Robert Bruce at Bannockburn.[33] Mary Jarvey took great pride in her lineage. She was quiet, deeply devout and a gentle loving mother, but she never forgot that she was descended from Scotland's ancient gentry and she was determined that her son James should recover for her family the position in society that she felt she had lost.

James was brought up almost as a single child. When he was born his brother Thomas had already left home to found his own business as a merchant in the busy port of Grangemouth, and his sister Mary had gone with him and later became his housekeeper. Alexander and John were well launched on their careers in Bathgate. David had been at school for three years, and George died when James was still an infant. James was a much cherished child, a 'rosy bairn with a laughing mouth and dimpled cheeks'.[34] During his earliest years his mother was able to spend much of her time with him and to direct the first steps in his education. It soon became clear that he had a keen intelligence, a remarkable memory and an appetite for everything he was taught. For the family, even in these early years, he was their 'wise wean'. His mother decided that he was the son who should become famous and raise the family's position in society, and she had no difficulty in extracting a promise from his brothers and sisters that they would play their parts in helping to promote her ambition.

His mother had intended that James should be educated at home with the assistance of a private tutor. But suddenly in 1815, the village school in Bathgate became one of the best endowed and most generously and professionally staffed parish schools in Scotland.

Bathgate's benefactor was John Newland. Born in the village in 1737, he had served an apprenticeship as a carpenter. But at the age of seventeen, perhaps because of a quarrel with his stepmother, he left home. He found employment as a carpenter at the Royal Naval Dockyard at Chatham at a time when the Royal Dockyard was the largest industrial enterprise in the Empire.[35] A few years later he was transferred to the Royal Naval Dockyard at Port Royal in Jamaica. He remained there for the rest of his life and became a successful businessman and planter with over 100 slaves and a property valued at £30,000. He took one of his slaves, Elizabeth, as his common-law wife and lived happily with her for over thirty years; they had two sons. When he became terminally ill in 1799, he made a will but he was prohibited from bequeathing his fortune to Elizabeth or his two sons since, by Jamaican law, they were still slaves. When he died in 1800, he had done what was legally possible to provide for Elizabeth and his sons, but the greater part of his estate of £48,000 was left to be divided among his surviving relatives in Bathgate, none of whom he had ever met. However his will contained a crucial provision: his relatives were not to receive their legacy, £29,527 2s 3d, for ten years, and during those years his trustees were to 'pay and apply the interest of the whole of such principal money in the erection of a free school in the parish of Bathgate'. As his trustees, he nominated the lairds of three estates in the parish, Alexander Marjoribanks of Balbardie, Andrew Gillon of Wallhouse and William Baillie of Polkemmet, along with the parish minister, Mr Jardine.

The special provision in his will was disputed by the relatives, but it was vigorously defended in the courts by the trustees. It was not until 17 August 1815 that the Privy Council ruled that the provision should stand. The trustees now had at their disposal the accumulated interest of ten years, a sum of approximately £14,000 (equivalent to £1,050,000 now). It was decided to allow the major part of the sum to continue to gather interest until it became sufficient to build the school that Alexander Marjoribanks, the most active of the trustees, now had in mind.[36] But it was also decided that some part of the available funds should be used immediately to make better provision for the education of the children of the parish.

In the early years of the century, the parish school in Bathgate had been a one-room affair with a single teacher. Families had paid the teacher 'for teaching their sons to read, write and sometimes arithmetic and their daughters to read and often to sew and to write'.[37] The changes effected in 1815 by Newland's trustees were dramatic. Classrooms were opened at seven sites across the parish.[38] A headmaster was appointed at the then very handsome salary of £90 per annum; seven university-educated assistant masters were appointed at correspondingly generous salaries of up to £56 per annum. Within a very short time, Bathgate Parish School, at its seven sites, had a total roll of over 500 pupils. Most of Bathgate's children still left school as soon as they were old enough to find work and contribute to the family income; in their short time at school they could only be taught to read and write and to have some skill in arithmetic, although now to a higher standard. The others could now continue at school and be taught English, Latin, mathematics and perhaps some Greek or French. James Simpson became one of the first to benefit from the free schooling now offered to children in the parish of Bathgate.

When he first went to school he was short and stocky with a remarkably large head, made even more striking by his shorter than average frame. At home he was described as a 'child of cherubic innocence', 'gentle as a girl, quiet and affectionate'.[39] As a very young boy in the family bakery he was often to be seen contentedly tracing his letters and numbers in the flour on the shop counter. Later he helped from time to time in the delivery of scones and baps (bread rolls) to his father's customers, but he spent the greater part of his time in the family shop where he was able to ignore the noise and bustle and read quietly on his own; customers became accustomed to seeing 'the baker's lad at his Latin'. But at school the red-headed James Simpson was considered steerin' (aggressive) in both the playground and the classroom[40] and had always a great 'readiness for conflict'.[41] He was fiercely competitive with a keen but intolerant critical intelligence. These contrasting patterns of behaviour that were to be so characteristic of the adult were already apparent in the child – gentle, affectionate and considerate within the circle of family and friends, but fiercely combative and unrelenting when exposed to the competition of potential rivals.

When he was nine, his mother died after a long illness. His sister Mary, now aged twenty, returned from Grangemouth and took her place in managing the home and in providing James with continuing care and affection. His great-uncle, George Jarvey, a brewer and innkeeper in Bathgate, became his chief mentor, encouraging and adding new directions to his studies. George Jarvey was an enthusiastic student of natural history and archaeology, and James acquired an interest in both that lasted for the rest of his life. At school he continued to find the work easy: his memory was prodigious and his industry remarkable; he was, by far, the outstanding pupil. To his family he had once been their 'wise wean'; now he was their 'young philosopher'.[42] When he reached the age of fourteen, they were agreed that he must continue his education at university. They set him no clearly defined objectives. As had been directed by his mother, his family had simply commissioned him to be famous.[43] He chose to make himself famous in science and medicine.

TWO

A Sense of Exclusion

*The moving power in this species of government is
of necessity Corruption.*

Tom Paine

Plump, rosy and resplendent in his corduroy suit, Simpson set out for Edinburgh at the beginning of the new academic year in 1825. Edinburgh University had no residential colleges. The university's governing body, the Town Council, had long since decided that it was to the advantage of both the town and the students that they should not be cloistered within the university but should live as members of the general population of Edinburgh. His family had arranged for the fourteen-year-old Simpson to share lodgings with an old school friend in Stockbridge, an ancient village on the Water of Leith that had become one of Edinburgh's most handsome and fashionable suburbs, linked by way of Royal Crescent to the city's elegant New Town.[1] He arrived at 1 Adam Street, accompanied by a quantity of luggage and a generous supply of food, on the carrier's cart that plied regularly between Bathgate and Edinburgh.

From the beginning his family made every effort to ensure that Simpson should live comfortably for as long as he chose to continue his studies at Edinburgh. He was kept generously funded by his brother Alexander, now both manager of the family business and an agent of the Royal Bank of Scotland, and by his brother John, now a lawyer and an agent of the new Standard Life Assurance Company. Simpson could therefore easily afford the three shillings he paid each week for his lodgings. The record that he kept of his expenditure shows that he could also afford such minor luxuries as cake, fruit and fresh fish, and even extravagances such as a plentiful supply of snuff. In his first days at Edinburgh he was able to buy not only the books that he required for his studies but also Byron's *Childe Harold,* a volume of Milton's poems, Paley's *Natural Theology,* Adam's *Antiquities* and Sir Walter Scott's *Fortunes of Nigel.* Later that year, in preparation for his studies of anatomy, he was able to buy all four volumes of Fyfe's

Anatomy, Alexander Monro's *Elements of the Anatomy of the Human Body in its Sound State* (both volumes), *The Anatomy and Physiology of the Human Body* by J. and C. Bell, *The London Dissector: A System of Dissection Practised in the Hospitals and Lecture Rooms of the Metropolis* and *The Economy of Human Life* by Robert Dodsley.

Simpson's style of living might have been envied by many of the students at Edinburgh. Of the several thousands who enrolled for classes there, only 2,260 were matriculated students studying for degrees in Arts, Medicine or Divinity.[2] The great majority had no plan to take a degree. They paid the required class fees directly to the professors whose classes they wished to attend but did not matriculate and become members of the university unless they wished to have access to the university library. Some of those who chose to matriculate were affluent young men who had travelled to Edinburgh to complete a liberal and polite European education at what was widely recognised as one of the leading centres of learning of the time; others were studying for a short time at Edinburgh before moving on to Oxford or Cambridge. A number were grammar or parish school boys who meant only to acquire the command of Latin, Greek, and mathematics and moral philosophy that was expected of those who wished to matriculate as students preparing for a career in one of the learned professions (medicine, the law or the church). But the great majority of the 8,000 or so non-matriculated students were boys or young men who hoped to acquire, in the shortest possible time and at the least possible expense, the knowledge of Latin, Greek and mathematics that the Church of Scotland required of candidates for its licence to teach at a parish school.[3] Most were barely able to afford their class fees and, for their sustenance, they had only the sacks of oatmeal and whatever other supplies that they could carry with them when they walked to Edinburgh at the beginning of each term.

The friend that Simpson joined in lodgings in Stockbridge was John Reid, the son of a well-to-do cattle dealer and farmer at Bathgate. Like Simpson, he had been a pupil at the village school in Bathgate and there they had become close friends. Two years older than Simpson, John Reid had already completed his preliminary studies of Latin, Greek, moral philosophy and mathematics at Edinburgh and was now in his second year as a matriculated medical student. Their lodgings were in the top flat of a house owned by Dr Alexander MacArthur.

MacArthur had come first to Edinburgh as an impecunious student making his own way without financial help from his family. After his first year, he had left university for a time to earn enough to allow him to complete the remaining years of study required for a degree in medicine. He had become an assistant schoolmaster at Bathgate, and there he had taught both Simpson and John Reid. By 1825, he had taken his MD degree but was still supporting himself by teaching, now at a public school in Edinburgh. He had also been engaged by Simpson's family to act as his personal tutor and mentor.

Simpson very quickly became profoundly influenced by MacArthur's political views. Simpson was only fourteen years old and had grown up in a family and in a community in which the processes of government and the niceties of political allegiance seemed to have no relevance to everyday life. The impact of MacArthur's convictions shaped Simpson's years as a student and had a lasting influence in colouring his political allegiances. MacArthur was a committed Radical, fiercely opposed to the political system that had enabled a corrupt regime to keep a firm grip on power in Britain for over half a century. This system of 'Old Corruption', as it became known,[4] had always been particularly strong in Scotland where, as Lord Cockburn recorded in his *Memorials,* it 'engrossed almost the whole wealth, and rank and public office of the country'.[5] In Edinburgh, it had subverted every one of the city's great public institutions. In 1825, MacArthur resented it as an intolerable and shameful anachronism.

Edinburgh was now a modern city that had broken out from its ancient walls. The elegant squares and terraces in its New Town made Edinburgh one of the most admired cities in Europe. Its modern piped water supply now ensured high standards of cleanliness in public places. The existence of gas lighting in its streets and a police force[6] created a new sense of safety and order. New roads connected Edinburgh with Scotland's growing towns, and a new canal linked the capital with the heartland of the country's flourishing industries in the west. Stage coaches still ran between Edinburgh and London, but most passengers now preferred to travel on the new steam packets that sailed regularly from Leith. Edinburgh had become a modern nineteenth-century city. But, in 1825, its institutions were still governed by a political system that belonged to a different age.

The system had been designed in the aftermath of the Jacobite Rebellion of 1745. In a drive to destroy the Highlands as a source of military power, the clans had been disarmed and the hereditary jurisdictions, which supported the authority of the clan chiefs, had been withdrawn. Even the office of Secretary of State for Scotland had been abolished. In Scotland it was feared that the government in London might go even further and abolish the few remnants of independence that had been left to Scotland in the Treaty of Union in 1707. The political factions in Scotland[7] now buried their differences and joined together to ensure the survival of Scotland's national institutions – the Law, the Universities, the Royal Burghs and the Kirk[8] – by demonstrating their loyalty to the crown and their readiness to conform to the demands of the government in London. This they achieved by acquiescing in a system of government in which patronage from above was traded for loyalty from below. At the heart of the system was the election of Scotland's representatives at Westminster. Scottish peers had the power to elect sixteen of their number to the House of Lords, but before each election the government of the day issued a King's List of the peers whose election would be most acceptable and a subservient peerage accepted that there was nothing to be gained by voting against the wishes of the government. Scotland's towns sent fifteen members and the counties thirty members to the House of Commons. In the towns only the town councillors had the right to vote. In the counties only those landowners who held the feudal superiorities could vote, and in very many cases their votes could be influenced by the wishes of one or other of a very small number of great feudal magnates. Ultimately, only a small and manageable number of men determined who was to represent Scotland in Parliament, and their loyalty could be secured by the patronage of the Crown, the Treasury or other government-controlled institutions. And the government not only created a reliable body of support in Parliament, it also established its control of Scotland's 'independent' public institutions by ensuring that only those whose loyalty could be relied on, or whose loyalty could be secured, were elected to office.

This corrupt system became fully effective in 1775, when the distribution of all government patronage in Scotland was delivered into the hands of the Lord Advocate, Henry Dundas. As he rose in the hierarchy of government in London – becoming at various times Treasurer of the Navy, First Lord of the Admiralty, President of the Board of Control of the East India Company, Lord Privy Seal in Scotland, Home Secretary and, for twenty years, the constant and much valued colleague of William Pitt, the First Lord of the Treasury and the King's chief minister[9] – his command of patronage increased until his power in Scotland became all but complete. He could command members of the political classes by the promise of advancement in the peerage, generous pensions, lucrative or prestigious public office, or personal influence or support; for their sons he could provide commissions in the armed forces or cadetships in the East India Company. For the professional classes in Scotland he could secure advancement in the judiciary, the church and the universities. This unofficial but accepted arrangement ('Old Corruption') ensured that every national institution, and every appointment made within them, was subject to the approval of Dundas. This 'Dundas Despotism',[10] although quite evidently corrupt, was very generally accepted in Scotland since it provided strong, consistent and competent government.

By the mid-1780s, government fears of another Jacobite rebellion had subsided, but when revolution toppled the government of France in 1789 government fears revived; this time, fears of a much more popular and dangerous rebellion. The events in Paris had been widely and enthusiastically welcomed across Britain and disturbingly large numbers of the population formed societies (notably 'The Society of the Friends of the People, Associated for the Purpose of Obtaining a Parliamentary Reform' in London, and 'The Friends of the People'[11] in Scotland) to campaign for similar radical reform in Britain. In 1792, the Prime Minister, William Pitt, instituted a system of terror that was pursued with 'vigour beyond the law';[12] it was conducted with the greatest severity in Scotland, where Dundas' already despotic powers enabled him to clamp down with particular harshness. During 'Pitt's Terror', political activists were pilloried, shipped off to Botany Bay or sentenced to years in prison; a few were hanged. In 1806, Pitt died and Dundas was forced from office but the 'Terror' continued under their successors.

As the fear of invasion by the French began to recede, Pitt's Terror was conducted at a somewhat lower intensity. But it did not stop; it was judged that a measure of repression was still required to maintain civil order. Until 1815 wartime scarcities and poor harvests led to high food prices, public demonstrations and occasional rioting. When the war came to an end, a short period of relative prosperity was soon followed by economic decline, unemployment, poverty, food shortages and further public protests. These were brutally crushed by troops of cavalry. The most notorious 'slaughters' were at Peters Field near Manchester[13] and later at Bonnymuir near Falkirk.[14] The government and its loyal supporters (now generally called 'Tories'[15]) argued that, to maintain civil order, all those advocating reform (now commonly referred to as 'Whigs') should be excluded from positions of influence. This was readily achieved in Scotland where, under Henry Dundas, every appointment to office within every national institution had already been brought under the control of government ministers or their appointees. In the 1820s, candidates for public office, even within the universities, required Tory patronage or strong personal influence if they were to be successful.

While Dundas was 'manager' of Scotland he had used his powers largely to Scotland's benefit. Edinburgh's professors of history, moral philosophy, literature and political economy – William Robertson, Adam Ferguson, Hugh Blair and Dugald Stewart, among others – were appointed, or retained in office, and were able to attract students from Europe and America as well as from every part of Britain. And William Cullen, Alexander Monro II, Andrew Duncan, John Gregory, Joseph Black and John Hope, the professors of medicine, surgery and anatomy, public health, medical ethics, medical chemistry and botany, made Edinburgh University the leading medical school in the Western World. But after Dundas' resignation, government patronage was not used with such attention to merit, and the teachers who had made Edinburgh's reputation were succeeded by lesser men who, in many cases, owed their appointments entirely to family influence and political favour.

Simpson's first two professors provided him with two quite different illustrations of the exercise of this administrative corruption within the university. His professor of Greek, George Dunbar, had been a gardener until, at the age of twenty, he suffered an injury that precluded him from any occupation that involved physical labour. His employer in Berwickshire paid for him to become a student at Edinburgh where, after two years, he had mastered enough Latin, Greek and mathematics to be granted a licence to teach by the Church of Scotland. He was immediately employed as tutor to his son by Sir William Fettes. Originally a tea merchant in Edinburgh, Sir William had been the contractor for the provisioning of every military establishment in Scotland during all the years of the wars with France. He had become rich with country estates in the Borders and elsewhere in Scotland; he was made a Baronet, Lord Provost of Edinburgh and therefore, *ex officio*, Chancellor of Edinburgh University. In 1805, when he no longer required George Dunbar's services as tutor to his son, he arranged for him to be appointed as professor of Greek at Edinburgh. As a professor he was not a success. His classes, held every morning at eight o'clock, were not popular; during the winter months he 'sat with pale composed visage betwixt his two dingy tallow candles while snores and yawns, with practical jokes of diverse kinds, wore through the long hour'.[16] Ineffective in the classroom, he produced volumes of printed summaries of his lectures which his students were obliged to buy.

James Pillans, Simpson's professor of Humanity (Latin), had been appointed by the exercise of special interest of a very different kind. Born in Edinburgh in 1779, he had been an outstanding pupil at the High School when Alexander Adam was Rector. At Edinburgh University, he had been taught by Alexander Dalzel, John Playfair and Dugald Stewart. He had established long-lasting friendships with the most distinguished of his contemporaries at Edinburgh: Francis Jeffrey,[17] Francis Horner,[18] Henry (Lord) Cockburn, Henry Brougham[19] and the future Marquess of Londonderry all, in their time, prominent Whigs; later he contributed to the Whig *Edinburgh Review*. After graduating MA at Edinburgh in 1801, he had taught at Eton until, in 1810, he was persuaded by his Edinburgh contemporaries to apply for the post of Rector of the High School. In his memoirs Lord Cockburn wrote: 'It seemed hopeless. His superiority to the other candidates was never doubted but the black spot of Whiggism was upon him. This would certainly have been conclusive in the [Tory] Town Council had not some of his friends proposed a reference to a few of the judges, including President of the Court of Session Blair, who quashed his brethren and warmly recommended Pillans.'[20] Ten years later, Pillans again enjoyed the same influential support and was elected, without opposition, as professor of Humanity.

Unlike Dunbar, James Pillans was an excellent teacher, but even he found Simpson a strangely difficult and unresponsive student. Simpson's performance showed that he had lost all appetite for work. MacArthur reported to his family in Bathgate that he could not persuade him to keep to a proper routine of study. His written work was never graded higher than 'tolerably good' and, at least once, it was described as 'very bad'. He was dismissive of the teaching he was offered by his professors. He took a carefully written record of every lecture he attended, producing texts that were liberally sprinkled with ? and ! and derogatory comments that marked the many passages that he found unsatisfactory. When his essays were returned to him he would indicate the few criticisms that he was willing to accept and then add 'I object to the rest'.

The causes of Simpson's negative behaviour at this time are perhaps uncertain. It has been suggested that, while at school in Bathgate he had always been the prize pupil, at Edinburgh he was disturbed to find himself only one of many equally talented students. However, it is much more probable that he was disheartened and depressed by the threat of Old Corruption[21] that MacArthur had revealed to him. Many years later he said that at this time he had felt 'poor and almost friendless'.[22] Certainly he could not command the wealth that had established Professor Dunbar's career or the influential friends who had secured prestigious appointments

for Professor Pillans. It must have seemed that, unable to satisfy the requirements of 'Old Corruption', he was inevitably doomed to failure.

However, encouraged by Professor Pillans, he did not abandon his
studies. At the end of his first year Pillans advised him to enter the competition for the Stewart Bursary. The bursary had been established by the
Rev. James Stewart of Carolina and was open to students named Stewart
or Simpson (his wife's name). There were few applications and the examination was not rigorous; Simpson was duly awarded a bursary of £10 for
each of the following three years while he continued to attend lectures on
Arts subjects.

For his second year, Simpson enrolled again with Dunbar and Pillans
for their senior classes in Greek and Humanity, and now also with Professor
William Wallace for mathematics and Professor John Wilson for moral
philosophy. Simpson was inspired by neither. William Wallace was a self-
educated man who had begun life as an apprentice bookbinder. He had
taught mathematics at Perth Academy and at the Royal Military College,
Sandhurst, before being elected professor of mathematics at Edinburgh
(in preference to Charles Babbage, the inventor of the first computer, the
'automatic calculating engine'). He was a poor teacher and was best known
for his contributions on mathematical subjects to the fourth edition of the
Encyclopaedia Britannica. John Wilson was famous as 'Christopher North',
author of 'Noctes Ambrosianae', a long series of articles published in *Blackwood's Magazine* in which literary reviews and amusing commentaries
on the people and books of the day were presented as conversations in a
tavern. Although professor of moral philosophy, Wilson had little interest
in the subject; but since he was a fascinating talker on the many subjects
that did interest him, his students were ready to forgive him for teaching
them no moral philosophy at all.

Simpson's second and third years as a student of the Arts were no more
distinguished than his first. However, in the autumn of 1826 and at the
beginning of his second year as an Arts student, he had recovered some
degree of confidence and had also enrolled as a medical student. Candidates for the degree of MD were required to produce evidence that they
had attended the classes given by the professors of Botany, Chemistry,
Anatomy and Surgery, Institutes of Medicine, Practice of Medicine,
Clinical Medicine, Midwifery and Materia Medica, as well as three-month
courses on two of the optional subjects taught by the professors of Medical
Jurisprudence, Clinical Surgery, Practical Anatomy and Natural History.
In his four years as a medical student he duly attended these university

lectures, but university professors were not the only teachers in Edinburgh offering classes on medical subjects. For many years before the Town Council of Edinburgh agreed to the establishment of a medical faculty within its university, it had been its practice to license a very limited number of physicians and surgeons to teach medical subjects elsewhere within the city. After the university faculty was founded in 1726, this practice ceased; the Town Council appointed no more extramural lecturers, but successions of able and ambitious young physicians, surgeons, anatomists and chemists at the beginning of their careers had continued to make their mark by teaching every aspect of medicine at private schools, usually in houses in Brown's Square or in Surgeons' Square near the Royal Infirmary. For the most part those attending these extramural classes in the first decades of the nineteenth century were not university students but young men preparing for the examinations for the licentiate diploma of either the Royal College of Surgeons of Edinburgh or the Royal College of Physicians of Edinburgh; in the 1820s the number taking the diploma of one or other of the Royal Colleges each year was always more than twice the number being awarded the university degree of MD.[23] But a number of those who enrolled in Edinburgh's extramural classes were not candidates for the diploma of an Edinburgh college. Some were from abroad and had chosen to come to Edinburgh for only part of their professional medical training; a few had chosen to study anatomy or chemistry in Edinburgh as part of a liberal rather than a professional education. Lastly there were those university students who were either attracted by the reputation of an extramural lecturer or dissatisfied with the standard of teaching offered by one or more of the professors of the university's Faculty of Medicine.

James Russell, the professor of clinical surgery, for example, was an uninspiring lecturer who had the 'inveterate habit of yawning while he spoke and continuing to speak while he yawned'.[24] Many university students chose to supplement his teaching by attending the extramural lectures of Robert Liston, an outstanding lecturer and the finest and most dextrous operator of his generation in Britain. The university professor who, year after year, was found wanting by almost every one of his students was Alexander Monro *tertius*. He was the grandson of Alexander Monro *primus*, who had become the university's first professor of anatomy in 1720, and the son of Alexander Monro *secundus*, who had succeeded to his father as professor in 1758. Alexander Monro *tertius* had 'inherited' the chair in 1798 but had proved to be a great disappointment. The well known story that, for forty-eight years, he did no more than read his grandfather's lecture notes verbatim to his class is probably apocryphal,[25] but he was certainly a very poor lecturer. Sir Robert Christison wrote in his *Recollections* that 'his manner betrayed an unimpassioned indifference, as if it were all one to him whether his teaching was acceptable and accepted or not. He lacked neither ability nor accomplishments but apathy in a teacher cannot stir up enthusiasm in a student. He lost command of his class which in his later years became the frequent scene of disturbance and uproar.' Almost every one of Monro's students who could afford to pay two sets of class fees also attended classes at the school of one of Edinburgh's three extramural lecturers in anatomy, John Lizars at No. 1 Surgeons' Square, John Aitkin at No. 4 or Robert Knox at No. 10. Both Simpson and his friend, John Reid, chose to become pupils of both Robert Liston and Robert Knox.

By 1828, John Reid had attended Knox's lecture course three times and had become Knox's assistant and demonstrator in the dissecting room. Simpson completed Knox's course twice and, like John Reid, he became not only one of Knox's student assistants but also his friend. It was his association with Dr Knox that was to draw Simpson into the most notorious scandal ever to descend on the medical profession in Edinburgh. The scandal and its aftermath confirmed and deepened Simpson's distrust of the network of power and influence that could make or, more probably, break his own career.

On Christmas Eve 1828, William Burke was condemned to death for a series of murders carried out specifically to supply bodies for anatomical dissection. The bodies of the victims had been sold to Robert Knox but, since he had played no part in the murders, Knox was not tried along with Burke in the High Court. But he was tried and found guilty in the court of public opinion and abandoned by Edinburgh's medical establishment.

Robert Knox was born in Edinburgh in 1793. When still an infant he suffered a severe attack of smallpox which destroyed his left eye and badly disfigured his face.[26] Because of this deformity he was not sent to school but, until he was twelve, he was taught at home by his father. His father, a mathematics teacher at George Heriot's School, was deeply in sympathy with the principles of the French Revolution and he had been a founder member of the Society of the Friends of the People in Scotland. To escape prosecution and dismissal from his post as a teacher, he had made his peace with Henry Dundas and abandoned his open political activities,[27] but not before he had passed on his political principles to his son. From 1805, Robert Knox was a pupil at Edinburgh's High School where he was an outstanding pupil, becoming Dux of the school and Gold Medallist in

1810. He then became a medical student at Edinburgh. There he was taught anatomy by Alexander Monro *tertius* but learned so little that he failed to satisfy the examiners in anatomy when he presented himself for the degree of MD. For the next year he attended the classes of John Barclay, then the foremost of Edinburgh's extramural teachers of anatomy; by 1814, when he was awarded his MD, he had already been inspired by John Barclay to become an anatomist.

After graduating, he went to London to study under John Abernethy at St Bartholomew's Hospital, but within a few months war broke out again with Napoleon's armies in France. Knox joined the Army Medical Department and in June 1815 he was sent to Brussels to assist in the management of the thousands of casualties from the battle of Waterloo. Knox was then posted to South Africa where, from 1817, he was heavily involved in the treatment of the casualties of both sides in the Kaffir Wars between the Xhosa people and the British settlers supported by British troops. In 1820 he was released from the army on half-pay and returned to Scotland.

During his five years of army service he had carried out a great many post-mortem examinations and had begun what later became a large and important collection of skilfully dissected pathological specimens. He had also widened his interests to include comparative anatomy, dissecting and studying the sharks and dolphins caught on the voyages to and from South Africa as well as the animals he had shot as game while there; his observations had been published in the *Edinburgh Medical and Surgical Journal* and the *Edinburgh Philosophical Journal*. In 1821, still on half-pay from the army,[28] he travelled to Paris, and for a year he continued his anatomical studies with Professors Boyer and Roux at La Charite.

Back in Edinburgh he was elected a Fellow of the Royal Society of Edinburgh. He continued to build up his collection of anatomical specimens and exhibits without which a teacher of anatomy would be 'in the state of a man without a language'.[29] In 1825, he became a partner in John Barclay's Anatomy School at 10 Surgeons' Square and a year later he was appointed by the Royal College of Surgeons of Edinburgh to be conservator of its museum. There he quickly brought together over 15,000 pathological anatomy specimens, making it the second largest collection in Britain.[30]

When John Barclay died in 1826, Knox became the sole proprietor of the school at 10 Surgeons' Square. In Barclay's last year some 300 medical students attended his lecture course; when Knox succeeded him the number enrolled for his lecture course increased to 504, 'the largest anatomy class ever assembled in Britain'.[31] In the advertisements for his school Knox promised that for those attending his somewhat smaller practical class of anatomical dissection, arrangements had been made 'to secure as usual an ample supply of anatomical subjects'.[32] In the dissecting room, one body was allotted to each group of students and as many as twelve students might be working together at any one time.[33] Securing this 'ample supply' of cadavers became even more difficult when anatomical dissection was made a compulsory subject for both the university degree of MD and the licentiate diploma of the Royal College of Surgeons. By 1828, the number of students enrolled for Knox's practical anatomy class had risen to 355 and there were also other medical students enrolled at John Lizars' school, at John Aitkin's school and at Professor Monro's school at the university. To supply all four schools with adequate numbers of cadavers had now become very difficult indeed. To do so legally was impossible. The law allowed Edinburgh's anatomy schools to have for dissection only the bodies of criminals who had died in custody, stillborn infants, found-lings who had died before school age and suicides who had no friends or relatives to take charge of the body. This legal source of subjects for dissec-tion had been quite inadequate since the middle of the eighteenth century and trafficking in bodies had become tacitly accepted as a necessary evil by everyone not directly involved, and conveniently ignored, whenever possible, by the city's magistrates.

A handful of merchants in bodies made a precarious living from the trade. When a friendless pauper died in one of Edinburgh's sordid lodging houses these merchants would present themselves as long-lost relatives and remove the body for a 'family' burial; or when they heard of a death, or even an impending death, among the desperately poor in Edinburgh's crowded tenements, they would offer to buy the body for some paltry sum from a family grateful to be relieved of the cost of a funeral. Wherever acquired, the body could be sold on to one of the anatomy schools for £8 in the summer or £10 in the winter.[34]

Bodies of the recently buried could also be removed from their graves. Usually during the hours of darkness, professional grave robbers ('resur-rectionists') could quickly dig down through the recently disturbed earth, break open the coffin, remove the body and carry it off in a sack. Very often the grave robbers were not professional resurrectionists but medical students in urgent need of 'subjects' for dissection, an essential part of their own training. Students who robbed graves did little or no damage to their reputations or their careers; some of Knox's 'grave robber' students later achieved positions of the greatest respectability – including William Fergusson, later Professor of Surgery at King's College, London and Sergeant Surgeon to the Queen; Robert Liston, later Professor of Clinical Surgery at London University; Thomas Wharton Jones, later Professor of Ophthalmic Medicine at University College, London; and Simpson's friend John Reid, Professor of Anatomy at St Andrews University. While there is now no documentary evidence that Simpson took part in grave robbing, it must be assumed that he did. As Knox's assistant, John Reid took it on himself to lead grave robbing expeditions to procure the necessary number of cadavers for Knox's practical classes in dissection, and he relied on his friends to take part.[35]

For more than 100 years the families of the recent dead had dreaded the depredations of medical students and professional 'resurrectionists'. From as early as 1711, there had been a number of public protests, yet successive governments had done nothing to suppress their activities. There was therefore a long-subdued anger to fuel the public outrage that erupted when in November 1828 it was discovered that William Hare, his wife Margaret, William Burke and his partner Helen McDougal had killed sixteen lonely and friendless strangers and sold their bodies for dissection. They had plied their victims with whisky until they were rendered helpless and then suffocated them so carefully that they left none of the signs of physical violence that might have raised suspicion of murder. They had first intended to sell the bodies to Alexander Monro at the university but a student, whom they met only by chance, had advised them to take their dead victims to Robert Knox's school at Surgeons' Square. There the bodies had been logged in by one or other of Knox's student assistants – John Reid, William Robertson, Thomas Wharton or Alexander Miller – and had been paid for by Knox's laboratory manager, David Paterson. There was no suspicion that they had been unlawfully killed until, eventually, one of the bodies delivered to the laboratory was recognised.[36] At an autopsy carried out on the body on 2 November 1828, Robert Christison, the professor of Medical Jurisprudence, found that 'death by violence is probable', although 'I do not think that the medical circumstances could justify a more certain opinion'.[37] By then Burke, Helen McDougal, Hare and Mrs Hare had already been arrested. However, the legal evidence against them continued to be so thin that a prosecution only became possible when Hare agreed to confess and give King's Evidence against Burke and McDougal in return for freedom for himself and his wife. At the trial, the case against Helen McDougal was found Not Proven; Burke was found guilty and on

28 January 1829 he was hanged.

There was never the slightest evidence that Knox had instigated or even known of the murders committed by Burke and Hare before Hare confessed. However, in the weeks from the discovery of the murders until the execution of William Burke, the people of Edinburgh were in a frenzy of rage whipped up by extra editions of the newspapers and by specially published news sheets. In the public mind, Knox was found guilty of murder by association. His house in Newington was besieged, and in the street he was hanged in effigy. At his school in Surgeons' Square, teaching was made almost impossible by the disturbance caused by the crowd picketing the building.

Knox was able to withstand the attentions of the mob; he told his students of 'how little [he] regarded these ruffians in spite of daily warnings and the destruction of [his] property'. However, he found it impossible to shrug off the disparagement and humiliation he was to suffer from leading members of both the Senate of Edinburgh University and the Council of the Royal College of Surgeons.

Knox was a distinguished medical scientist, acknowledged as one of the leading philosophical anatomists in Europe.[38] He was also the most brilliant and effective teacher of anatomy of his time in Edinburgh. But he was also a Radical in his politics and a public advocate of the principles of the Society of the Friends of the People in Scotland. While his lectures displayed 'a rare union of scientific precision and literary elegance', they were also enlivened by flashes of satirical wit at the expense of the Tory medical establishment; for many months his hilarious gibes had been winning loud applause from Edinburgh's medical students. The dignitaries of the Council of the Royal College of Surgeons and Senate of the University were unforgiving. A committee that included the professors of Clinical Surgery, Institutes of Medicine and Military Surgery pronounced that the part that Knox had played in the crimes of Burke and Hare must be a matter of deep and lasting regret to all those interested in the promotion of the study of anatomy. The professor of moral philosophy was even more damning. In March 1829, he wrote in *Blackwood's Magazine*: 'Dr Knox stands arraigned at the bar of the public, his accuser being human nature. He is not the victim of some wild and foolish calumny; the whole world shudders at his transactions; and none but a base, blind, brutal beast can at this moment dare to declare that Dr Knox stands free from all suspicion of being accessory to murder.'

His students, however, were unfailing in their support for Dr Knox.

In April 1829, as a token of their undiminished respect, they presented him with a handsome gold vase. Throughout the whole affair, Simpson played a prominent part in every demonstration of sympathy with Knox as his reputation and his career continued to be deliberately undermined by Edinburgh's medical establishment.

It was perhaps inevitable that, during this time, Simpson should identify strongly with Knox. As a student, he had been on unusually close friendly terms with Knox. At the height of the Burke and Hare affair, Knox had received warm and sympathetic welcome at Simpson's family home in Bathgate.[39] Since his introduction to politics by Alexander MacArthur, Simpson had shared Knox's Radical principles. And, like Knox, he had no wealthy or political patron to promote his career or even to protect his interests. From his first months as a student Simpson had feared that advancement in his career would be made difficult, if not impossible, by the same forces within the College of Surgeons and the university that, led by James Syme, now seemed intent on the destruction of Robert Knox.

James Syme seemed an unlikely person to parade contempt for Knox, largely because of his own somewhat shady practices in purchasing cadavers. Like Knox, Syme had once taught anatomy at an extramural school. From 1823, he had offered practical tuition and experience at his dissection room in a house in Brown Square. He had overcome the difficulty in finding an adequate supply of cadavers from local sources in Edinburgh by importing bodies from London and Dublin in packing cases labelled 'Perishable Goods'; at Leith docks in the summer of 1826, the stench caused the packing cases to be opened and all was revealed. Syme was obliged to resign from his school in Brown Square, and he moved to Minto House to teach surgery. Now, in 1828, Syme was still struggling to establish himself in practice as a surgeon against the competition of the established men in Edinburgh: Liston, Lizars, Fergusson, Thomson and Russell. Knox was not only a teacher of anatomy, he was also a practising surgeon and yet another very accomplished rival for Syme.

As one of the curators of the museum of the Royal College of Surgeons, Syme was in a position to undermine Knox's standing with the college and the university and thus indirectly damage his practice as a surgeon. First he contrived to oust Knox from his post as conservator of the museum of the Royal College of Surgeons; in September 1829, he declined to accept Knox's routine report that the college's collections were in a good state of preservation and informed him that the curators had decided to make their own annual inspection of the museum's collections and publish their own report.

Other such pinpricks continued thereafter until, in March 1831, Knox was instructed to present for inspection all the pathological and anatomical preparations that he had so generously added to the museum in the preceding ten years. When this operation was not completed at once, Syme complained that Knox had failed to show a proper willingness to meet the views of the curators. Asked to give an explanation Knox refused and, in June 1831, he resigned as conservator of the museum. Thereafter Syme began to orchestrate a systematic denigration of Knox that soon became widespread within the university as well as the College of Surgeons. While Knox's reputation continued to be eroded, no one in office in any of Edinburgh's great institutions dared raise his voice to protect him.

Knox continued to teach at Surgeons' Square and continued to attract large numbers of students. In July 1837, his obvious success encouraged him to apply for the newly created Chair of Pathology at Edinburgh. In his letter to the Lord Provost he gave a full account of the years of achievement that had earned him his 'scientific status among the most enlightened body of men in the world'.[40] Bitterly, but unwisely, he added that 'the determined opposition and hostility of numerous individuals and even of associated public and corporate bodies in my own country present the best proofs which those acquainted with the world can require that the individual so strenuously opposed must at least have attainments and a status in science which could not with safety be overlooked'. His application was rejected. In 1842, Knox applied to succeed W. P. Alison in the Chair of the Institutes of Medicine. Again his application was rejected and, at the age of forty-nine, Knox left Edinburgh to rebuild his career in London.

When Knox was eventually forced to leave Edinburgh, Simpson had not only survived, he had made outstanding progress in his career. It was a success that he had not foreseen or even dreamed of in 1829. In that, his last year as a medical student, he had become obsessed by the idea that the prejudices and interests that were then being ranged against Knox would also be ranged against him and would preclude any prospect of a successful career. And he had also concluded that Syme, who had been Knox's enemy, would always be his enemy.

In December 1829, his father became terminally ill and Simpson returned to Bathgate to be at his bedside. When his father died three weeks later, Simpson did not return to Edinburgh. He was still too young to present himself for his MD degree but his family had expected that, as planned, he would take the necessary examinations and become a Licentiate of the

Royal College of Surgeons. However, he insisted that it would be quite pointless for him to go before James Syme and the other examiners at the College of Surgeons since he would undoubtedly be 'plucked' (failed). For months he remained at home, convinced that he could never achieve the eminent place in society that his mother had hoped and planned for him.

THREE

Revival

Fain would I climb, yet fear I to fall
Walter Raleigh

I conceive now that I have a capital chance
James Y. Simpson

Throughout his life, Simpson experienced recurring periods of depression during which he retired to his room and his bed. But he never again suffered the deep and prolonged depression that afflicted him in the winter and spring of 1829–30. Nothing seemed to rouse him. His great-uncle, George Jarvey, tried to rekindle his interest in archaeology and botany. His brother, Alexander, arranged for him, at an exceptionally early age, to be admitted as a Freemason at the lodge in Bathgate. Eventually, and with the greatest difficulty, in April 1830 his brothers bundled him off on the coach to Edinburgh to sit his exams at the College of Surgeons. There, to his surprise, he encountered not the least evidence of prejudice against him and he passed without difficulty.

Now licensed to practise as a surgeon, Simpson applied for the Poor Law post of surgeon for the Renfrewshire parish of Inverkip on the Clyde coast. The salary was small[1] but the parish included the village of Gourock and the burgh of Inverkip, both flourishing communities, and the post seemed to promise an opportunity to build up a private practice. Many years later he wrote that 'if chosen I would probably have been working there still'. However he was not chosen and for eighteen months, again depressed and disheartened and with no other appointment in view, he remained in Bathgate, occasionally assisting the local surgeon, Mr Dawson, and, from time to time, offering his services at the Public Dispensary at Falkirk.

In the summer of 1830, Simpson was sadly resigned to a future as an obscure country surgeon. His family, however, believed that he could still achieve greatness if only he could be roused from his depression and persuaded to complete his university training. His brother Thomas, now a very successful merchant in the busy seaport of Grangemouth, discussed Simpson's difficulties with a second cousin, Walter Grindlay, who, some years before, had transferred his shipping firm from Grangemouth to Liverpool. And later, on 3 June, Simpson's brother John wrote to Walter Grindlay:

'I understand from my brother in Grangemouth that he had mentioned to you that our youngest brother, James, wished to get to be a surgeon of a ship going out on a voyage of twelve or fifteen months. He has been five years studying at the College of Edinburgh and passed surgeon in April last. His ultimate intention at present is to take a degree as physician and practise somewhere in Scotland or England; but he cannot obtain that until he is twenty-one and is only nineteen this month. As to his medical proficiency I am no judge but a friend of mine, Mr Dawson, surgeon here, speaks favourably of him and I know he is a good scholar, steady, upright and attentive and I think would be a good surgeon of a ship. He will require to attend the College another session before taking a degree and his great anxiety at present is to procure a situation which will yield him a little and where he can at the same time see some practice. He is the youngest of us all, and a favourite, and we would be averse to his going in a ship designed for any unhealthy shore, but if you thought your extensive influence could procure him the situation of surgeon in an East Indiaman, or any ship somewhere in that quarter I would take it most particularly kind and hope you will keep him in view should you hear of any suitable situation.'

Walter Grindlay was very willing to help but his ships were engaged in trade with the notoriously unhealthy west coast of Africa and the almost equally unhealthy West Indies. He was not immediately able to find a suitable berth on any ship sailing from Liverpool to India or the East Indies. Simpson meanwhile seemed to settle into life as an assistant in the practice of Mr Dawson, the local surgeon in Bathgate, and for sixteen months he showed no inclination to do as his family wished and return to his studies at Edinburgh. His family, however, did not mean to give up.

In October 1831, just as they had done in April 1830, his brothers again bundled a reluctant Simpson into the coach for Edinburgh. They had undertaken to cover whatever funding he might need to finish his studies and take his degree. It was also arranged that Simpson should lodge with his brother David who, earlier that year, had been set up in business as a baker in Stockbridge, near Simpson's first lodgings in Adam Street. Once more at Edinburgh, Simpson enrolled for the courses that he still had to attend before he would be allowed to present himself as a candidate for the

MD degree. But he still had no expectation of success; he bluntly informed his brothers and sister that he had returned to Edinburgh 'just to please you all'.

To please himself, he proceeded to prepare for what he believed must inevitably be his future as a country surgeon. In the months that he had spent assisting Mr Dawson in Bathgate, he had discovered that midwifery was a major part of a country surgeon's practice; he had also been made very aware that his own knowledge of obstetrics was sadly deficient. As a student he had attended Professor Hamilton's classes on midwifery, but midwifery was then only an optional subject in the curriculum and was not included in the examinations for the MD degree. Professor Hamilton's classes were held at the end of what had usually been busy days and Simpson had regularly fallen asleep during the lectures. Now, in 1831, he enrolled in the extramural classes on obstetrics held by John Thatcher; he went on to attend Dr Thatcher's lecture course no less than three times.

He also took up again his association with Edinburgh's Royal Dispensary for the Poor. He had assisted in the work of the dispensary during his earlier years as a medical student. At that time Dr W. T. Gairdner, the director of the dispensary, had 'been so much satisfied with Mr Simpson's abilities and pains in the discharge of his arduous duties' that he had asked him on several occasions to act as his deputy at the dispensary and in his private practice. Now, in October 1831, Gairdner was happy to award him the formal appointment as his first assistant.

However, Simpson's immediate task was the preparation of his thesis for his MD degree and he chose to write on inflammation. It was an astute choice. The most important contribution to medical science to come from Edinburgh in the early years of the nineteenth century had been John Thomson's *Lectures on Inflammation* published in 1813. The book had quickly sold out and copies were soon changing hands at four times the original price. Translations had been published in France, Germany and Italy and, within a few years, two new English editions were produced in America. Thereafter, Thomson had continued his studies on inflammation and in 1820 he had commissioned the artist (and medical student) Robert Carswell[2] to visit the leading hospitals and medical museums in Europe to make accurate illustrations of the best available pathological specimens relevant to his work on inflammation. After five years, Thomson's collection of over 1,500 drawings, watercolours and engravings had become the finest in existence.[3] In 1831, John Thomson had just been appointed to a new chair of General Pathology and both Thomson and his collection were in Edinburgh. For a medical student at Edinburgh there could be no more appropriate, conveniently accessible and topical subject for study and discussion than inflammation. As his thesis Simpson wrote *De Causa Mortis In Quibusdam Inflammationibus Proxima* ('of the immediate cause of death in certain inflammations').[4]

On 5 June 1832, Simpson reached the required age of twenty-one and in July he presented himself for examination for the MD degree. The examination was in three parts, all conducted in Latin.[5] First, at the home of one of the professors, the candidate was questioned on subjects in the classical medical literature and on various current aspects of both medicine and surgery. Later, in the presence of several of the members of the medical faculty, the candidate was examined by two professors on two aphorisms of Hippocrates and on his written reports on two clinical cases. Lastly, on the day of graduation he presented his thesis and defended it at a public ceremony within the university. Simpson satisfied his examiners and graduated MD on 12 July 1832.

Professor Thomson had read Simpson's thesis when it was first submitted to the university and he was present when it was formally read and examined in public. He was impressed both by the originality of the thesis and by Simpson's skill in defending it on the day of his graduation. He immediately offered Simpson the position as his first assistant at a salary of £50 per annum. Simpson just as promptly accepted.

This was one of the most critical moments in Simpson's career. From childhood he had had behind him a devoted family constantly encouraging in him an acute sense of ambition and a craving for success. However, he had had no one in his family to help him focus his ambition and guide him towards the achievement of success. In his earliest years as a medical student, he had looked to Robert Knox as his mentor but the failure of Knox's career had only made him despair of his own. John Thomson, however, had been born into greater poverty than Knox and had even fewer advantages during his childhood, and he had succeeded where Knox had failed. Thomson had made himself one of the most eminent physicians and medical scientists in Britain. Later, he became known as 'The Chairmaker'[6] having managed the creation of a number of new academic chairs which were immediately filled by Thomson himself or by one or other of his protégés. He had made the careers of a number of these young men and Simpson was to be the greatest of his young protégés. And since he had overcome so many of the difficulties that Simpson expected to encounter in his own career, Simpson adopted Thomson as his model and mentor.

John Thomson was born in 1765, the son of a bankrupt silk weaver in Paisley. From the age of seven, he was employed as a casual labourer by other silk weavers in the town until the family business had recovered. At the age of eleven, he was able to begin a seven-year apprenticeship with his father and, his apprenticeship completed, he continued for a further two years as a journeyman in his father's workshop. He had never been to school. He had been taught to read by his father and had read his father's books (chiefly works on divinity); he had also borrowed books from friends. At a time when his total free income was a penny a week,[7] he had subscribed to a circulating library; and for a year he had paid a tutor to teach him Latin.

At the age of twenty, he was accepted as an apprentice by Dr White, a physician practising in Paisley. While with Dr White, 'his zeal in acquiring medical knowledge was ardent and unremitting, reading the best authors on every medical subject'.[8] He became particularly interested in botany, and early in his apprenticeship he succeeded in making a comprehensive collection of the flora of Arran. It was this collection that won him his first important patron.

One of Dr White's wealthiest patients was Robert Alexander, a descendant of Claude Alexander, who had been paymaster general of the East India Company in the middle years of the eighteenth century. Robert Alexander was an amateur botanist with a large scientific library and a rich collection of plants at Southbar, his house near Paisley. Dr White invited him to inspect his apprentice's new collection. When the collection was enthusiastically admired, John Thomson at once presented it to Robert Alexander; in return, Alexander allowed Thomson to use his library and provided him with all the equipment he required to pursue his new interest in experimental chemistry. When Thomson's two years as Dr White's apprentice came to an end, Robert Alexander arranged for him to attend classes on anatomy and chemistry at Glasgow University. After a year at Glasgow, and with further financial assistance from Robert Alexander, he moved to Edinburgh University to continue his studies of anatomy and chemistry during the academic session 1789–90. Robert Alexander died in 1789, but his patronage did not come to an end. At his funeral, Mr Hogg, manager of the Paisley Bank (and later manager of the British Linen Bank in Edinburgh) informed Thomson that out of respect to his friend Alexander, he would 'endeavour to supply to him the loss he had sustained in Mr Alexander's death'.[9] Until he too died, Mr Hogg continued to be John Thomson's generous patron.

In 1790, Thomson was appointed to the staff of Edinburgh Royal Infirmary, first as assistant apothecary and later as a house surgeon. With the financial support of Mr Hogg, he joined the Royal Medical Society and within a year he had been elected one of its presidents. In 1792, and again supported by Mr Hogg, he resigned from the infirmary and travelled to London where he studied surgery and anatomy at John Hunter's school in Leicester Square. In the summer of 1793, he returned to Edinburgh and, with the continuing financial support of Mr Hogg, he became a Fellow of the Royal College of Surgeons and set up in private practice in Gray's Close in partnership with his friend John Allen.[10] Even as he built up his busy surgical practice, he found time to continue his work on chemistry. He published his edition of *Fourcroy's Elements of Chemistry and Natural History with the Philosophy of Chemistry* in three volumes in 1798, 1799 and 1800.

It was also at this time that John Thomson found his all-important political patron. The Earl of Lauderdale (born James, Viscount Maitland in 1759) was educated at Edinburgh High School and at the universities of Edinburgh, Paris, Oxford and Glasgow. In 1780 he became an advocate in Edinburgh and, as Viscount Maitland, was elected to the House of Commons as member for Newport in Cornwall. After he succeeded to the earldom of Lauderdale in 1789, he was elected as a Scottish representative peer in the House of Lords. Throughout his parliamentary career he was a Radical. In 1783 he spoke against the King's appointment of William Pitt as First Lord of the Treasury (Prime Minister) and thereafter consistently opposed his policies; he was also a fierce critic of Henry Dundas, both as Pitt's closest ally in the Commons and as the government's 'manager' in Scotland. In 1789, he became an outspoken and flamboyant supporter of the French Revolution, styling himself 'Citizen' and wearing Jacobin costume in the House of Lords. Although his enthusiasm for the Revolution faded, he remained a vigorous opponent of the repression of civil liberties that the government, in fear of revolution at home, had imposed in Britain. In 1792, he was a founder member of the Society of the Friends of the People.

In the winter of 1799, Lauderdale was at home in Scotland. In Edinburgh at this time, while 'the middle aged talked of nothing but the French Revolution and its supposed consequences, younger men of good education were immersed in the new chemistry that Lavoisier had made fashionable'.[11] Lauderdale decided to take up this fashionable interest and John Thomson was recommended to him as an appropriate teacher. In 1799 and again in 1800 Thomson gave a series of lectures to Lauderdale and his group of like-minded friends. Thereafter Lauderdale and Thomson founded a Chemistry Society that included in its membership Francis Horner, Henry Brougham, John Allen and other young liberal Whigs. In the months that followed, Thomson himself became politically active. At this time almost all those openly campaigning for Parliamentary reform and against the government's policy of repression were lawyers. Alone among the medical profession were Thomson and his friend John Allen;[12] they, however, 'were active and fearless'.[13] Thomson's activities were noticed; the Secretary of State's Office recorded a *caveat* against him ever receiving any public appointment.[14] This might have brought his career to an end but his tactical agility allowed him once again to overcome the obstruction.

First he managed to advance his position as a surgeon at the Royal Infirmary. For many years surgical services at the infirmary had been provided by the Royal College of Surgeons, every Fellow having the privilege of acting as an attending surgeon on a two-monthly rotation. This system conspicuously failed to provide patients of the infirmary with proper continuity of care or the services of the most experienced surgeons. In 1800, Thomson published proposals for change in a pamphlet *Outlines of a Plan for the Management of the Surgical Department of the Royal Infirmary*. Had he submitted his scheme to the College of Surgeons, Town Council or the managers of the infirmary it is probable that it would have been immediately rejected. But aware that among those who had been treated at the infirmary there was widespread discontent with the existing arrangement, he had submitted his scheme directly to the public. Under the resulting public pressure, the managers of the infirmary abandoned the two-monthly rotation and appointed six surgeons on a more permanent basis. Thomson was one of the first to be appointed.

Three years later, Thomson was appointed to his first chair. When the war with France broke out again in 1803, there were proposals that a military hospital should be established in Scotland. Thomson immediately travelled to London to apply in person to Robert Keate, the Inspector General of Hospitals, for an appointment in the Army Medical Department. He was granted the lowly rank of Hospital Mate but with a promise that he would be given a more senior appointment at the Military Hospital in Scotland should it be established. Back in Edinburgh, Thomson, who had already established himself as an extramural lecturer in surgery, added an additional course of lectures on military surgery which medical officers of the army and navy were allowed to attend *gratis*. This venture proved to be so successful that the College of Surgeons became eager to be associated with it; in 1804 the college established a Professorship of Surgeons. Thomson was universally considered to be better qualified for the position than any other Fellow of the college and was appointed Professor of Surgery at the Royal College of Surgeons of Edinburgh.

Thomson's second appointment to a chair came only two years later. In 1805, Dundas was forced to resign from office in Pitt's 'Tory' administration,[15] and a few months later the whole administration came to an end when Pitt died. In 1806, Charles James Fox was appointed as First Lord of the Treasury at the head of a Whig government at Westminster; in Scotland, Thomson's friend, Lord Lauderdale, became Keeper of the Great Seal and succeeded Dundas in his role as manager of government patronage in Scotland. One of the first to benefit from Lauderdale's patronage was John Thomson. With Lauderdale's support he petitioned the Secretary of State for the creation of a new regius chair[16] of military surgery at Edinburgh University; his petition was successful and he was subsequently appointed to the new professorship. For the next fifteen years, Thomson was both Professor of Surgery at the Royal College of Surgeons and Professor of Military Surgery at Edinburgh University.

In 1810, Thomson's career began to suffer a series of setbacks. His operating skills had been found wanting by his surgical colleagues and he had been forced to give up surgical practice and retire from the staff of the Royal Infirmary. Thereafter he concentrated on advancing his reputation as a medical scientist and adding to his experience and expertise in the study and teaching of medical disciplines other than surgery. In 1815, he applied for the Chair of Botany and Medicine at Edinburgh, but the Whigs were once again out of office and he no longer had any political support; his application was rejected. In 1821, he applied to succeed James Gregory as Professor of the Practice of Physic but once again he was unsuccessful. Then, in 1821, as military establishments in Britain were reduced, his appointment as surgeon to the forces was discontinued and he resigned from both his university chair of Military Surgery and his chair of Surgery at the College of Surgeons. He now set out on his own as an extramural lecturer on medicine and pathology.[17] His courses on pathology, superbly illustrated by the drawings of Robert Carswell, attracted large numbers of students, including many from the university, until 1829 when he handed over the teaching of pathology to his son in order to devote all his time to his research work.[18] However, at the general election in 1830, a Whig government was elected for the first time in a quarter of a century. Thomson immediately petitioned the new Secretary of State for the establishment at

Edinburgh University of a chair of General Pathology and a separate chair of Surgery.[19] Six years earlier, he had made similar proposals to the Secretary of State in a Tory government but they had been rejected. In 1830, his proposals had the support of Lauderdale and his other Whig friends and they were quietly adopted by the Whig Secretary of State, Lord Melbourne. In 1831, John Turner, who had been Thomson's protégé and his successor as Professor of Surgery at Edinburgh's Royal College of Surgeons, became the new Professor of Surgery at Edinburgh University and Thomson himself became the first Professor of General Pathology.

When Simpson was appointed as his assistant in 1831, John Thomson had shown that it was possible to circumvent the barriers that, for half a century, Old Corruption[20] had put in the way of those born without wealth or family influence. Simpson now looked to John Thomson for support and inspiration.

From the autumn of 1831, Simpson acted as Thomson's academic secretary, re-writing and updating his lectures and editing his publications. The greater part of his time, however, was given over to research. For many years, Thomson had studied and taught 'external' pathology as it related to surgery; from 1821 he had extended his work to include 'internal' pathology as it related to medicine; now in 1832, having undertaken to profess the whole range of General Pathology, he set his new able and articulate assistant to work on pathology as it related to midwifery.

Soon Simpson was being encouraged to include the results of his own studies when preparing revised versions of his professor's lectures on obstetric pathology. Simpson's confidence, already re-awakened by his appointment as Professor Thomson's assistant, was further boosted by this endorsement of his work by Edinburgh's foremost medical scientist. The insecurity and bitter disenchantment that had dogged his undergraduate years evaporated, and the uncharacteristic diffidence that had surprised and distressed his family during those years now disappeared. All thought of a future as an obscure country surgeon was abandoned; Simpson was now determined to make his name as a medical scientist. He petitioned for membership of the Royal Physical Society[21] and became one of its most active members. He joined the Royal Medical Society and within two years he had been elected as one of its four presidents. And, with Thomson's encouragement, he made it his business to meet and talk to the most distinguished members of every branch of his profession.[22]

In the spring of 1835, armed with letters of introduction from John Thomson, he set out to visit the leading medical schools in London, Paris and the newly created kingdom of Belgium. He was accompanied on his tour by Douglas Maclagan,[23] a junior colleague at the Royal Dispensary whose father had served with distinction as physician to the forces during Wellington's Peninsular Wars. Maclagan was able to introduce Simpson to some of the most eminent men in London and Paris.

Throughout his tour, Simpson maintained a lively correspondence with his brothers and sister, who followed closely every step of his progress and kept him constantly and generously supplied with funds. Simpson had never before travelled beyond Scotland or even beyond the Lothians. His letters record the impressions of a somewhat unsophisticated but nevertheless self-confident tourist:

> The neatness and cleanliness of the English cottages is greatly superior to all we have in Scotland. The little patches of garden ground before, behind and around them set them off amazingly. I wish the Scotch peasantry could, by some means or other, be excited to a little more love of cleanliness and horticulture. I did not see above two or three dirty windows along the whole line of road. The snow-white smockfrocks of the peasantry do actually look well.

On the cross-channel ferry from Southampton:

> The company on board was partly French, partly English. I never before saw so well the verification of the remark that speaking French consists 'in making mouths', and it was easy to point out all our French party individually by observing, from even the greatest distance, how much they used their poor hard-worked orbicularis oris.

On arriving in France:

> Everything in Havre was new and striking, the town itself being a very neatly built Norman one. The coifs or headdresses of the ladies would have surprised you, I am sure. At least they surprised me. Many of them had no such things as bonnets on but a cap as high or even higher than a sugarloaf made of muslin and lace and as white as driven snow.

In Paris:

> We have got the most excellent bread. It is beautifully white and costs sixpence the 4 lb. loaf or rather I should say the 4 lb. roll for all is in the form of roll from four inches to more than four feet and

more long. They are the most unearthly rolls you ever saw. I have never seen in a bakehouse but I saw two bakers emerge from one a few days back; they had only a shirt and a petticoat on and no such article as trousers.

Wherever he went he found time to visit the cathedrals, art galleries and the places of interest to any tourist. However, his tour had a different and even urgent professional objective. He had been appointed at Edinburgh as an assistant in general pathology on the strength of a single undergraduate dissertation on inflammation. To justify his appointment it was necessary for him to acquire a proper command of the subject that he was expected to promote and teach. The immediate purpose of his tour was to learn everything he could from some of the best pathological collections and museums of the time.

On arrival in London, Simpson called first on Robert Carswell, John Thomson's former colleague and collaborator who was now Professor of Pathological Anatomy at London University. He visited the university's museum and spent several hours studying its collection of pathological specimens, inquiring into techniques involved in their preparation and display and carefully recording every detail in his journal. In the following five weeks he interviewed the curators and studied the collections in the museums of London's foremost hospital medical schools – the North London, St Bartholomew's, St Thomas's, Guy's, St George's and the Middlesex – and, finally, Sir Richard Owen, Professor of Anatomy at the Royal College of Surgeons of England (who famously resisted Charles Darwin's ideas on natural selection) and William Clift[24] introduced Simpson to the college's great collection in the Hunterian Museum at Lincoln's Inn Fields. On 5 May he crossed to France to continue his studies in the museum of the School of Medicine in Paris and thereafter in the museums of the universities of Liège, Louvain, Brussels and Ghent.

On 21 June, Simpson returned to London. There he spent a few more days before travelling to Liverpool and from there, by sea, to Glasgow. On 10 July 1835, after fifteen weeks of study in a dozen and more of Europe's best pathological museums and with everything he had learned carefully recorded in the two sturdy volumes of his journal, he was back in Edinburgh. He was now well prepared to fulfil his obligations to John Thomson and go on to build a career as a pathologist. His friend John Reid had already decided to give up clinical practice to become a dedicated medical scientist,[25] but Simpson was not ready to make such a decision. During his tour he had taken every opportunity to meet leading clinicians in London, France and Belgium and to learn what he could from those at the forefront of medicine and surgery.

In Scotland, bloodletting was still practised in the treatment of 'simple' fevers such as colds and pneumonia. Simpson learned from Dr William Somerville that, in London, bleedings of 16 oz, 12 oz and even 8 oz were considered to be excessive. (Simpson thought it possible that such bloodletting could not be tolerated by Londoners because the constitution of the people of London had been weakened by their 'drinking so much porter and gin'.[26]) In Paris, Pierre Louis, using statistical analysis ('numerical methods') in his clinical trials had already shown that bloodletting made no difference to the outcome in cases of pneumonia whether the volume of blood drawn was large or small or whether the bloodletting was performed early or late in the illness.

For centuries, and everywhere in Europe, mercury had been regarded as a safe medicine that could be included with confidence in the routine treatment of almost every ailment. In London, Simpson discovered that Robert Liston, now Professor of Surgery at King's College, had recently treated several of his patients without including mercury and they had come to no harm. Later, in Liège, he saw the ill effects of mercury when he was introduced to the pharmacologist Professor Fohmann. Fohmann had a tremor and walked with a staggering gait; he informed Simpson that his disability was due to *tremblement metallique* contracted as a result of his having worked for many years making up mercury preparations.

Britain had been at war for over twenty-five of the previous forty years, and advances in surgery and medicine are always among the very few gains of war. In London, Simpson had several discussions with Sir James McGrigor, FRS, director general of the Army Medical Department, and with Samuel Clarke, the army's inspector general of hospitals; and he made lengthy visits to the military hospitals at Chelsea and Chatham. At the *Hopital des Invalides* in Paris (where the wards were 'the most elegant' he had ever seen) he met and toured the wards with Baron Dominique Larrey. Larrey had been surgeon-in-chief to Napoleon's armies in all his campaigns from Italy in 1797 to Waterloo in 1815 and since then had been widely regarded as the father of military surgery.

In 1805, Philippe Pinel at the Salpetriere in Paris had launched a revolution in the management of the insane. It had long been the practice in France and in Britain that 'lunatics' who could not be tolerated at large in the community or managed at home were confined to asylums, where they were routinely restrained in chains, bedded on straw and 'treated exactly as if they had been beasts'.[27] Pinel, and later his pupil Jean-Etienne Esquirol, had introduced what became known as the 'Moral Treatment' of the insane: physical restraint was used only when absolutely necessary; asylums were to be comfortable and as unlike prisons as possible; patients were to be cared for by suitably trained staff 'in whom mildness and command of temper are indispensable'; and in these circumstances the patients might be expected to be 'dissipated by judicious intercourse with others'.

In Paris, Simpson met Esquirol at his Charenton Asylum, where he was able to see for himself that no 'coercive treatment under any form' was being used. And in June, at the asylum in Ghent, where Dr Guislain had adopted the new 'Moral Treatment', all the patients 'were at work on something or other; none were idle except those who were utterly furious. Some patients were so comfortable and happy that they were with difficulty induced to leave.' However, in 1835, 'Moral Treatment' was still very controversial in Britain. In London, Simpson had visited the Bethlehem Hospital (Bedlam) where he could 'fish out little or nothing about the management of the institution or the treatment employed'; but 'there seemed to be too many bolts about the windows and rooms', all of which suggested that the new Moral Treatment was not being practised.

Back in Edinburgh after an instructive and, in parts, inspiring tour, Simpson was confident enough of his immediate future to leave his brother David's house in Stockbridge and set up on his own near the infirmary at 2 Teviot Row. Only four years before he had been living with his family in Bathgate, an inexperienced young man of nineteen with a licence to practise surgery, but in an overcrowded profession and unable to find regular employment. Now he was a Doctor of Medicine with an appointment at one of the most prestigious medical schools in Europe and with the real prospect of achieving success in any branch of the medical profession that he might happen to choose.

John Thomson had rescued Simpson's ambitions and directed the first steps of his career. And as that career continued, Simpson was able to look back for inspiration to the history of Thomson's success. Thomson had not confined his interests to one branch of his profession but had read widely in the medical literature and had been ready to shift from one discipline to another as his career demanded. By his outstanding professional and personal skills, he had attracted the attention of the wealthy and powerful and had gone on to enjoy and cultivate their friendship and support. When facing obstruction by the medical establishment he had been ready to appeal to the general public. Simpson was to follow Thomson's example.

FOUR

Professor of Midwifery

Never mind. I have got the chair in despite of them, professors and all.
James Y. Simpson

At the beginning of the academic year in the first week of October 1835, Simpson was elected president of the Royal Medical Society.[1] His inauguration address was to be given at the meeting of the society on 20 November and he planned to seize the occasion to present himself, not only to the society but also to the medical world, as an authority on obstetric pathology. He chose as his subject 'Diseases of the Placenta'. Although the lecture was to include some work of his own, it was planned as a comprehensive review of everything that had been written on the subject and every aspect of it that was currently being explored. It was an ambitious project, and while he prepared a concise version for presentation to the Royal Medical Society he also prepared a full and extended version for publication in the British and the European medical press. In the short time available, he made use of every available archival source; he wrote to consult medical scientists and obstetricians whom he had met during his tour of London, Paris and Belgium, and recognised authorities in Germany and France whom he had never met. On the day of his address, he wrote to his brother Sandy: 'It is five o'clock in the morning and I am confoundedly tired. I have been up all night correcting the last printed sheet of my paper. I was up all night on Monday, never in bed and have done with three or four hours sleep for several others.'

At the meeting that evening, however, he appeared the confident master of events. A guest of the society later wrote: 'The chair was occupied by a young man whose appearance was striking and peculiar. As we entered the room, his head was down to enable him, in his elevated position, to converse with someone on the floor of the apartment and little was seen of him but a mass of long tangled hair partially concealing what appeared to be a head of a very large size. He raised his head and his countenance at once impressed us. Massive brows from which shone eyes piercing as it were to your inmost soul and mouth that seemed capable of being made at will the exponent of every passion and emotion. Even if we had never seen him again he would have remained indelibly impressed on our memory.'[2]

His address was very well received by the Royal Medical Society. The extended version, 'Pathological Observations on the Diseases of the Placenta', was published in the *Edinburgh Medical and Surgical Journal*[3] early in 1836, and later that year translations appeared in journals published in Paris, Berlin, and Milan. It was a major work and Simpson had intended that it should mark the beginning of a distinguished career as a pathologist. But, even before it was published in Europe, his future in pathology was already in doubt, perhaps ended, before it had really begun.

In the summer of 1835, John Thomson had suffered a number of bouts of illness. He announced that he would no longer visit patients in their homes but would 'confine himself to such consultative practice as could be pursued at his own residence'. He hoped that by reducing his clinical commitments he would be able to continue as Professor of General Pathology. However, at the beginning of the academic year in October 1835, as he was still quite unwell, he obtained permission to delegate his professorial duties until he had recovered his health. He arranged for the presentation of his lecture course to be shared equally by his son William and Simpson.[4]

Later that winter, as Thomson continued to be unwell, the university authorities decided that it had become necessary to make a formal appointment of a deputy professor. Thomson feared that if his son showed that he was willing to accept a position that carried only the status of a deputy professor, this might damage his prospects of eventually succeeding to his chair. Thomson therefore offered the appointment as his deputy to Simpson, and Simpson accepted. But in doing so he was aware that he was allowing William Thomson to emerge as, by far, the stronger, more prestigious and overwhelmingly the more likely candidate for succession to the chair of General Pathology.

William Thomson was thirty-three years old and for much of his life he had been his father's companion, pupil and assistant. At his father's direction, he had studied medicine at Edinburgh and Glasgow for a total of four years. In 1825, he had become a Fellow of the Royal College of Surgeons of Edinburgh, in 1828 an MD of Aberdeen University and, in 1833, a Fellow of the Royal College of Physicians of Edinburgh. He had been surgeon to the New Town Dispensary and had lectured at his father's extramural schools, first on the Institutes of Medicine and later on the Practice of

Physic. While still a student he had been sent to Paris to assist Robert Carswell in collecting the illustrations for his father's famous lectures on inflammation, and since then his father had continued to direct the greater part of William's attention to the study of pathology and pathological anatomy. Even as he had contrived the establishment of the chair of General Pathology at Edinburgh in 1831, John Thomson planned that his son William should succeed him.[5]

In 1836, John Thomson was seventy-eight years old and therefore unlikely to continue much longer in his chair. Neither John Thomson nor Simpson was in any doubt that William would very soon be appointed to succeed him as Professor of General Pathology. There would then be no need for a deputy and Simpson's post would be abolished. Since no other senior academic posts in General Pathology had yet been created in Scotland, it seemed clear that if Simpson hoped to continue in an academic career in Scotland he must change to some other discipline. On the advice of John Thomson, he chose clinical obstetrics; James Hamilton, the Professor of Midwifery at Edinburgh, was sixty-eight years old and likely to retire within the next few years, and he had no obvious successor.

Simpson had attended four courses of lectures on the theory and practice of obstetrics but he had no clinical experience other than the few deliveries he had attended with Dr Dawson in Bathgate in 1830 and 1831. However, at the request of John Thomson, Professor Hamilton agreed to accept Simpson as a house surgeon at his Lying-in Hospital. Simpson was confident that in twelve months at the Lying-In Hospital he would see as much midwifery as he would otherwise see in twenty years. On the promise of the appointment he moved from his brother David's house in Stockbridge to rooms near the hospital at 2 Teviot Row. There he set up in private practice and, even before he took up his appointment at the Lying-In Hospital in June 1836, he was already beginning to attract patients. In a letter to his brother Sandy he wrote that 'the patients are mostly poor it is true, but still they are patients'. When he took up his promised place as house surgeon at the Lying-In Hospital, the number of his private patients began to increase and, as he told Sandy, they were 'now not the poor alone'.

Simpson had intended to spend at least a year gaining practical experience in obstetrics before offering himself as an extramural teacher. However, when news of his forthcoming appointment to the staff of the Lying-in Hospital became known in May 1836, John Mackintosh, then the leading extramural lecturer on midwifery in Edinburgh, offered to take him into partnership. The proposal was that Simpson should first buy Mackintosh's museum[6] at valuation and then, for a maximum of four academic sessions, Simpson and Mackintosh should share the teaching duties; thereafter, Mackintosh would retire leaving Simpson in sole charge of the school. Simpson hesitated. As he explained in a letter to Sandy, Mackintosh's offer had come too soon: 'It brings me so suddenly into the field. I am by no means as well prepared as I could wish.'

However, Professor Thomson and Professor Hamilton both advised him to accept Mackintosh's offer. His friend, John Reid, took charge of the early stages of the negotiations, even writing to Simpson's brother John, to ensure that the necessary funds would be available. John, who was to act as Simpson's lawyer, replied that the family would, of course, leave the question of whether or not the offer should be accepted entirely to Simpson himself. But whatever he decided, John promised that: 'I should support him to the extent of all my abilities and so will Sandy. Sandy and I can easily raise £200 or £300 meantime and pay Mackintosh by instalments. I am sure that I have told him again and again, both verbally and in writing, that he might consider mine as the joint-stock purse of the family ... If my presence in Edinburgh is required on the occasion, and although the coaches are very throng just now, I can easily "mount my bold grey for there's life in his hoof-clank and hope in his neigh".'

Simpson allowed negotiations to continue for many months. When Mackintosh proposed that, as a partner in his extramural school, Simpson should teach medical jurisprudence as well as midwifery, Simpson could not be persuaded to agree. There was also some very protracted haggling over the purchase price of the museum. But, in the end, John Simpson, as he had promised, drove up in his gig to Edinburgh where he conducted the final negotiations, drew up the contract and completed the sale. Simpson delivered his first course of lectures on obstetrics at his extramural school in the session 1838–9. By then he had the experience in clinical obstetric practice that he had lacked when Mackintosh first offered him a partnership.

Many years later, Simpson wrote that it was at this time that he decided to settle down as a citizen of Edinburgh and 'fight the hard and uphill battle of life for bread and name and fame'. But in the years during which he worked to establish himself as an obstetrician, Simpson's life was not the impoverished and joyless struggle that his somewhat theatrical phraseology might suggest. Even while still acting as Thomson's deputy in General Pathology he was only required to lecture at the university once a day during the months of the academic year. As the co-owner of an extramural school of midwifery in Surgeons' Square, he shared the teaching duties with John Mackintosh. At Teviot Row, the funds provided by his brothers allowed him to live comfortably while he gradually built up his practice and his reputation. He could not afford a carriage and was therefore obliged to walk to every part of the city to attend the few patients he had yet acquired; his sister Mary provided him with a regular supply of excellent and suitably studded boots.

As always throughout his professional life, he read widely in the medical literature and began to make contributions of his own. Translations of his *Pathological Observations on the Diseases of the Placenta* continued to be published in European journals: following its appearance in Belgium he was elected a Corresponding Member of the Medical Society of Ghent. In 1838, he published 'Notes on Cases of Peritonitis in the Foetus',[7] the first part of his book, *Contribution to Intrauterine Pathology*. The second part, 'On the Inflammatory Origin of Some Malformations in the Foetus',[8] appeared in January 1839. The results of his experimental work on hermaphroditism were published in the *Cyclopaedia of Anatomy and Physiology* in the summer of 1839.[9]

Their many professional commitments did not prevent Simpson and his friend, John Reid, from being taken up by Edinburgh society. Both had been elected as Fellows of the Royal College of Physicians in 1836 and both were already showing great promise in their careers. Although neither was yet able to earn a living, they were both able to maintain an agreeable life style. John Reid was living in Edinburgh with his widowed sister and was generously financed by his father. Simpson lived in his rooms at Teviot Row until September 1837, when he moved to more convenient and comfortable apartments at No. 2 Deanhaugh Street. His brothers, Sandy and John, settled his accounts with his bookseller and were always ready to provide whatever other money he required; his sister Mary, who had married in 1831, sent him occasional luxuries, and her husband, John Pearson, sent him a regular supply of ale from his brewery. Simpson and John Reid were considered to be eligible young men by the mothers of equally eligible daughters and they were made very welcome at many dinner parties and balls in Edinburgh's fashionable New Town.

Simpson had several transient and light-hearted flirtations. But his relationship with a Miss Girdwood ('a sweet and lovely girl' whom he referred to in his correspondence as 'Cinderella') went rather deeper. In the early summer of 1836, her friends had come to believe that everything was settled between them; her aunt even let it be known that, should he propose, his proposal would be welcomed by her family.[10] But Simpson did not propose. As he explained in a letter to Jessie Grindlay, his cousin in Liverpool: 'Cinderella is, I confess, a lovely young lady but somehow or other I have come to think this summer that there is a great difference between the beauty and ornament of the drawing room and ballroom and that of the domestic fireside, between a companion in a dance and a companion in life. I have no doubt that Cinderella will make a good wife to anyone who is able to maintain her; but I have my strong doubts if she could make anyone happy where there were many domestic cares and concerns to annoy.'[11]

Simpson was not always so content with himself and his life. That summer, he suffered one of his recurring periods of depression. In another of his regular letters to his cousin Jessie, he wrote: 'Yesterday I was sadder than ever. If I were superstitious, and who is free from some little taint of it, I would almost regard yesterday as darkly ominous to me. All day long I was in the blues. I could not get my mind to look at the sunny side of this world and its struggles. It was one of those days, those fitful days of gloom in which the past appears to me to be almost lost, the future a labyrinth of vexations and disappointments and poverty and dependence.'

Simpson soon emerged from his depression and, as always after such spells, he became buoyant and exuberant. Life was again 'a strange blend of working and romping, of studying and idleness, of pleasure and pathology, of lecturing and laughing, of diseases and dinner parties, of agues and quadrilles, of insanity and coquetry everything in excess except sleep.'[12] As always when in such a high state of mind, he wrote poetry.

One of his early poems, written in 1829 when he was a student, was his 'Farewell to Loch Vennacher'. Simpson had never visited the Highlands; his poem was inspired by the notorious clearances of Sutherland that had taken place only a few years before, and it describes the feelings of a young Highlander forced to leave his home and his country. The subject, the setting and the style in which the poem was written all seem to show the influence of Simpson's favourite author, Sir Walter Scott.

> Ye scenes of my childhood, a long, long adieu,
> Adieu my all-happy, my sweet Highland home.
> For in far distant climes, far from pleasure and you
> In life's mazy paths I am doomed now to roam
>
> And thee I must leave too, my fair Highland maid!
> But think on me, Mary when distant afar,
> And remember the sweet, sweet words that you said
> On the heather-bell brae of Loch Vennachar

Later, when again in rhyming frame of mind, he sent a friend the breast bone of a chicken accompanied by a verse carrying distant echoes of Robert Burn's 'Address to the Haggis':

> My noble, lordly, high born chicken
> Well wert thou worth a gentleman's picking
> Thy savoury flesh so sweetly pure
> Would have charmed the veriest epicure
> Thou sacred bone that guards the breast
> I summon thee from midst the rest
> Let not one instant now be lost
> But speed thee through the Penny Post

In his bachelor years of the 1830s, his poems were addressed to various young ladies of his acquaintance. The verse quoted here was written as a preface to an album of songs collected by Miss Maria Bauchope of Kinneil, the daughter of the Duke of Hamilton's factor:

> Oh! Once a lonely nightingale
> Stray'd afar to our northern strand
> Lured by a love of upland and dale
> And charms of our mountain land
> 'Twas neither far nor long he sought
> For soon the minstrel's glancing eye
> The object of his fond wish caught
> As e'en Maria's self was nigh!
> Then straight he poured into her soul
> That racy flood of living song
> By which, with siren like control
> The lady thralls her listening throng
> By whose strange soothing witchery
> O'er the still'd heart a charm is thrown
> Forcing the spirit of man to own
> The spell of magic melody

At times throughout his very busy and difficult career Simpson continued to write poetry. In his maturity his poems were published privately and distributed to his large circle of friends.

Simpson was still in a buoyant and poetry-writing state of mind in September 1839 when James Hamilton resigned as Professor of Midwifery. Simpson was immediately determined to succeed him. An almost insuperable barrier to his election that would have confronted him only a few years before had already been removed. He was a known Whig and, as a student, he had consorted with Radicals, taking part in every public demonstration against the policies of the Tory administration. Since then he had become the protégé of that most prominent of Whigs, John Thomson. But the political climate had changed since Whig sympathies had effectively barred the appointment of John Thomson (in 1815 and again in 1821) and Robert Liston (in 1833) to university chairs at Edinburgh. Since the late 1820s, new young men who had not been brought up in fear of the revolution in France spreading to Britain had been elected to Parliament, and green shoots of liberalism had begun to grow within both the Tory and Whig parties. In 1828, the Tory government had been unable to find enough support to deny a Whig Bill to repeal the Test Act and the Corporation Act.[13] In 1829, an embattled and divided Tory government had consented to the passing of the Catholic Emancipation Act. Of much greater relevance in Scotland, in 1832 the Reform Act increased the electorate from 4,239 to over 65,000, making it impossible for the established government to determine the outcome of elections as it had done during the long years of the Dundas Despotism and its aftermath. And of particular relevance to Simpson's ambitions to succeed James Hamilton, the Royal Burghs Act of 1833 had reformed the election of the town councils of Scotland's royal burghs. Everyone qualified to vote in Parliamentary elections under the Reform Act was now entitled to vote in the election of a town council; the self-perpetuating oligarchies, drawn only from the city's ancient merchant and craft guilds, that had made up Edinburgh's Town Council for centuries were now abolished. From 1833 the reformed council was made up of thirty-three elected members, the majority of whom were 'ordinary traders of the middling mercantile orders'. It was to these thirty-three that Simpson would now have to direct his application. His carefully printed and skilfully presented application was sent to 'the Right Honourable the Lord Provost, the Magistrates and Town Council of the City of Edinburgh, Patrons of the University' on 15 November 1839 after weeks of hectic preparation.

The *Times* described what still had to be done: 'Every candidate for a chair in the University of Edinburgh, except those which are under the patronage of the Crown,[14] must personally canvass all of those individuals [Town Councillors] and bring influence to bear upon each one of them. He must publish volumes of testimonials and have a committee constantly in action to promote his claims. It is needless to expatiate upon the trouble, expense and moral degradation of such a process. The patrons, as they delight to be styled from their position in society, have no means of knowing the merits of candidates except through testimonials as the respective value of which they are no less incompetent to judge. They are in consequence exposed to private solicitation and the influence of sectarian prejudices.'

The first part of Simpson's submission to the patrons of the university was a list of his qualifications, his previous and current professional appointments, and the learned bodies of which he was a member, together with a catalogue of his 'museum', the collection of pathological specimens and other material that he would use in teaching his students. The main body was made up of printed copies of his testimonials. From every possible quarter, Simpson had collected over seventy testimonials, including some that had to be translated from French or German.[15] And as was then the accepted practice, he had had them sympathetically edited and then printed and distributed not only to the thirty-three electors, but also among the general public, all at a cost of £168 2s 1d[16] (the equivalent of £12,600 in 2005[17]). Simpson also personally canvassed every member of the Town Council. And, since the members of the council were generally unable to assess the true value of medical testimonials, it was to be expected that they would seek the guidance of medical men they knew and trusted; Simpson therefore assiduously canvassed a very large section of the medical profession in Edinburgh.

Although the town councillors respected the views of members of the medical profession, they also had their own requirements of a successor to the 72-year-old James Hamilton. James Hamilton had been a Professor of Midwifery since 1800 and Professor of Medicine, Midwifery and the Diseases of Children since 1830.[18] He still dressed in the breeches, silk stockings and buckles of the eighteenth century and was the last Edinburgh physician to be conveyed in a sedan chair when visiting his patients. He was short, plump and irritable, 'a man of war, pugnacious and uncompromising'.[19] But for over forty years he had been Edinburgh's most fashionable obstetrician and, unlike every other successful physician of the time, he refused to attend his wealthy patients at their places in the country but had them come to him in Edinburgh. Having his many wealthy patients in Edinburgh was good for business, and it was business that the tradesmen and shopkeepers of the Town Council did not intend to lose. They hoped to find a successor for Hamilton who would follow him in building a large and lucrative private practice within the city.

Simpson and his small 'committee' of supporters canvassed vigorously but not always tactfully; more than one ill-considered approach brought a stinging rebuff.[20] And, very early in his canvass, Simpson was made aware of a major problem. In a letter to his brother Sandy he reported: 'I have been told by a number of the Council that they have no objection to me except my youth and my celibacy.' His youth could not be helped, but he could correct his celibacy.

When passing through Liverpool on the way home from France in July 1835, he had spent an evening with his father's cousin Walter Grindlay and his family. In a letter to his brother Sandy at that time he reported that 'one of the Misses Grindlay has a resemblance to Mary, much more like a sister than a second or third cousin'. Simpson, of course, had a sister but Mary had always been his deeply devoted 'mother' rather than the friend and ally that a sister might have been. The Miss Grindlay who was 'more like a sister' was Jessie Grindlay and, as we have seen, in the years that followed he had written regularly to Jessie and had come to expect a letter in reply every Monday. His letters were friendly and playful and no more affectionate than they might have been to a sister. He discussed books that they had read and exchanged. He told her something of his work but much more of his lodgings, his domestic arrangements and his financial affairs. He wrote freely of his social life, including the nuances of his relationship with Cinderella.

They met for only the second time when Jessie spent part of the summer of 1837 with relatives at Cameron in Fife and visiting friends in Bathgate and Edinburgh. While she was there, Simpson and John Reid had to travel briefly to London on business and on the way north they spent a few days with the Grindlay family in Liverpool. After he returned home, in his letter to Jessie's sisters in Liverpool, Simpson wrote: 'I have been most abundantly teased since I came back. Everybody about Bathgate and many in Edinburgh knows a great deal more about Jessie than I myself do. I was told since my return the number of silk gowns she had when she was in Edinburgh by one person, the number of bonnets by another, the shape of her mouth by a third, the colour of her face by a fourth, the exact amount of her fortune by a fifth. What shall I be next year at this date if I am here to write to you again? Shall I be married think ye? And shall I have the pleasure of calling you sister?'[21]

However, Jessie returned to Liverpool and her correspondence with Simpson continued as before for a further two years. In September 1839, Simpson had a meeting at Queen's College, Dublin. On returning through

Liverpool, he again called on the Grindlay family at Toxteth Park in Liverpool. In his letter to Sandy giving a full account of his expedition to Dublin, he commented only that 'Mr Grindlay's people were all very kind'.[22] There was no mention of an engagement or of Jessie.

But now, suddenly, in October, Simpson wrote to Walter Grindlay asking for his daughter's hand in marriage. On receiving a favourable reply to his first letter, Simpson immediately wrote a second.

> Last Friday, I wrote to solicit what I had long set my heart on, your daughter's hand in marriage. At present, though my friends tell me my chance for the professorship is excellent, yet I believe myself that I shall not get it just now as possibly Dr Lee or Doctor Kennedy will be preferred over me. In asking then your daughter's hand I ask it, not with any certainty of being elected and thus having a future at once at my feet. I ask it for better or for worse whether I succeed or what is more probable, do not succeed. But taking it at the worst I do think that I shall be enabled by my practice alone to maintain a wife respectably. At the same time I am sure you will pardon me if I tell you – indeed it is my bounden duty to tell you – that I am in debt.

Having set out the extent of his debts (giving a very modest estimate of £320), he made it clear that he could only retrieve the situation and make his fortune by 'my pen and my lancet'. But because he was unmarried he was already losing patients and his celibacy was now the chief objection to his being appointed to a chair at Edinburgh. These, he explained, were his reasons for asking for consent for his marrying Jessie.[23]

Having received a second letter of consent from Walter Grindlay, Simpson immediately interrupted his canvass to travel to Liverpool, where on 26 December 1839 Dr J. Y. Simpson was married to Miss Jessie Grindlay. There was no honeymoon. The couple returned at once to Edinburgh to continue the canvass. Jessie wrote her husband's many letters to his dictation but her main task was the preparation of the catalogue of his museum. The museum was made up of over 700 items: obstetric forceps and other instruments, 'obstetric machinery' (leather models of foetuses and the bones of pelvis used to demonstrate obstetric manoeuvres), plaster casts, pathological specimens in bottles, paintings, drawings and statistical tables. While Jessie continued hard at work at home in Dean Street, Simpson was able to concentrate on calling on town councillors and those who might be able to influence them in his favour.

Simpson had the backing of John Reid and a number of his other contemporaries, but he found little support among the more senior ranks of the medical profession in Edinburgh. Robert Christison, James Syme and the majority of the members of the university's Faculty of Medicine thought him too young and inexperienced, even presumptuous, in applying. Only two years before he had been employed as a deputy to the Professor of Pathology. In all he had a little less than three years of practical experience of obstetrics and he was still scarcely able to make a living from his practice. 'He may know midwifery well enough as many old women throughout the country do but his knowledge of medical science and its literature is meagre.'[24]

There were, in all, six applicants for the chair (Campbell, Kennedy, Lee, Renton, Simpson and Thatcher) but Simpson's chief rivals were John Thatcher, Robert Lee and Evory Kennedy. In a letter to Walter Grindlay he wrote that his rivals had 'come forward on the ground of their local or political interest and my present object is to break down these fortifications and to leave the decision to be made on the ground of merit alone. They have all either family or fortune influence and I have neither.'

Simpson was still obsessed by the idea that the network of prejudice and power that had destroyed his friend Robert Knox was still at work and had even been strengthened by the appointment of his enemy James Syme to the Faculty of Medicine.[25] He was also being disingenuous. John Thatcher had been a successful extramural lecturer on midwifery for many years; Simpson had attended his course of lectures three times. Robert Lee was an Edinburgh graduate who had become a prominent obstetrician in London and had been elected a Fellow of the Royal Society. Evory Kennedy, Professor of Midwifery at Queen's College, Dublin, had an international reputation and was greatly respected by the medical profession everywhere in Britain, including Edinburgh. All three had claims to merit at least equal to Simpson's. And to break down his opponents' supposed 'fortifications of family and fortune influence' Simpson had recruited to his informal election committee four of the most influential figures in local politics in Edinburgh: John Ritchie (Whig), the proprietor and editor of the *Scotsman*; Duncan McLaren (Whig), the City Treasurer who had recently rescued Edinburgh from bankruptcy and was now also MP for Edinburgh; Sir William Drysdale, the leading Tory member of the Town Council; and Baillie Grieve (Whig), the Dean of Guild.

The competition was fierce. By the middle of January, Robert Lee and John Thatcher had withdrawn from the contest. To the end, the outcome was impossible to predict but on 4 February 1840, when the issue was

put to the vote, Simpson was the winner by 17 votes to 16. His decision
to seek the help of key local politicians had proved vital. Yet on the day of
his election, he wrote to his father-in-law that 'all the political influence of
both the leading Whigs and Tories here were employed against me; but
never mind – I have got the chair in despite of them'.

Simpson's sister Mary and her husband John Pearson had left Bathgate
to emigrate to Australia, but they were still on board ship in the English
Channel when they received the news of his success. Mary immediately
wrote:

> My dear, dear and fortunate brother,
> I have taken up the pen to wish you joy, joy, but I feel I am scarcely
> able to write. I never believed till now that excess of joy was worse
> to bear than excess of grief. I cannot describe how, but I certainly
> feel as I never did all my life. I hope we will still be here to learn all
> the particulars of this happy event. My dear, dear James, may God
> Himself bless you and prosper you in all your ways.

His brothers were equally delighted. Since he was a child they had nurtured
his ambitions. For almost twenty years they had financed his education and maintained him in a secure and comfortable life style. As they
had prospered in their professions, their generosity had increased. His
campaign to be elected a professor at Edinburgh University alone had cost
them some £500 (the equivalent of £37,500 in 2005). But all their years of
investment of faith, encouragement and money had been rewarded.

FIVE

Physician to the Queen

Fame is the spur that the clear spirit doth raise
to scorn delights and live laborious days

Milton

Within hours of the announcement of his election to the Chair of Midwifery, Simpson wrote in triumph to his father-in-law that 'all the political influence of both the leading Whigs and Tories here were employed against me; but never mind – I have got the chair in despite of them, professors and all'. Since his first bitter and disillusioned years as a student, Simpson had believed that as a liberal, even mildly radical, Whig, his ambitions must inevitably be frustrated by the established network of power and privilege that had kept a firm grip on the administration of Edinburgh and its institutions since the middle of the eighteenth century. But by 1840, that fiercely reactionary regime, with its blatantly corrupt processes of government, had been brought to an end. Nevertheless, when, during his election to his university chair, Simpson found no support from among the leading members of the university Senatus and the Faculty of Medicine, he concluded that the old prejudices were still ranged against him. In 1825, when he was a student, the threat of such prejudices had disheartened him; now in 1840, and Professor of Midwifery, the belief that they still continued infuriated him. After taking his place as a member of the Faculty of Medicine, every minor vexation or suggestion of further opposition provoked his defiance.

At his first meeting of the Faculty of Medicine, Simpson was asked to take on the duties of Secretary (Dean) of the faculty. However, he felt slighted by the manner in which the offer was made; it seemed to him that, in spite of his election to equal membership of the faculty, he was still to be treated as the 'son of a baker'. He therefore refused to be made Secretary. Almost at once he became aware that in doing so he had given particular offence to Robert Graham, the urbane and normally cordial Professor of Botany. That evening he wrote to Graham what was offered as a placatory letter but which nevertheless showed that he meant to have peace only on his own terms.

> . . . You are one of the last of the medical faculty whose good opinion I should wish to forfeit. It is probable that you may continue to look upon my line of conduct today as an unfortunate one. It possibly may have been so; but if you had been placed in the same position in all respects as I have during and since my election, I fear you would have found yourself under the necessity of acting in the same manner. At least, now that the matter is over, I do feel that I have done the right thing in refusing the Secretaryship under the extraordinary circumstances in which it was offered to me.

Professor Graham's reply was formal and crushing:[1]

> 19 May 1840
>
> Dr. Graham has received Dr. Simpson's letter of this date. He will not again argue the matter to which it relates and he has now neither the right nor inclination to advise. He cannot think his own conduct requires explanation; he merely begs to state the position in which, in his opinion, matters stand and are likely to remain.
>
> Dr. Simpson alludes to circumstances during his election. These are that his colleagues preferred another candidate for the Chair of Midwifery and used their best endeavours to procure his election. They may have been mistaken, and after the election every one of them wished to find it so.
>
> Dr. Simpson alludes to circumstances after his election. These are the subjects of the present discussion which Dr. Simpson thinks were derogatory to him and meant to be so. He persists in asserting this notwithstanding a solemn denial from every one of his colleagues. He ought to know that this is flying in the face of the ordinary courtesies of life, the common rules of civilised society and cannot but render utterly nugatory the desire of every member of the University that the right hand of fellowship given in all sincerity to Dr. Simpson after his election should be the pledge of kindly feeling and constant exertion for the mutual benefit and prosperity of the medical school.

Simpson replied in the same formal manner. His letter briefly restated his case as he saw it, but it ended:

Dr. Simpson considers it beneath his dignity as a gentleman to rebut the insinuations made against him in Dr. Graham's note regarding his want of knowledge of 'the ordinary courtesies of life' and the 'common rules of civilised society'. If Dr. Graham's conduct yesterday and his note of this morning are specimens of the ordinary courtesies of life as understood by Dr. Graham they are, Dr. Simpson must confess, very different from any that he has hitherto been accustomed to.

In winning the chair of Midwifery, Simpson had made no friends among the Faculty of Medicine and, as Robert Graham predicted, his refusal to accept the friendly overtures of the members of Faculty created a lack of sympathy that was to continue for many years. In 1840, his failure to establish a satisfactory relationship with his colleagues in faculty may well have influenced the senior physicians and surgeons who made up the board of management of the Royal Infirmary in making their decision not to appoint him to the staff of the infirmary or to allow him to teach there.

However, there was no opposition to his succeeding Professor James Hamilton at the Lying-In Hospital. The hospital had been opened in 1793 as a charitable foundation promoted by Professor James Hamilton's father, Alexander Hamilton, as a service for the poor but also to provide practical experience for his pupils, both trainee midwives and medical students. Alexander Hamilton's plan was for a hospital to be supported by public subscription and managed by a board of directors chaired by the Lord Provost. The Town Council agreed, and the charity was given incorporated status and founded as the Society for Relieving Indigent Pregnant Women.[2] The society did not attract popular support[3] and was never able to fund the project or even to buy a building to house it. To establish his hospital Alexander Hamilton therefore bought the handsome Park House[4] himself, and thereafter he financed the activities of his hospital by the sale of 'tickets' to students wishing to attend for instruction and by frequent donations and loans from the proceeds of his very successful private practice.

The patients at Park House were invariably poor. On discharge each one was given a small maternity grant (usually of tea, sugar and money[5]) so that she 'may not feel immediate distress from her change of situation'. Park House had two floors and a basement. On the ground floor there were two wards, each of seven beds, a delivery room and a small laboratory. On the upper floor there were six rooms each with two beds. Initially, one ward on the ground floor was reserved for married women, while all other accommodation was designated for unmarried women and prostitutes.

However, in time, the number of married women seeking admission steadily increased and unmarried women were admitted only 'under very particular circumstances of distress' or if their lives were thought to be in danger.

From 1793, Alexander Hamilton was assisted at his Lying-In Hospital by his son, James. In 1800, James took over the hospital from his father and continued to finance it just as his father had done. In 1836, he appointed Simpson as his principal assistant and when he retired (and later died) in 1839, Simpson became his obvious successor. However, for years the hospital had been falling more and more deeply in debt to Professor James Hamilton and when, in 1842, his daughters were obliged to realise his estate they ordered that Park House should be sold.

In a letter to his brother Sandy, Simpson wrote: 'Dr Hamilton would blush to see what his family have done.' Simpson could not afford to buy Park House or continue to help finance the hospital as James Hamilton had done. However, from Sandy he borrowed enough to buy the furniture and equipment from Park House and arranged with the Town Council for the patients to be housed temporarily in Queensberry House in the Canongate. From 1815 until 1833, Queensberry House had been used during epidemics as a fever hospital and since then it had been a House of Refuge for the destitute. At best, it could only be used as a temporary and unsatisfactory expedient. Without a permanent home or an adequate source of funding it seemed inevitable that the Lying-In Hospital would soon have to be disbanded. However, in 1843, the Town Council decided to set up a new charity and founded a new hospital, the Edinburgh Royal Maternity Hospital. Simpson and John Moir were appointed as consultant obstetricians with a staff of two obstetricians, a consultant surgeon, a surgeon, two assistant medical officers, two house surgeons, an apothecary, a matron and a hospital secretary.

Unfortunately the new charity, like its predecessor, attracted very few subscribers. From the beginning there had been a 'good deal of feeling against supporting the Maternity Hospital',[6] since many of the patients were unmarried and a significant number were prostitutes. In Edinburgh, even until the end of the century, it was widely held that to help provide for the care of prostitutes was to sponsor immorality.[7] In its first years the annual income of the hospital amounted only to some £500. A little over £100 came from private subscriptions; two parochial councils in Edinburgh each subscribed £30; a third Edinburgh parochial council and a parochial council in Leith each contributed £10. The greater part of the hospital's income was made up by the fees paid by the pupil midwives, the proceeds of the sales of 'tickets' to medical students, the income from the board and lodgings of the midwives and the fees paid by the two house surgeons in training. There was never any possibility of financing a new purpose-built hospital. In 1844, the Edinburgh Royal Maternity Hospital opened (with fewer beds than the old Lying-In Hospital) in makeshift quarters in St John Street, moving later to Milton House and later still to Minto House. It was not until 1856, when Simpson was able to lend the hospital £1,000[8], that the directors were able to buy Chapel House[9] and provide the hospital with satisfactory accommodation.

Until his death Simpson served as one of the nine directors of the Edinburgh Royal Maternity Hospital and as a trustee of Chapel House. During these years he was 'a kind and liberal benefactor of the hospital'. The directors also acknowledged that 'the hospital derived great advantage from the estimation which the fact of [Simpson] being one of its chief office bearers caused it to be held by the medical profession and the public'.[10] However, Simpson took little part in the day-to-day clinical work of the hospital. During his years as consultant obstetrician, he was called for only in cases of extreme difficulty, and then often only when the case was beyond help. In twenty-six years, he is recorded as having conducted only twenty-two of these traumatic deliveries; six of the twenty-two mothers died and seventeen of the infants.[11] There had been long periods during which he had not been available and, after 1855, there is no record of his having attended any deliveries in the Royal Maternity Hospital. Yet it was during these years that he built his reputation as the leading obstetrician in Britain and perhaps the foremost in Europe. That reputation was made in his private practice and by his frequent publications in the medical press, each of these very successful activities feeding off the other.

When Simpson first set up in practice at his lodging at No. 2 Teviot Row in the early spring of 1836, it was as a general physician. His practice was among the poor of Edinburgh's Old Town and it grew slowly until he was seeing, at best, fourteen patients each day and very few of these were obstetric cases. But after taking up his appointment as house physician at the Lying-In Hospital in the summer, the number of obstetric cases increased. His rooms on an upper floor of a tenement building became inadequate and especially inconvenient for patients in the later stages of pregnancy. He moved to larger apartments at 9 Deanhaugh Street, near his old lodgings in Stockbridge; his practice continued to grow and by early 1839 his income had reached approximately £300 per annum. His landlady now complained of the number of patients who had to be greeted at her front door and the number of urgent messages she was expected to pass on to her troublesome tenant. In April 1839, he rented a house in the newest part of the New Town at No. 1 Dean Terrace at £28 per annum and employed a housekeeper.[12] A few days later he confessed to Jessie that he felt that he had been rash: 'I was frightened after I did it.' But from Bathgate, his sister Mary reported that 'every visitor from Edinburgh brings us word of your prosperity or rather of your industry and your just reward'. His acquisition of a house and consulting rooms in a fashionable part of the city may have been rash but it soon became evident that the outcome had justified the risk. His practice increased even more rapidly than before and his patients were no longer the poor of Edinburgh's Old Town but the prosperous residents of the New Town.

Within only a few months, the testimonials that made up the large part of his application for the chair of Midwifery were widely circulated in Edinburgh and they proved even more effective in promoting his reputation and his practice than his house in Dean Terrace. He reported to his brother Sandy that, while he might have no hope of being appointed to the chair of Midwifery, the campaign and the public attention 'will make me as a practitioner though not as a Professor'. Now, more confident than ever of building a large and fashionable practice, he moved from Dean Terrace at the periphery of the New Town to 22 Albany Street at its heart, an address even more convenient for the patients he hoped to attract. And he bought a coach;[13] in applying to his brother Sandy for yet another loan, he explained that a coach would be 'expensive to buy as well as keep but I have no alternative but to get one, both to support my rank among my wealthier compeers and to save my body from excess of work'.

However, his success in being elected to his chair in February 1840 led him into one of the most difficult periods of his career. In the acrimonious weeks of campaigning he had made many enemies, especially among the more senior members of his profession. A more immediate difficulty was that his weeks of campaigning had left him in even greater debt to his brother Sandy and now also deeply in debt to Walter Grindlay. Simpson wrote to his father-in-law that he was 'most anxious there should be a marriage-contract, the tenure of life, particularly medical life being so uncertain that all contingences should be guarded against as far as lies in our power'. The contract was drawn up by Walter Grindlay's lawyers in Liverpool and delivered to Simpson in Edinburgh; Simpson approved it and passed it to his banker and financial advisor, his brother Sandy, for his signature.[14] It was a long and detailed document of eighteen pages. Among its many provisions it laid down that Simpson's life should be insured for a very large sum and that, should he die, the loans that he had received from Walter Grindlay should be repaid first and in full from his estate. However, the contract made no provision for the repayment of the much larger loans he had received from Sandy and his other brothers. Sandy refused to sign the contract and sent Simpson a sharp letter of protest. Simpson was surprised and deeply distressed by Sandy's reaction. He had always taken Sandy's generosity and his unquestioning support for granted. As he was to do at other times during his career when he felt that he had lost control of events, he retired to bed for four days complaining of palpitations and pains in his head and side. Meanwhile his wife wrote to her father objecting to the whole idea of a contract and protesting that: 'The long rigmarole would lay down the law for what it has no business with and for what it was never asked to interfere in.' Sandy was persuaded to accept Simpson's explanation that he had not read the contract before approving it and passing it on. Family harmony was restored, but the contract was abandoned.

However, Simpson's financial difficulties continued. Many of his patients were slow to pay his fees; he was writing frequent articles on medical history and archaeology but the returns from his publisher were very modest and, of course, his appointments as consultant physician at the Royal Dispensary and the Lying-in Hospital carried no salary. At the same time his household and personal expenses were mounting. Interest had to be returned on the loans he had received from his father-in-law; large premiums had to be paid on the insurance policy he had taken out on his life, and he was spending considerable sums on his library and exhibits for his museum. Sandy, who now had a wife and three children, had made new business investments and was very reluctant to provide further financial support. So, for more than three years after his appointment to his chair, Simpson continued be dependent on further loans from his father-in-law.

Some slight relief came in November 1840 when students enrolled for his first session of undergraduate lectures. His class proved to be the largest at the university at that time. At his first lecture many of those who had enrolled could not find seats and arrangements had to be made for his lectures to be repeated to an overflow audience. Simpson was triumphant. In a letter to his sister-in-law he wrote:

> It is very satisfactory to have beat in the race not only all my 'friends' of the Medical Faculty but all the thirty bald and grey-headed Professors. Dr. Alison, who changed his hour to lecture at the same

one with me, has a very small class. Don't he deserve it. He has
broken his own head and missed mine.

Student fees for his first university session brought him over £600. He
was at last able to think of repaying to his family something of the money
that they had been so unstinting in investing in his career for more than
fifteen years. However, he and Jessie now had had their first child and his
household expenses continued to increase; at the end of December he was
obliged to borrowed a further £100 from Sandy.

Simpson's ambition was to make himself known to the world as a
medical scholar, scientist and teacher, but first he meant to provide for the
security and comfort of his family and himself. This he aimed to do as a
clinician in fashionable private practice. In the months that followed his
appointment as Professor of Midwifery, Simpson was to be seen driving
his curricle with great panache around the more fashionable parts of
Edinburgh. The large number of patients who flocked to Edinburgh to see
him provided excellent business for the city's hotels, shops and services.
The Town Council was soon content that the loss of Simpson's predecessor, James Hamilton, had not led to any loss of business for the town.
But whereas James Hamilton had insisted that all his patients should come
to him in Edinburgh, Simpson made it clear that he was ready to travel
long distances to attend members of the upper ranks of Scottish society at
their country seats.

In time, his fashionable practice extended from Keith in the north
to London in the south. His reputation did not depend on his office as
Professor of Midwifery at Edinburgh but on his personal reputation as
a clinician. He had an imposing presence. He was short in stature, but
his unusually large head, crowned with a shock of auburn hair reaching
to his shoulders, was (according to his new friend William Makepeace
Thackeray) the head of Zeus. At rest his expression was very often
somewhat melancholy, but in conversation he had a warm and ready smile
and 'that arrow to the heart, a pleasing voice'.[15] He spoke quietly and confi-
dently, reassuring his patients that they had his sympathy, that he fully
understood their troubles and that he could be relied on to do whatever
was necessary to relieve their complaints.

As an obstetrician he stood apart from his rivals. In the 1840s those who
practised obstetrics in Britain were, almost without exception, physician-
accoucheurs without surgical training. Their approach was conservative
and essentially supportive. Their chief instruments were their hands: they

might use forceps, but any intervention that might cause an increase in the mother's pain was avoided whenever possible. Since caesarean sections carried a very high mortality, they were rarely performed except as a last resort, and they called for the services of a surgeon. Physician-accoucheurs (and even fully committed obstetricians) did not perform the operations themselves. Even the damage caused in traumatic or mismanaged labours often left patients with distressing disabilities for much of their adult lives. Tears of the perineum were not at all uncommon, but the conventional obstetrician simply tied his patient's legs together and hoped that the tear would mend by itself. However, Simpson was never content to leave such matters to nature. He was quick to intervene and since he was a licentiate of the Royal College of Surgeons of Edinburgh, trained in surgery by Robert Liston, one of the greatest surgeons of the time, he was confident that the procedures that he saw as so obviously necessary in the practice of obstetrics were not beyond his skills. He was a courageous and competent, if not brilliant, operator and he was careful in the selection of his cases. He was ready to repair not only the unfortunate consequences of traumatic deliveries that occurred in his own practice, but also those that occurred in the practices of other obstetricians. His services as a gynaecologist were soon as much in demand as his services as an obstetrician. Even so, at least half his practice continued to be as a physician caring for the medical disorders of women and children. A colleague later commented:

> Nothing baffles his intellect, he sticks at nothing, he bungles nothing. From all parts not of Britain only but of Europe do ladies rush to see, consult and fee the little man. He is bold but not reckless, ever ready but never rash. What other men would speculate as to the propriety of for hours, Simpson does.[16]

Simpson's remarkable confidence was founded on his powers as a diagnostician. Traditionally physicians had relied on a 'functional' diagnosis based on the patient's own account of his symptoms and disabilities. Scotland's greatest physician of the eighteenth century, William Cullen, had conducted much of his vast practice entirely by correspondence, prescribing treatment regimes for patients whom he had never met. For much of the nineteenth century, in addition to listening carefully to the full history of the illness, physicians would observe the patient's facial expression and behaviour, feel his pulse and perhaps examine his urine and faeces. But experience had convinced Simpson that a diagnosis made in this way by a physician was less likely to be accurate than one made by a surgeon;

a surgeon's diagnosis was always made after a careful physical examination of the patient. Simpson not only followed the surgeons' example in making a visual and manual examination of his patients, he also used the newest technical aids. He was among the first in Scotland to use the stethoscope invented by Laennec in 1816; he used the percussion technique re-introduced by Skoda in 1836;[17] he designed his own version of the uterine sound devised by Samuel Lair in 1828;[18] and he developed more efficient methods of using the vaginal speculum.

The strength of Simpson's diagnosis allowed him to select the most appropriate of the treatments already available. It also gave him the confidence to try new procedures to meet the problems as he had discovered them to be. Less certain of the exact diagnosis, his rivals hesitated to go beyond standard practice; they denigrated Simpson's display of confidence and condemned his ventures as reckless. However, patients were attracted by Simpson's confidence and his courage in offering forms of treatment that his rivals were unwilling to try.

In his frequent letters to his family, Simpson was able report on the progress of his practice, particularly on the growing number of members of the aristocracy who had become his patients. Soon after moving to Albany Street he wrote: 'Saw yesterday one Countess and three Ladies. Good for one day among the nobility'; and months later: 'I had a letter from the Earl yesterday stating how greatly pleased he and the Countess were with my services . . . I was out two miles into the country this afternoon seeing professionally a niece of the Marquis of Lothian.' In December 1841 he wrote to Walter Grindlay: 'I have been very busy in practice for several weeks past. I often wish that the day were 30 hours long in order to get all done that ought to be done. Yesterday I had the honour of waiting professionally on several Honourable Ladies, on the three daughters of the Lord President, on Lady Dundas and in the evening on Lady Anstruther who had a nice little lively daughter after an hour or two of real suffering.'

By January 1843 Simpson's fees far exceeded even his highest expectations. He was able to send Sandy £300 to complete the repayment of a debt that had accumulated for almost twenty years; to mark the occasion he sent Sandy a box of silver spoons. In the summer, Simpson bought a new and much grander carriage, 'a very handsome affair and exceedingly comfortable, painted claret with red lining and eight windows in it'. He had already acquired a manservant and general factotum (Jarvis); now he engaged a coachman.

Six months later, in January 1844, he was summoned to the Palace of Holyroodhouse to see the nineteen-year-old Princess Marie Amelia of

Baden who had recently married the Marquis of Douglas, heir of the Duke of Hamilton.[19] Simpson told Sandy that he thought himself 'fortunate in getting the Princess as a patient because it quietly places me at the top of the practice on this side of the Tweed. She is the constant theme of talk here in our Edinburgh circles at present and crowds wait occasionally in the streets to see her.' For two months he remained in Edinburgh to look after his 'royal' patient and during that time he was also called to the palace to see the Duke of Argyll's daughter, the Countess of Lincoln, and the Marchioness of Breadalbane.[20]

In September 1844, and already engaged to 'bring in to the world no fewer than the heirs to three Earldoms' later that year, he was summoned to attend the Countess of Lincoln at Hamilton Palace in Lanarkshire. Having successfully relieved his patient's anxieties, he was invited to stay and dine with Prince George, Duke of Cambridge. Before he left he was invited to visit Brodick Castle on the Isle of Arran[21] for a few days later in the season to 'try to shoot grouse'. In due course, in March 1845, he travelled to London to deliver Princess Marie's first son and the Marquis of Douglas's heir. The Marquis later wrote to Simpson: 'I need not tell you all I feel on this occasion and I assure you that I feel great pleasure in writing to you as I can never forget your kindness.'

Simpson relished his time with the families of the aristocracy and they in turn found him an agreeable and interesting guest. He was an excellent and well informed conversationalist. He had read widely. In one not untypical period of six months, he made over thirty purchases from his bookseller. Only six were works on medicine; the rest included the *British Foreign Review*, *Thucydides* (two volumes), Whately's *History Doubts*, the *Antiquities of Denmark*, Carpenter's *Essay on Alcohol*, Stroud's *The Death of Christ*, Irving's *Columbus*, Disraeli's *Works* (two volumes), Goodsir's *Annals*, and Lyell's *Principles of Geology*. He also bought the controversial (and still anonymous) *Vestiges of the Natural History of Creation*, although still unaware that it had been written by his friend Robert Chambers. And he could always discuss the latest novels. As a youth he had eagerly bought the works of Sir Walter Scott, and in the 1840s he was enjoying (and quoting from) the early works of Anthony Trollope. He could amuse as well as interest his hosts and the relationships that he cultivated with the families of his prestigious patients often became personal as well as formally professional. Long after he had first been consulted he continued to correspond with their families and to keep them informed of new forms of treatment. He became particularly friendly with the 7th Duke of Argyll, a Whig politician, an eminent amateur scientist and a Fellow of the Royal Society; and with the scholarly Marquis of Lorne who, after he succeed his father as the 8th Duke of Argyll in 1847, served in a number of Liberal governments as Lord Privy Seal and Secretary of State for India; he was also a close friend of Prince Albert.

Simpson had many patients among the friends and relatives of the dukes of Argyll, Hamilton and Sutherland and other members of Scotland's aristocracy, but an ever-growing number of less prestigious patients continued to crowd into his waiting room, and more and more young couples in Edinburgh engaged his services for the delivery of their anxiously expected infants. In 1845, he had spent £2,150 on the purchase of a large house at 52 Queen Street and he had hired an apprentice, the last physician's apprentice to be indentured in Edinburgh. His practice had continued to grow. The house in Queen Street had a large dining room and two smaller rooms on the ground floor, two drawing rooms and bedroom on the first floor, four bedrooms and nursery on the second floor and four smaller bedrooms on the third floor. By 1846 it was already too small and Simpson had it enlarged to provide accommodation for two new assistants, George Keith and James Matthews Duncan. But the waiting rooms were still always overcrowded. And Simpson continued to travel to see his important patients in distant parts of the country.

His relationship with the Duke of Sutherland's family had become almost that of a friend rather than that of an attending physician. When, in the autumn of 1846, he felt 'in need of a long rest and a complete change of scene'[22] he was invited by the Duke's son-in-law, Lord Blantyre, to spend a few weeks at his splendid new Erskine House on the southern shore of the Clyde, opposite Dumbarton Castle. For three weeks, Simpson was able to shoot on the Erskine estate to the south of the Clyde and explore Strath-leven, Loch Lomond and the Gair Loch to the north. At Erskine House the party included Lord and Lady Blantyre, the Duke and Duchess of Sutherland, the Marquis and Marchioness of Lorne and the Duke's two sisters, the Ladies Gower. Simpson reported to Sandy that they had all been exceedingly kind to him and that he had felt quite at home among them, although the only untitled person at the table. His wife and children spent these three weeks in the north-east of Scotland at St Cyrus in Kincardineshire.

Some time later that winter, the Duchess of Sutherland, the Mistress of the Robes, suggested to Queen Victoria that Simpson might be appointed as Physician to the Queen in Scotland. On 18 January 1847, the Duchess wrote to him:

Dear Sir,

It was great pleasure to me to receive yesterday a letter from the Queen telling me that she would have much pleasure in complying with the request 'which his high character and abilities make him fit for'. The Queen adds that it will be officially communicated to you.

I remain, dear sir, yours very truly,

Harriet Sutherland.

Simpson immediately wrote to Sandy to tell him of the appointment. At the same time he informed him that he had recently been in London and that in one day he had not only dined with the Mistress of the Robes, he had also breakfasted with the Secretary of War, Earl Grey, and had tea and an egg with the Prime Minister, Lord John Russell.

Simpson's family had reason to be content and quietly proud. Their grandfather had been a landless cottar who had experienced extreme poverty and famine. Now Thomas was a successful merchant in Grangemouth; Alexander (Sandy) had expanded and developed the family bakery but had since appointed John Brodie to manage the business, with its four journeymen and four apprentices, while he made a new career as a banker;[23] John had been a much respected lawyer and an agent of the Standard Life Assurance Company before he died at the age of forty-seven in 1841; Mary and her husband, John Pearson (who had inherited a fortune, it was said, of £40,000) had emigrated to Australia and bought a large sheep station at Casterton, in Victoria; and David had followed his sister to Australia and had established his own business in Hamilton, Victoria.

Simpson himself had reached the top of his profession. He and his wife and three sons[24] enjoyed a very comfortable and expansive style of life in his large and well staffed house in Edinburgh's New Town. He also owned Viewbank, a small country house near the fishing village of Newhaven, where his family could escape the smoke and bustle of Edinburgh. He had made his mark in society and, within the medical profession, he was already greatly respected and admired in Scotland.

But to be respected in Scotland was not enough. He had been commissioned by his mother to be a great man. He now turned his attention to making an international reputation as a medical scholar and critic, and as a clinical innovator.

SIX

Experimental Medicine:
Galvanism and Gynaecology

If a man will begin with certainties he shall end in doubts but if he will be content to begin with doubts he shall end in certainties.

Francis Bacon

Simpson's election to the chair of Midwifery at Edinburgh established his position as the leading obstetrician in Edinburgh. But he had greater ambitions. He planned to win a place on the world stage as one of the leading obstetricians of his time. To that end, he made it his practice to be constantly alert to news of any new obstetrical procedure that seemed to offer a prospect of being an advance in clinical practice. He then courageously (many said rashly) tried out such procedures in the treatment of his own patients and published reports of his trials in the medical press.

In such a strategy, Simpson was seizing an advantage that had not been available to previous generations of medical scientists. For his plan to succeed it was essential that he should have the earliest possible notice of every new procedure being tried or even suggested anywhere in Europe or North America; it was equally essential that he should be able to publish the results of his trials as quickly and widely as possible. For this he was dependent on the medical press. In 1800 there had been only eight medical journals published in Britain; by 1840 there were over fifty.[1] The number and the variety of interests of these many journals allowed Simpson to be quickly aware not only of possible advances in his own professed subject of obstetrics, but also in every other related field of medicine.

As he built his international reputation, Simpson published scores of clinical reports. His earliest works were published in the *Edinburgh Medical and Surgical Journal*, then the most prestigious medical journal in Britain.[2] But to ensure that his views would reach an even wider audience in Europe and America, he later joined with John Rose Cormack to found *The Monthly Journal of Medical Science*, published in Edinburgh by Sutherland and Knox and in London by John Constable. And everything he wrote in these and other journals he had reprinted and published (and sold, price

6d) as pamphlets in Edinburgh, London, Dublin and Philadelphia.[3]

His 'Observations Regarding the Influence of Galvanism upon the Action of the Uterus during Labour' provided an example of the style and method that Simpson had developed by the 1840s and put forward as an example that others should follow. This trial in July 1846 followed from the publication of Hermann Kilian's *Operative Midwifery* in 1845. In his book, Kilian had reported that his attempts to enhance uterine contractions during labour by electrical stimulation had 'fallen short of his expectations'. This unexpected admission had revived a debate in the medical press on whether or not electrical stimulation of the uterus had any place in the management of labour. Simpson decided to settle the issue by conducting a trial of his own.

His report, published in July 1846,[4] began with a review of everything than had been published on the subject from 1803, when Gottfried Herder, in Leipzig, had first suggested that electrical stimulation ('galvanism') might be helpful in cases of slow and tedious labour,[5] until 1844, when Thomas Radford in Manchester had reported on his success in using galvanism to control uterine haemorrhage.[6] Simpson found all the reports unsatisfactory. He pointed out that the obstetricians who had published them had tried galvanism on only a few random cases, had failed to distinguish between *post hoc* and *propter hoc* and had not taken account of the fact that 'the uterus, particularly during labour, is well known to be very readily, and sometimes very powerfully, influenced in its parturient action by mere states and emotions of the mind alone'. Simpson conducted a formal trial designed to overcome these deficiencies. It was a trial that was intended not simply to confirm that galvanism had a stimulant effect on the pregnant uterus, but also to 'ascertain and fix its actual amount'.

The procedure that he followed was based on that described by Radford in his article in the *Provincial Medical and Surgical Journal* in 1844. A metal conductor attached by a wire to one terminal of a galvanic machine (a battery the power of which could be increased or lowered) was inserted into the vagina and advanced to make contact with the cervix; an external conductor connected to the second terminal of the galvanic machine was placed in contact with the skin of the abdomen over the fundus of the uterus. The galvanic machine was capable of producing a current that could not be tolerated even by a very determined person holding a conducting wire in each hand. The trial was conducted in the Edinburgh Royal Maternity Hospital on six patients experiencing prolonged labour; several other patients had to be excluded from the trial because they found that

Table 6.1 Observations on Case I

Before application of wires		Wires applied but galvanic circle incomplete		Wires applied and galvanic circle complete		After removal of wires	
Duration of pains secs	Duration of intervals secs	Duration of pains secs	Duration of intervals secs	Duration of pains secs	Duration of intervals secs	Duration of pains secs	Duration of intervals secs
30	30	40	80	45	75	45	165
33	267	38	22	40	170	37	368
31	200	40	50	35	145	45	300
33	147	38	172	30	120	40	95
35	205	45	135	45	195	30	103
30	150	40	140	32	163	25	95
35	325	35	205	30	195	28	182
35	175	50	190	33	117	35	145
32		42		40		28	
Avr: 33	Avr: 188	Avr: 41	Avr: 124	Avr: 37	Avr: 147	Avr: 56	Avr: 125

Table 6.2 Summary of Observations of Cases I, III, IV & VI

Case	Before application of wires		Wires applied but galvanic circle incomplete		Wires applied and galvanic circle complete		After removal of wires	
	Duration of pains secs	Duration of intervals sec	Duration of pains secs	Duration of intervals secs	Duration of pains secs	Duration of intervals secs	Duration of pains secs	Duration of intervals secs
No. I	33	188	41	124	37	147	35	182
No. III	51	155	43	152	43	177	52	194
No. IV	56	76	46	94	55	70	54	68
No. VI	77	48	75	77	82	63	83	59
Average of Whole	54	117	50	112	54	114	56	125

they could not tolerate the pain caused by the galvanic current. For all six patients the procedure was carried out during the first stage of labour, since stages two and three did not allow sufficient time for the apparatus to be assembled and set up.

In presenting his results Simpson was guided by Jules Gavarret's *Principes Generaux de Statisique Medicale* which had been published in 1840. After reading Gavarret's book, Simpson always insisted on using statistics ('arithmetical methods') when presenting the results of his investigations.

The first patient in his trial, Case I, was a young woman of twenty having her first child. The galvanism was applied between the third and sixth hours of a nine-hour first stage of labour. The duration of the contractions and the intervals between were carefully measured by stopwatch and recorded by the house surgeon. The trial was witnessed by a number of medical students and a few other spectators. The results he presented in tabular form, as shown in Table 6.1.

This procedure was completed only in Cases I, III, IV, and VI. In Case II, when galvanism was applied the duration of the labour pains became distinctly shorter than in any of the other periods and the trial was halted. In Case V there was only one pain after galvanism was applied, and thereafter uterine action disappeared entirely throughout the twenty-three minutes during which the galvanism was continued; the pains again became regular as soon as the galvanic apparatus was removed. A summary of the results in Cases I, III, IV and VI is shown in Table 6.2.

Simpson conceded that a trial on only four patients was unsatisfactory, but it had been impossible to find a larger number to take part because of the pain caused by the passage of the galvanic current. Nevertheless, the data collected showed that neither does the duration of the pains always go on increasing as labour continues, nor does the duration between pains always go on decreasing as authorities on obstetrics often claimed.[7] And the limited evidence that had been gathered did not show that either the frequency of labour pains or their duration was affected in 'any appreciable or direct manner by the employment of galvanism'. Simpson avoided giving undue significance to the results of his trial:

> It would be hasty and logically incorrect to deduce from these observations that under no modification and under no manner of application does galvanism possess the power of directly exciting or increasing the contractile activity of the uterus. Forms or methods of employing it may yet possibly be detected or devised, affording a different result. But I believe I am justified in inferring from the inquiry that as employed at the present time, and in its present mode, it is not a means which can be in any degree relied upon for the purpose in question; and is so far practically and entirely useless as a stimulant to the parturient uterus.

In stating these conclusions as a result of my own experience I, of course, by no means wish to impugn, in any way, the validity of the observations made in one or two cases by others and in which the opposite effect was supposed to be obtained under the employment of galvanism during labour. Uterine contractions may certainly have become occasionally increased while galvanism was being used but I strongly question if that increase was the result of the galvanic agency.

At the end of his report he added:

As a concluding remark, I would beg to take the liberty of suggesting that perhaps the plan of investigation which I pursued in the present inquiry is one that might be usefully and successfully applied to test the validity, or fix the value, of other supposed measures besides galvanism.

After succeeding James Hamilton as Professor of Midwifery, Simpson had quickly built up a large and fashionable private practice. His remarkable success was due largely to his courage and skill as a pioneer of the new and related speciality of gynaecology; even the word 'gynaecology' did not come into use until 1847.

In England, even the obstetricians with appointments to London's great teaching hospitals, were still physician-accoucheurs with no formal training in surgery.[8] As noted earlier, tears of the perineum caused during difficult deliveries were not immediately repaired; all that was thought possible was to approximate the sides of the tear by tying the patient's legs together and 'to hope for the best'; attempts to suture the tear at some later time were most often unsuccessful. In Alabama, Marion Sims had treated one patient with urinary incontinence due to a vesico-vaginal fistula, but it had taken thirty-three operations to complete the repair; in Britain in the first half of the nineteenth century, no attempt was ever made to close the vesico-vaginal fistulas produced by the mismanagement of deliveries, leaving many women suffering an intensely distressing condition for the rest of their lives. Prolapse of the uterus, one of the commonest disabilities to afflict women after repeated pregnancies, was relieved only mechanically by pads and pessaries, and the result was rarely satisfactory.

Nothing was then known about other gynaecological disorders, such as the causes of cancer. In 1845, Marc Colombat de L'Isere, a prominent medical figure in Paris, wrote that cancer of the cervix occurred in women 'of an erotic temperament who, tormented by venereal desires, gave themselves up with excess to masturbation or venery or passed their lives in crowded parties'. In Britain there were very few attempts at surgical intervention; patients were treated by bleeding and purging, and restricted to a semi-starvation diet.

Physician-accoucheurs did treat a few 'diseases of women', but these were only the disorders of menstruation, displacements of the uterus and the pains usually attributed to inflammation of the uterus. The treatments available to them were pessaries, clysters, blisters, setons, cauterisation of the cervix and acupuncture.[9] Even in Scotland, where obstetricians were more likely to have had some formal training in surgery, major procedures, including caesarean section, were carried out only by licensed surgeons.

The first major gynaecological operation of modern times was carried out in Rockbridge County, Virginia, by Ephraim McDowell. McDowell's father, who had emigrated from Argyll, had attended medical lectures at Edinburgh University and had been trained in surgery in Edinburgh by John Bell. His son, Ephraim, performed the first successful removal of an ovarian cyst in 1809,[10] and he went on to perform a further twelve such operations; four of his patients died. In Britain no ovariotomy was carried out successfully until 1842 when, in Manchester, Charles Clay, an Edinburgh graduate and a licentiate of the Royal College of Surgeons of Edinburgh, removed an ovarian cyst weighing 36 lbs. But in spite of this remarkable success, most cases in Britain continued to be treated by the insertion of a needle and cannula through the wall of the vagina or the abdomen to tap the cyst and withdraw as much as possible of its content; iodine, port wine and water, rose leaves in wine, muriate of lime or even pure alcohol was then injected into the cyst in an attempt to prevent the further accumulation of fluid.

Three years after the publication of Charles Clay's report, the reluctance of surgeons to follow his lead was discussed by Simpson at a meeting of the Edinburgh Medico-Chirurgical Society.[11] As reported later, he suggested that one factor was the understandable reluctance of surgeons to perform a hazardous operation based not on their own diagnosis but on the basis of a diagnosis made by an obstetrician. He also argued that surgeons did not appreciate the relative merits of treatment by tapping and treatment by ovariotomy. Treatment by tapping and injection was only palliative, at best allowing the patient some temporary relief. Almost invariably the procedure had to be repeated again and again. He had no belief 'that iodine or aught else was capable of absorbing and removing the structure and contents of a cystic tumour of the ovary. He would as soon believe that the head could be absorbed and removed by medicine.' And in the longer term the prognosis for patients treated by tapping was very poor indeed. In one reported series of twenty cases, four patients had died of 'inflammation' (infection) within a few days of the first tapping. In all, fourteen died within nine months of the first tapping; two more died within eighteen months; and four lived for periods varying from four to nine years.

Simpson conceded that the risks of removing the ovarian cyst by ovariotomy were high. So far, one in three patients had died but he believed 'that would betimes become rectified'. In any case, surgeons accepted greater risks almost daily in performing amputations; even in the best of hospitals the mortality was over 35 per cent[12] and could be more than 50 per cent.[13]

Many surgeons also claimed that it was unwise to subject patients to ovariotomy when 'the process of reparation after the operation was too great to accomplish with health and safety'. Simpson gave 'a direct and practical denial to this theory by demonstrating the reverse to be true'. He cited what was known of the outcomes of all the earliest ovariotomies on record. Ephraim McDowell's first patient had gone on to have five living children. Of Charles Clay's first patients, one 'continues well and follows her household duties with ease'; 'one is at this time perfectly well and capable of greater exertion than most women of her age, viz., 60'; one complained 'of a polypus of the nose – [but] in every other respect she is quite well'; one was 'in better health than in any part of her former life'. Indeed, all of Clay's patients were reported to be well.

Simpson had found that some surgeons attributed their reluctance to perform hazardous ovariotomies on patients with ovarian cysts to the high probability that the disease would recur. This argument he also dismissed. The other ovary might be minimally affected and might require removal along with the first, but the 'pathological nature of multilocular disease of the ovary was such that it had no tendency to spring up again in the same locality or in distant and different organs of the body'. Again he pointed out that these surgeons were being inconsistent; they were always ready to remove carcinomatous disease from any external part of the body even though recurrence was almost inevitable.

Simpson suggested the real reason for surgeons' reluctance to operate on ovarian cysts was their dread of opening the abdomen and exposing the peritoneum. But recent experience had shown 'that the exposure of the cavity of the peritoneum was not so dangerous as was formerly dreamed of by pathologists. The success of Caesarian section in the hands of Continental accoucheurs might have taught us a different lesson, the peritoneal cavity in that operation being of necessity opened up; and we may daily see the same done upon the females of some of our domestic animals, with remarkable impunity in the coarse operation of spaying.'

As his career progressed, Simpson became even more ready to venture beyond the recognised limits of his expertise as an obstetrician. His pronouncements often gave offence to experienced practitioners in other branches of the profession; the reactions of the surgeons present at this meeting of the Edinburgh Medico-Chirurgical Society in December 1843 are not recorded.

Simpson had published a report in 1841 on his own first contribution to gynaecology.[14] In it he gave an account of a radical operation that had not been performed before in Britain. The patient was a woman aged thirty-three who had been married for thirteen years and had borne five children. In May 1838, she began to have a red-tinted vaginal discharge. From October the discharge increased and was soon seen to contain blood. After many weeks she became pale and so debilitated and exhausted that she was bedridden. She was first seen by a doctor in May 1839; he found that she had a large tumour of the cervix. He examined her a few days later and he was able to describe the tumour as a firm, red and painless mass with a rough granular and lobulated surface. He decided that 'the free amputation of the cervix offered by far the most probable means of success'. This was an adventurous decision. Only a few months before Dr Fleetwood Churchill had reported that he was 'not aware that any attempts have ever been made in Great Britain to excise the cervix'.

Simpson had informed the patient and her husband that even if the operation were successful the tumour would probably recur. At first they refused to have the operation but after three weeks, during which she became increasingly weak and ill, they at last consented. Simpson carried out the operation with the assistance of Dr Lewins and a surgeon, Mr Zeigler. In 1839 it was, of course, performed without any form of anaesthesia. The patient was positioned by the assistants face down on her bed with her legs falling over one side. By long forceps, Simpson 'was enabled to pull down the tumour cautiously until it was entirely protruded beyond the external parts'. The tumour and the whole of the vaginal part of the cervix were then excised. 'The patient bore the operation well and complained wonderfully little during it.' After the operation the patient was free of symptoms and rapidly regained her strength.

Simpson was able to examine the histology of the tumour using a new and powerful microscope owned by his friend John Reid. The appearances were exactly those that had been described by Sir Charles Clerke 'under the quaint but expressive name of Cauliflower Excrescence from the *os uterus*'. The nature of such Cauliflower tumours was still uncertain. Simpson quoted four authorities (Richard Gooch,[15] Robert Hooper, David Davis[16] and Robert Lee) who believed such tumours to be cancerous, and three (Sir Charles Clerke, John Burns and John Waller) who regarded them as being composed of morbid tissue that was not necessarily malignant. Simpson believed that, since it was known that such tumours could occur in patients as young as twenty, progressed only very slowly and were not accompanied by deposits of disease in other parts of the body, they should not be regarded as malignant, at least in their early stages. However both Gooch[17] and Boivin[18] had found that the tumour could recur if only partially removed and Davis[19] had found that even some years after the tumour's apparent removal it could reappear as a cancerous ulceration. Simpson concluded that if a radical operation for the cure of a Cauliflower tumour was to be attempted, the radical excision of both the tumour and the whole of the vaginal part of the cervix appeared to be 'the only measure which can at all be hoped to insure ultimate success'. In the diligent search of the medical literature that was always part of Simpson's routine practice, he found that, contrary to Churchill's statement in 1838, this had already been done in France on three occasions. Since 1828, Colombat de L'Isere,[20] Boivin[21] and Hervez de Chegoin[22] had each treated a patient suffering from Cauliflower Excrescence by amputation of the cervix, and all three patients had thereafter remained well. Simpson's was the first such case in Britain, and over a year later he was able to report that his patient had not only remained well but was now pregnant.

The publication of his report on his 'Case of Amputation of the Neck of the Womb followed by Pregnancy' in the *Edinburgh Medical and Surgical Journal* in 1841, and its later re-issue as a pamphlet by Sutherland and Knox in Edinburgh, gave early notice of Simpson's readiness to use new and radical measures in the treatment of gynaecological conditions previously thought to be untreatable.

SEVEN

Library Medicine:
Evolution of Disease

*The highest wisdom has but one science, the science explaining
the whole creation and man's place in it.*

Leo Tolstoy

*So much perverse misjudgement on these points is simply owing
to intellectual obtuseness.*

Anon (Vestiges of Creation)

Although, in 1840, Simpson had been appointed as a Professor of Midwifery, it had never been his intention to confine his ambitions to the study and teaching of obstetrics. He meant to make his name not only by contributing to the advance of clinical practice but also by making his voice heard in the debates on all the great issues in the medical science of his time.

His literary powers and energy were remarkable. Before writing on any subject it was his practice to make a comprehensive and perceptive review of all the relevant literature from the works of the classical Greek physicians and the physicians of the great Arabian school of the tenth century onwards to include those of even the most obscure writers of his own time. He searched the archives of every institution where neglected information might possibly be found. He then presented his conclusions, at length and supported whenever possible by statistical analysis, in a publication and in a style calculated to appeal to his target audience.

The issue that disturbed and divided scientific opinion in Britain and attracted Simpson's attention in the 1840s was the question of 'Evolution'. In Scotland, the concept of evolution had been debated since James Hutton presented his Theory of the Earth to the Royal Society of Edinburgh in the spring of 1785.[1] After almost half a century, the phenomenon, if not the mechanism, of evolution had been quietly accepted by the scientific community in Scotland. In England, however, the universities and scientific bodies such as the Royal College of Physicians of London were still unshaken in their loyalty to the Biblical story of the Creation.[2] And among even the educated members of the general public in Britain, Hutton's ideas were still virtually unknown.

James Hutton was born in 1726, the son of a merchant and City Treasurer in Edinburgh and the owner of a farm in Berwickshire. He was educated at Edinburgh's High School and Edinburgh University, and in 1743 he was apprenticed to an Edinburgh lawyer. After three years, he abandoned the law to study medicine at Edinburgh, Paris and Leyden. He took his MD at Leyden, but during his studies he had become more interested in chemistry than in medicine. He decided not to practise as a physician but to use his knowledge of chemistry to improve the fertility and productivity of the farm that he had inherited from his father. He travelled in England and in the Netherlands to study the best of their modern farming practices and within a few years of his return to Berwickshire he had developed his father's antiquated farm into a successful commercial business. He had also invented and patented a chemical process for the production of sal ammoniac from soot and, together, the profits from his farm and from his invention had made him, if not conspicuously wealthy, at least financially independent and secure.

During his tours of the farms and lands of Scotland, England and the Netherlands he had added the study of geology to his continuing interests in chemistry and medicine and, at the age of forty-two, he left his farm in the hands of a manager and moved to Edinburgh to devote himself to science. In 1783, he became one of the founder members of the Royal Society of Edinburgh and one of the *literati* of the Scottish Enlightenment. His friends and associates in Edinburgh were Adam Smith,[3] Joseph Black, William Robertson, Hugh Blair, Adam Ferguson and Robert Adam.

In 1785, he wrote two papers on his Theory of the Earth. As he was not a confident speaker, the first of his papers was read to the society by his friend Joseph Black, Professor of Chemistry at Edinburgh; the second paper he read himself at another meeting.[4] It was not until ten years later that he wrote a full account of his work in his *Theory of the Earth with Proofs and Illustrations*; the first two volumes of the book were published in 1795, but he died in 1797 before the third volume was completed.

His theory was based on his many years of study of the form, appearance and chemical composition of rocks and their distribution over the surface of Britain. He had concluded that the rocky surface of the earth is being constantly eroded; that the resulting debris is carried by the rivers to the seabed, where it becomes mixed with other rock debris and various specimens of marine life; that the mixture is then melted and consolidated by the heat of the earth's interior into new rock; and that the new rock is slowly uplifted, again by the energy of the earth's heat, to renew the earth's crust. He believed that it must be assumed that this process, observed at work now, had been always at work in times past (his 'Principle of Uniformitarianism'). He therefore denied that the earth had been created by a sudden cataclysmic event as described in the Bible. He claimed that the surface of the earth was being constantly re-created by repeated cycles of erosion, igneous activity and uplift, and since the resulting changes in the shape and distribution of the earth's rocky surface proceeded so slowly as to be almost immeasurable in a single human lifetime, each complete cycle must take thousands of years. The whole process, continuing over billions of years, must belong in a time span for which there was 'no vestige of a beginning, no prospect of an end'.

Hutton's purpose in writing his *Theory of the Earth* was to present this concept of geological time. But he added a momentous rider that, then and since, has attracted less notice. He envisioned an earth on which it was not only the crust, but every living thing on the surface of that crust, that was slowly and constantly evolving. And he briefly speculated on the mechanism by which evolution of living things was achieved. He wrote that in considering 'the infinite variety among individuals of the same species we must be assured that those which depart most from the best adapted constitution will be most liable to perish while those organised bodies which most approach to the best constitution for the present circumstances will be best adapted to continue in preserving themselves and multiplying the individuals of their race'.

A year after the publication of the first volumes of Hutton's *Theory of the Earth,* Erasmus Darwin,[5] who had been Hutton's contemporary as a medical student at Edinburgh, made some further comment on how Hutton's 'best adapted constitution' might come about. In his *Zoonomia, or the Laws of Organic Life* he asked whether it would 'not be too bold to imagine, that in the great length of time since the earth began to exist all warm-blooded animals have arisen from one living filament possessing the faculty of continuing to improve by its own inherent activity, and of delivering down those improvements by generation to its posterity?' Here, in 1800, he makes an early statement of the doctrine of constant change and the survival of the fittest.

In these first years of the nineteenth century, there was no great public interest in Britain in theories of the evolution of the earth or of the generation of living things. (Even the word 'evolution' was not used in this context until 1826.) Hutton's *Theory of the Earth* had been so badly written that few had taken the trouble to read it, and it was not until John Playfair published his *Illustrations of the Huttonian Theory of the Earth* in 1802 that Hutton's concept of geological time was presented clearly and competently to the general public. In *Zoonomia*, Erasmus Darwin's main purpose had been to assign all forms of animal life into classes, orders, genera, and species, and that part of his book was favourably received. But his thoughts on the evolution of mankind had been received with scorn. In 1808, the *Edinburgh Review* announced its satisfaction that 'the days of Dr. Darwin's popularity of gnomes, sylphs, oxygen, gossamer, polygynia and polyandria have passed away'.[6]

However, James Hutton's concept of the evolution of the earth's crust had not been entirely forgotten. In 1833, Charles Lyell revived interest in his work in his book *Principles of Geology*. Charles Lyell belonged to a wealthy landowning family in Forfarshire (now Angus). In 1815, while studying law at Oxford, he had read both Hutton's *Theory of the Earth* and Playfair's *Illustrations of the Huttonian Theory of the Earth*. He was inspired to become an enthusiastic amateur geologist and, in 1819, he was elected to the Geological Society; three years later he became its secretary. His practice as a barrister had not prospered, but he had achieved considerable success in writing essays and book reviews for the *Quarterly Review*. In 1827, he decided to combine his interest in geology with his literary skills and write a book on geology. He produced the first edition of his three-volume *Principles of Geology* between 1830 and 1833; popular cheap editions followed in 1834, 1835 and 1837.

Lyell's *Principles* presented both a more readable version of Hutton's book and a more comprehensive account of Hutton's work than Playfair's *Illustrations*. Lyell accepted Hutton's idea of 'geological' time and his concept of geological cycles of erosion and igneous reformation. But he argued that, although these cycles restored and repaired the surface of the earth, they did not represent part of a system of constant change and endless progress. He also refused to accept the idea of evolution of living things; he believed that each species of plant and animal was an individual creation and was stable and unchanging. And he was particularly opposed to the idea of the evolution of man. In England, the several editions of his *Principles* reached a wide audience and his ideas became very generally accepted. He was appointed as the first Professor of Geology at King's College, London and was later knighted. But among the scientific community in Scotland, Lyell's views seemed retrograde and they stimulated a revival of interest in the whole subject of evolution.

John Pringle Nichol, Professor of Astronomy at Glasgow, disputed Lyell's assertion that, while the surface of the earth was constantly being repaired and renewed, it was not in a constant state of change. In his *Views of the Architecture of the Heavens*, published in 1837, Nichol set out clear and convincing evidence that the whole universe was constantly being irreversibly changed by the creation of new solar systems.

In 1841, Simpson and his friend the publisher Robert Chambers also decided, quite independently of each other, that they too must take issue with Lyell. In his *Antiquarian Notices of Leprosy and Leper Hospitals* published in the *Edinburgh Medical and Surgical Journal* in 1841 and 1842, Simpson disputed Lyell's claim that all living things were individually created and continued forever unchanged. Diseases, in his view, were living things and there were strong grounds for believing that the diseases suffered by man had changed quite markedly over the period of recorded history. Since the first observations of disease were recorded in Greece, various new human maladies had made their appearance: smallpox, measles and whooping-cough were well recognised examples. Other diseases, which had once been prevalent, had since disappeared completely: lyncanthropia (the werewolf mania of Burton's *Melancholia*), for example, and the sweating sickness of the fifteenth century. And there were diseases which had disappeared from one part of the world only to appear in another.

Simpson proposed to illustrate the changes that had taken place in human disease by making a detailed study of the history of leprosy. In the nineteenth century, leprosy was no longer an endemic disease in any part of Europe, yet from the tenth to the sixteenth centuries it had been prevalent almost everywhere across the continent. In the eleventh century an order of knighthood, the Knights Hospitallers, had been founded to protect them. In the twelfth century Pope Alexander III had issued Papal Bulls regulating the segregation and ecclesiastical separation of lepers, and establishing their rights while segregated. In the early thirteenth century, Matthew Paris had estimated that there were more than 19,000 'lazar houses' in Christendom. There had been over 2,000 leper hospitals in France alone.

Over these many years and in various parts of the world, the disease had been known by slightly different names. However, Simpson was satisfied that the disease had been the same everywhere during the whole period of its prevalence. The first signs of the disease appeared as tawny-red patches on the skin, especially on the nose, ears, lips and other parts on the face.

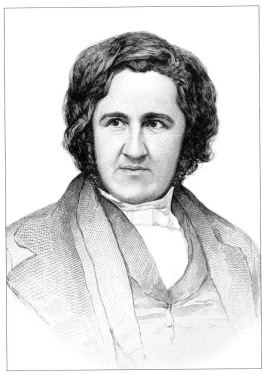

LEFT. Simpson, Fellow of the Royal College of Physicians of Edinburgh at the early age of 25.

BELOW. The Lawnmarket in 1825 as it was when Simpson arrived in Edinburgh as a student.

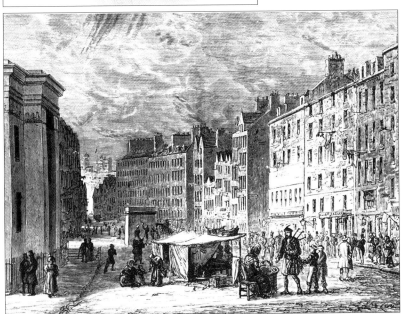

LEFT. Robert Knox (1779–1862), a distinguished comparative anatomist and medical scientist destroyed by his inadvertent involvement in the affair of Burke and Hare in 1828.

BELOW. Park House in which Professor James Hamilton established Edinburgh's Lying-in Hospital in 1793. When the building was sold by his heirs in 1842 Simpson transferred the hospital to Queensberry House.

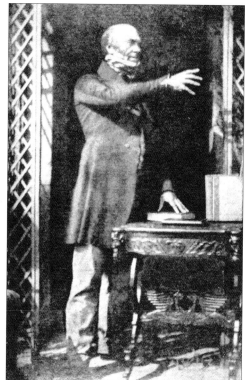

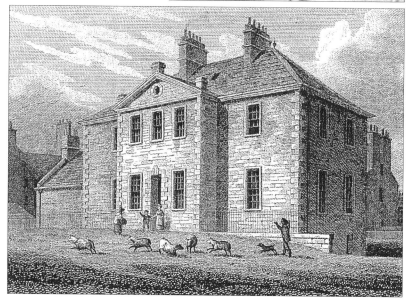

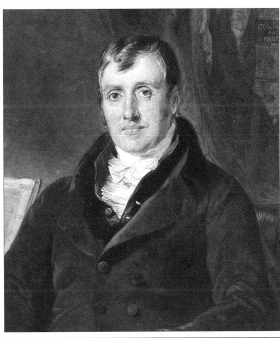

LEFT. John Thomson (1765–1856), Professor of Military Surgery and later of General Pathology. A prominent Whig, he was Simpson's first professional patron.

BELOW. Edinburgh University: the new college building (now Old College) designed by Robert Adam and completed after his death by William Playfair in 1827.

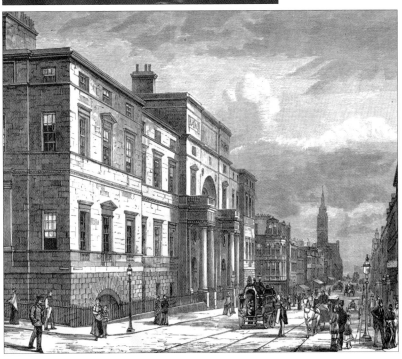

The Royal College of
Physicians of Edinburgh:
the New Hall designed
by Thomas Hamilton in
1844 and, after extensions
to the library, completed
in 1868.

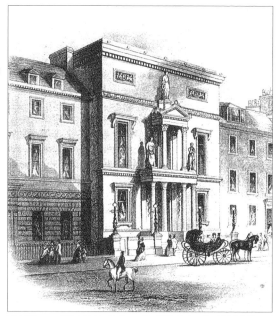

Simpson's house at 52
Queen Street, enlarged
to accommodate his
growing practice by the
still clearly visible
addition of a top floor.

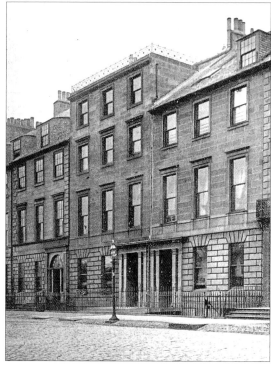

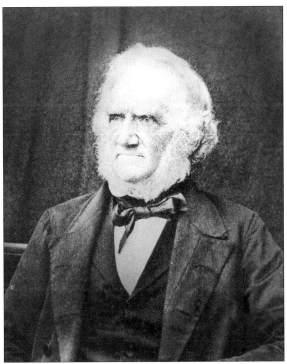

Alexander Simpson, Simpson's brother, born in 1797; banker and active proprietor of the family bakery and distilling businesses.

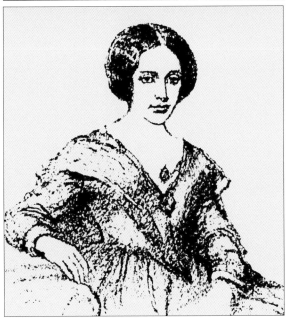

Miss Jessie Grindlay of Toxteth in Liverpool, Simpson's second cousin, soon to become his wife.

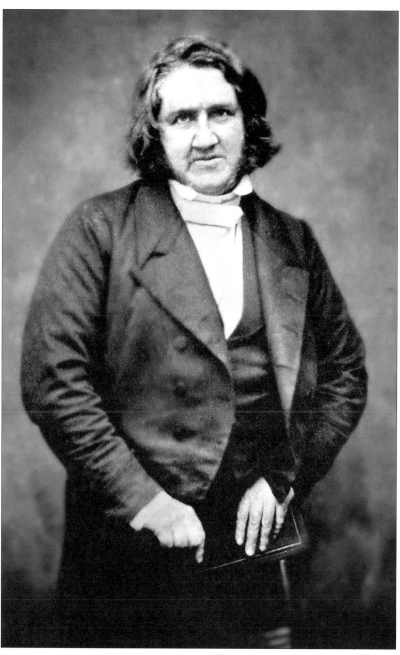

James Y. Simpson, newly elected Professor of Midwifery and the Diseases of Women and Children, in 1840.

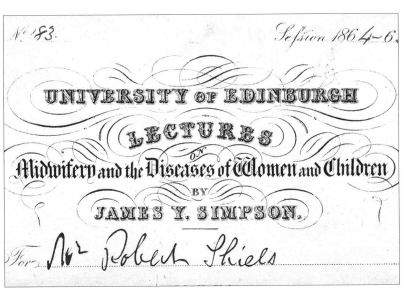

Nᵒ 83.   Session 1864-6.

UNIVERSITY OF EDINBURGH

LECTURES

ON

Midwifery and the Diseases of Women and Children

BY

JAMES Y. SIMPSON.

For Mʳ Robert Shiels

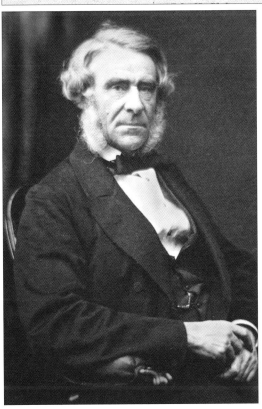

ABOVE. 'Class Ticket' for Simpson's lecture course.

LEFT. Professor Robert Christison (1797–1882), physician and toxicologist: the most influential member of the Medical Faculty when Simpson was appointed to his chair at Edinburgh.

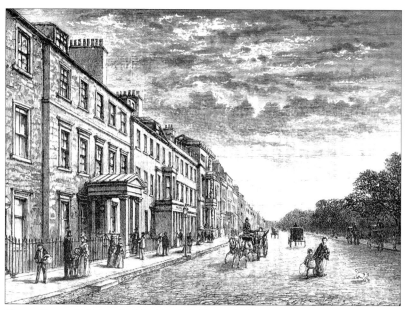

Queen Street, Edinburgh: The Royal College of Physicians at no. 9.

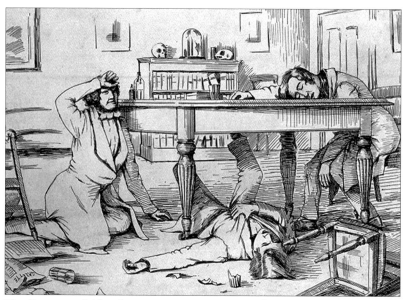

The discovery of chloroform. An artist's impression of Simpson, James Matthews Duncan and George Keith intoxicated by their first inhalations of its vapour.

The sensitivity of the affected part gradually diminished until eventually all feeling was lost. The discoloured skin thickened and became raised into roundish livid red tubercles. As they grew the tubercles split and ulcerated, forming discharging sores. In its last lethal stages, the disease extended into the lining of the intestine, producing large debilitating ulcers.

Simpson planned to establish when this dreadful illness had first appeared in Britain and when it had finally disappeared. There was, of course, no record of the number of individuals who had been afflicted by leprosy during those years. However, Simpson believed that he could produce indirect evidence of the increase and later the decline and fall in the prevalence of the disease by finding and examining the records of all the leper hospitals that had ever existed in Britain. It was a daunting task and it was typical of Simpson's quite extraordinary drive and industry that he not only attempted it but carried it out.

He had hoped to discover not only the number of leper hospitals that had existed in Scotland and England but also the dates of their foundation, the dates at which they were no longer judged to be necessary and the total number of patients that they had sheltered and cared for. However, he was disappointed to find that even for such a limited inquiry, the recorded evidence was 'exceedingly slight'. The charters and other documents to be found relating directly to leper hospitals were only the very few that had survived by chance and, without exception, they concerned grants made to the institutions at some very uncertain time after they had been founded. He therefore extended his research to include the examination of the archives of towns where it was believed that leper hospitals had once existed. This source also proved disappointing. In some cases the only evidence that a leper hospital had every existed was the persistence of 'liber', or other corruption of the word 'leper', in a place name (as in Liberton near Edinburgh).

In Scotland, he found worthwhile records of only the ten leper hospitals that there had once been at Aberdeen, Aldcambus (Berwickshire), Aldnestun (Berwickshire), Edinburgh (at Greenside and at Liberton), Glasgow, Linlithgow, Prestwick and Shetland (Lerwick and Papa Stour). The earliest had been founded in Berwickshire at some point before 1177, the last at Glasgow in 1330. None of the leper hospitals in Scotland had had accommodation for more than eight patients and never at any time could their existence give even the remotest indication of the incidence of the disease in the general population. He found no evidence that any of these hospitals had survived into the second half of the seventeenth century; the roof of the last leper house, at Greenside in Edinburgh, was finally removed in 1636. But he also discovered that the disappearance of leper hospitals did not mean that the disease had disappeared. He found reports that showed scattered cases of leprosy had continued to occur in Scotland long after the last leper hospital had been abandoned; in Shetland the disease had lingered into the nineteenth century. Simpson reluctantly concluded that, even after his most careful and diligent researches, the history of extent and prevalence of the disease in Scotland was still 'problematical'.

What he discovered of the leper hospitals in England was no more helpful. In his researches he found references to eighty-three hospitals, the first established in Kent at some time before the year 1000 and the last in London in 1472. In one there had been accommodation for sixty patients, but a more usual number was thirteen. Again he found it impossible to discover when exactly the prevalence of leprosy had declined to the point that these hospitals were no longer needed. In most cases the records had been irregularly maintained and, over the years, entries had been made less and less frequently until they gradually ceased completely. However it seemed from the rather uncertain evidence available that leper hospitals had been abandoned during the second half of the sixteenth century.

Simpson was intensely frustrated. His months devoted to the study of leprosy had only served to confirm what had already been known. Leprosy had appeared in Britain early in the eleventh century and had now all but disappeared. This he acknowledged in his presentation to the Medico-Chirurgical Society of Edinburgh in March 1841. But in the course of his studies he had accumulated a vast amount of detailed information on leprosy and had made some original observations. When he published his 'Antiquarian Notices of Leprosy and Leper Hospitals in Scotland and England' in the *Edinburgh Medical and Surgical Journal* in 1841[7] it included his observations on leprosy in essay form, in effect a monograph, of 93 pages and with references to 423 separate works in the medical literature.

First, Simpson did not share the generally accepted view that leprosy had been introduced to Europe by those returning from the Crusades. He produced evidence to show that leprosy had extended across the Continent of Europe as far westward as England long before the Crusade fanaticism had drawn converts from any part of Britain.[8] He also argued that the first relay of Crusaders from England had not returned until after 1095, and by then several leper hospitals had already been established in Britain.

Nor did he accept that leprosy was a contagious disease. He claimed that he knew personally of a boy of seventeen in Shetland who had leprosy but had never been in contact with any other victim of the disease. It was well known that cases of leprosy had occurred in places as remote as Madeira, the west of Ireland, Shetland, the Faroe Islands, Iceland and northern Norway. He wrote that 'few facts in the history of leprosy seem to be more universally admitted by all writers on the disease, both ancient and modern, than the transmission of the predisposition to it from parents to offspring'.[9] He went on to list a number of families in which more than one generation had been affected and pointed out that, like other hereditary diseases, leprosy could occur in only one or two members of a family and could lie dormant in one generation only to reappear in a subsequent one. He also noted that Louis IX of France, and Henry III of England and Robert II of Scotland, had made it a custom to embrace, kiss and wash the sores of lepers and had not contracted the disease. Quoting from Hector Boece's *History of the Scottish People*, he recalled that, in those earlier times, leprosy was accepted as an inherited affliction. To prevent its spread it had been the practice to castrate men suffering from the disease and to banish leprous women from the society of men; and when a woman suffering from leprosy was already pregnant, both she and her child were buried alive.[10]

Simpson's essay on leprosy continued with accounts of the disease as it occurred in England, Scotland, Shetland, Iceland and Norway, discussions of the age and sex of its victims, the 'external exciting causes' of the disease, the management of the diseases in leper hospitals and the measures that had been taken to prevent its spread. Since a person suffering from leprosy was, by various local enactments, deprived of the privileges and rights of citizenship, he was in effect legally and politically dead. Simpson ended his essay with a discussion of the position of lepers under civil law.

Simpson's 'Antiquarian Notices of Leprosy and Leper Hospitals in Scotland and England' failed to add substantial support for his hypothesis that diseases such as leprosy evolved over time like other living things. The article did include the most authoritative review of the causes, incidence, presentation, diagnosis and management of leprosy of his time, but as a contribution to the public debate on evolution, it was not a success. It was of very limited interest to the medical profession and did not attract the attention of the general public. In that, it was in sharp contrast to the counter to Lyell's *Principles of Geology* that his friend Robert Chambers was writing at that time.

Robert Chambers and Simpson were on very friendly terms, but it is unlikely that Simpson was allowed to know what Chambers had in mind. Chambers was a publisher and journalist who described himself as an 'essayist to the middle classes'.[11] He and his brother William were joint publishers of *Chambers' Edinburgh Journal*, which served a large and growing upwardly mobile section of the population that looked for upright, intelligent and informative reading at an economical price. Chambers planned to write a history of the Creation – not the *cataclysmic* history of the Creation as described in the Bible but the *natural* history of Creation. It was not a version of the Creation that was at all likely to be welcomed by the thousands who normally read his *Journal*.

During these first decades of the century, the general public had remained quietly indifferent towards the speculation of a few scientists on such remote matters as the age of the earth and the origins of animal life. But suddenly, from the late 1830s, any publication that seemed to question the absolute authority of the Bible provoked widespread hostility. There had been a great and rapid increase in the influence of Evangelicals in the churches of both Scotland and England; this had come as a reaction to the emergence in Britain of a new industrial society which seemed to answer only to the godless laws of physics and mathematics.[12] Thomas Carlyle was alarmed that 'not only the external and physical alone is now managed by machinery, but the internal and spiritual also'.[13] Evangelicals believed that man must answer directly to God. By an act of 'conversion' into such a relationship, one could receive the gift of faith, and with faith came the promise of salvation. But to maintain that relationship every action must be taken in the awareness of God and must be performed according to God's word as revealed in the Bible.

Soon up to a third of the clergy of the Church of England had been 'converted' to Evangelism and by the 1840s even the Archbishop of Canterbury was an Evangelical. The charismatic leading figure in the Church of Scotland was Thomas Chalmers, who 'impregnated' (his word) the nation with his Evangelical views and later, in 1843, led out over a third of the ministers of the established Church, and an even larger proportion of its members, to form an evangelical Free Church.[14] In the 1840s any attempt to deny the word of God as written in the Bible was anathema to a very large and very influential section of British society.

Robert Chambers therefore felt it necessary to write his book, *Vestiges of the Natural History of Creation*, in secret, and to publish it anonymously. In 1841, with his wife and family, he retired to Abbey Park, a country house near St Andrews, where he could write, free from the attention of his Edinburgh friends and colleagues and from his public. He used many of the same sources then being used by Charles Darwin. He was familiar with the medical and scientific terms used by Simpson and his other friends in Edinburgh, but he did not have the professional expertise of Darwin and he made occasional slips in his text. But he was writing for 'ordinary readers' and, for them, he wrote very well indeed. He carried the story of Creation from the coalescence of the planets, to the 'humble starting point in the evolution of Being and the reproduction of an individual',[15] to the early fossils (the '*Vestiges*' of his title), and finally to the emergence of man. But he did not deny God. He wrote in his introduction that 'there cannot be an inherent intelligence *within* the laws of nature. The intelligence appears external to the laws; something of which the laws are but as the expression of the Will and Power. If this be admitted, the laws cannot be regarded as a primary or independent cause of the phenomena of the physical world. We come, in short, to a Being beyond nature – its author, its God; infinite, inconceivable it may be and yet one whom these very laws present to us with attributes showing that our nature is in some way a faint and far-casting shadow of His, while all the gentlest and beautifullest of our emotions lead us to believe that we are as children in his care and as vessels in his hand. Let it then be understood – and this is for the reader's special attention – that when natural law is spoken of here, reference is only made to the mode in which the Divine Power is exercised. It is but another phrase for the *action* of the ever-present and sustaining God."[16]

Although Chambers had taken great care not to question the existence and Divine Power of God, he had nevertheless denied the word of God as it was revealed in the Biblical account of the Creation. He was therefore aware that his book would provoke protest, and he took extraordinary measures to ensure his anonymity. He had his wife copy out every part of his book. The text, in his wife's handwriting, was sent to his friend Alexander Ireland, a Scottish journalist who had recently moved to Manchester. Ireland posted the disguised text, under fresh covers, to the London publisher, John Churchill. The printer, Savill, later posted the proofs to Ireland, who sent them on to Chambers in Fife. The corrected proofs were returned by the same circuitous route.[17]

When *Vestiges of the Natural History of Creation* appeared in 1844, it was an instant success, attracting more public attention that any previous scientific book. It was reprinted three times in the first twelve months after its publication. It was warmly commended by the *Lancet*, the *Examiner* and other radically inclined publications, but it was condemned in the *Westminster Quarterly*, the *Athenaeum* and the *North American Review*. The

North British Review found it guilty of 'poisoning the fountains of science and sapping the foundations of religion'.[18] As Chambers had forecast, *Vestiges* scandalised a large and influential section of British society and prompted a witch-hunt by Evangelical Christians anxious to discover the author.[19] When, in November 1844, Charles Darwin first read *Vestiges* he was stunned.[20] He found the geology bad and the zoology worse, but the anonymous author had anticipated much of what he himself had intended to say. He had already written a draft of his *Origin of the Species*, but he did not immediately rush to publish his more scientifically sophisticated version of the natural history of Creation. He decided to delay publication, 'in order to preserve public order'. He did not publish until 1859, when much of the uproar caused by Chambers had subsided and the concept of evolution had been absorbed by the vast majority of educated people; he was also prompted by the knowledge that Alfred Russell Wallace was about to publish a version of the story of evolution that differed little from his.

Robert Chambers also decided to avoid the public controversy caused by the publication of *Vestiges*. Until his death in 1871 only five people were allowed to know that he was the author: his wife, his brother, Alexander Ireland, Robert Cox and Neil Arnott. His secret was at last revealed in 1884, in the introduction to the twelfth edition of *Vestiges*.

For Simpson also, the publication of *Vestiges* created a potential source of embarrassment. In his presentation to the Edinburgh Medico-Chirurgical Society, he had clearly accepted the reality of the transmutation of living things and had therefore indicated his readiness to accept the concept of evolution. But until 1841 he had not thought deeply, if at all, on religion, his relation to God or his own hopes for eternity.[21] However, in April of that year he had been drawn by his brother Sandy into a confrontation in the parish church in Bathgate between members of the Evangelical faction and representatives of the Moderate party within the Church of Scotland. He listened to the views of both sides, and after giving the matter long and careful consideration he found that his sympathies lay with the Evangelicals. When he published the results of his researches later in 1841 and in 1842, he did not include the word 'evolution' in the title 'Antiquarian Notices of Leprosy and Leper Hospitals'. And after his essay had been published, he abandoned his study of the evolution of diseases and never again wrote of evolution in any context. In 1843, he left the Church of Scotland and joined the new, Evangelical Free Church of Scotland.

EIGHT

Library Medicine:
On Cholera

If thou couldst, doctor, cast the water of my land, find her disease and purge it to a sound and pristine health, I would applaud thee to the very echo.

Shakespeare

From 1831 until 1854, Britain suffered repeated visitations of the great pandemic of 'Asiatic' cholera. For over twenty years, no community could feel completely safe, but its outbreaks in the rapidly growing industrial cities and towns were especially severe. There, thousands died a quick and miserably painful death. In the previous century it had been easily assumed that such sudden, debilitating and potentially fatal illnesses were acquired and spread by contagion. But in the first half of the nineteenth century, influenced by the powerful Evangelical Revival of that time, many eminent and influential doctors had come to believe that cholera and other such 'fevers' were the result of inflammation, a process intrinsic to the individual patient and therefore incapable of being transmitted to others. As Thomas Watson, later Sir Thomas Watson, President of the Royal College of Physicians of London, explained, such illnesses 'were the natural fruits of evil courses; of the sin of our fathers, of our own unbridled passions, of the malignant spirit of others'. They were 'judgements which are mercifully designed to recall men from the allurements of vice and the slumber of temporal prosperity, teaching that it is good for us to be sometimes afflicted'.[1]

Simpson had written the thesis for his MD degree on inflammation and had been assistant to Professor John Thomson, then the leading authority on inflammation. Simpson found it impossible to accept the view of the apocalyptic Evangelicals that the inflammation of cholera was a dispensation of providence, designed to turn the patient from sin. He therefore made his own study of the propagation of the disease.

The first news of what was to become a great pandemic reached Edinburgh on 2 March 1820 when the Royal College of Physicians of Edinburgh received from the Secretary of the East India Company copies of its reports on the progress of an epidemic of cholera that was then ravaging populations across India. The first cases had been reported in Calcutta in May 1817; three months later 3,000 of the company's 10,000-strong army in Bengal died from the disease. By July 1818, the disease had spread to the Presidency of Madras, and by August it had reached the third of the company's Presidencies at Bombay. An assistant surgeon at Bombay, on seeing his first cases, wrote:

> I never saw a disease where the debility came so soon or so suddenly
> and with such violence. It is common to find patients one hour after
> the first attack perfectly cold with no pulsation at the wrist.

The cause of the disease was unknown. Unable to discover any 'assignable connection between source and diffusion' of the disease, the medical staff of the East India Company had 'rejected at once the agency of contagion and ascribed it to the operation of a more general source'. That general source was assumed to be the weather; the case reports sent to the college were accompanied by full reports of local meteorological conditions and the phases of the moon.

As the epidemic began to subside in India it broke out in an even more virulent form in the Volga basin on the Caspian Sea, and from there it spread into Russia. In 1830, it reached Moscow and spread westward; by the spring of 1831 it had reached the coastal cities of the Baltic and north Germany. Since these were the entry ports for much of the country's trade with Europe, it seemed almost inevitable that the disease would soon spread to Britain. When the first cases were diagnosed in Sunderland on 23 October 1831, its arrival had long been expected and dreaded. And as the disease spread through England and Scotland, there was widespread bewilderment, terror and panic. A survivor wrote:

> To see a number of our fellow creatures, in a good state of health,
> in the full possession of their wonted strength and in the midst of
> their years, suddenly seized with the most violent spasms and in a
> few hours cast into the tomb is calculated to inspire dread in the
> stoutest heart.

The government body responsible for the prevention of epidemics was then the Privy Council; in practice its responsibility was delegated to its Clerk, Charles Grenville. When cholera reached Riga in the spring of 1831,

Grenville had ordered that all ships from Russia, the Baltic, the Cattegat and the Elbe should be detained for fourteen days at one of the designated quarantine stations around the coast of the country, from the Medway to Milford Haven, the Forth and Cromarty Bay. On 18 June, he set up a Central Board of Health to advise on what further measures might be required.[2]

From the beginning, the board was divided. Among themselves the members were unable to agree on whether or not the disease was contagious. They had therefore interviewed seven former army and civilian surgeons who had treated cholera in India; not one of them supported the idea that cholera was contagious or likely to be carried in the hemp, flax and other materials that made up the cargos in ships arriving from the Baltic. The board still had no clear view on how the disease was caused, spread or treated when, on 20 October 1831, it issued a *Public Notification Respecting the Cholera Morbus*. Nevertheless, it advised the public that it was of the utmost importance:

> to separate the sick from the healthy, one or more houses should be kept in each town or its neighbourhood to which every case of the disease might be removed, provided the family of the affected person consented to such removal, and in case of refusal a conspicuous mark ('Sick') should be placed in front of the house to inform persons that it is in quarantine and even when persons with the disease shall have been removed, the word 'Caution' should be substituted.

The houses from which the sick had been removed were to be cleaned, the 'walls from cellar to garret lime washed' and all 'papers, cordage, old clothes and hangings burnt'. As treatment the board advocated:

> White wine whey with spice, hot brandy and water, or sal volatile in the dose of a teaspoonful in hot water frequently repeated or from five to twenty drops of some of the essential oils as peppermint, cloves or cajeput in a wine-glass of water may be administered; where the stomach will bear it, warm broth with spice may be employed.

The *Lancet* was scathing:

> A Board of Health founded for the protection of England from the ravages, made to consist of men, not one of whom had ever been an eyewitness of the disease. As well might the Government seek

Simpson

information on the subject of Asian cholera from the old women of Wapping . . . Singular comicality! In the name of wonder who is to refer to them? The old dowagers and duchesses, we presume.[3]

Charles Grenville shared the views of the *Lancet*. The Board of Health was abolished, and on 22 November 1831 a new Cholera Board was appointed. However, by then the cholera epidemic was already spreading across Britain, and every town and village had been left to make its own arrangements.

The first cases of cholera in Scotland were diagnosed at Haddington on 17 December 1831. It was thought that the disease had been carried by three cobblers who had 'lodged in a low filthy part of the town' after walking there along the Great North Road from Newcastle. An explosive outbreak followed a few days later in Tranent. The disease then travelled along the south shore of the Firth of Forth to Leith; from there it passed to Edinburgh, where the first cases of cholera were reported on 27 January 1832.

In Edinburgh, planning had begun in August 1831. When the disease arrived in the city a Cholera Health Board was already in place. The services it had set up were modelled on those that had been introduced by the city's Fever Board in 1817 to combat an outbreak of 'contagious fever' (probably typhus). Soup kitchens were organised to feed the poor, as well as a store to provide them with free clothing. Restrictions were placed on the movement of vagrants and beggars into and within the city. Temporary cholera hospitals were established to accommodate a total of 270 patients. Arrangements were made for the fumigation of houses following the removal of cholera victims to hospital. Quarantine houses were designated to hold family members and others who had been in contact with the disease. The city was divided into thirty districts, each with its station for the supply of medicines. Small teams of two or three doctors[4] were assigned to make daily visitations within each of these districts. Posters were displayed throughout the city explaining the measures being put in place and justifying the restrictions that were to be imposed on the freedom of the individual citizen.

The disease rumbled on in the city for over nine months, twice seeming to die away before breaking out once again. The standard treatment was the administration of large doses of calomel (mercury chloride) and opium; the bloodletting that was then part of the standard treatment of contagious fever was often found to be impossible because the patients were already in circulatory collapse, cold to the touch and semi-conscious.

In spite of their best efforts, Edinburgh's medical men achieved very little. Almost all treated the cholera just as they had treated cases of contagious fever in the past, and 1,159 people died. A different treatment had offered some hope of better results. Dr W. B. O'Shaughnessy, an Edinburgh medical graduate, had investigated the changes in the blood of the early victims of the cholera outbreak at Newcastle.[5] He reported his preliminary results in the *Lancet* on 31 March 1831. His analyses revealed 'a great but variable deficiency of water in the blood in four malignant cholera cases; a total absence of carbonate of soda in two and a remarkable diminution of other saline ingredients'.[6] He concluded that in treating cholera it was necessary 'to restore the blood to its natural specific gravity' and 'to restore its deficient saline matters'. Thomas Latta, a doctor practising in Leith, had read O'Shaughnessy's report and attempted to follow his recommendations by administering the recommended fluid by mouth or per rectum. When these efforts failed he gave the fluid intravenously. The fluid was made up of 'two or three drachms of muriate of soda and two scruples of the subcarbonate of soda in six pints of water'. All six pints were injected through a major vein in an arm in thirty minutes. Of the first five patients treated, three survived.[7] Later, at one cholera hospital in Edinburgh, this new treatment was given to patients who had 'reached the last moment of earthly existence';[8] nineteen survived. No such 'miracle' had ever been seen before. However, Edinburgh's Board of Health was not convinced that the observed improvements and recoveries had been due to this new and very unconventional treatment, and they did not recommend the administration of intravenous fluids for routine use.

By the autumn of 1832 the epidemic of cholera had come to an end and interest in the nature and treatment of cholera had faded. Within a year Latta had died and O'Shaughnessy had departed to India, but their reports remained as further evidence that cholera was very different from the so-called contagious fever that had been so common in Scotland for generations. It had already been noted that, while in past epidemics of contagious fever the chief victims had been the very poor, the very young and the very old, in 1832 the victims of cholera were the badly housed poor in middle life, often the fathers and mothers of young families. Even after all the experience of a prolonged and widespread epidemic, there was still no agreement on the cause, nature and transmission of cholera.

Early in 1838, a second epidemic of cholera broke out in Italy, Malta and the Mediterranean coast of France, and there were soon fears that it would spread north to Britain.[9] Although Simpson had no personal experience of cholera, he took it upon himself to attempt to answer 'the *questio vexata* of the contagious or non-contagious nature of malignant cholera' by studying public and private records from the epidemic of 1832. He published his work 'On the Evidence of the Occasional Propagation of Malignant Cholera' in the *Edinburgh Medical and Surgical Journal* in the autumn of 1838.[10] First he commented on the 'long train of apparently very unnecessary discussion' that had taken place on the question of whether cholera was an aggravated variety of common sporadic cholera as described by Hippocrates in the fifth century BC, Aretaeus in the first century AD, and even up to the present, or a new disease that had originated in the Ganges Delta in India in 1817. He claimed that it was generally acknowledged that in all the years between those ancient times and 1817, the common sporadic cholera had never once spread in a general epidemic form over the different regions of the inhabited world. It was therefore 'contradictory and unphilosophical' to attribute the intermittent appearance of cholera in its mild endemic form during that long period to the influence of such supposed exciting causes of disease as irregularities of diet, temperature or moisture, and now to attribute its sudden appearance, in its new malignant and epidemic form, to these same supposed exciting factors. He wrote:

> I conceive that cholera, in its wide-spread epidemic form at least, is a disease that is specifically new, and one that has hitherto appeared only in certain places and for a limited time only in each place. Hence it seems impossible to avoid coming to the conclusion that the agencies or agency which gave rise to this new and specific form of malady must have been itself also of a new and specific character and that the human economy had been subjected to its operation only on those localities in which the disease prevailed and only during the temporary period of that prevalence.

He at once dismissed 'such fanciful theories' that had been suggested to explain the spread of cholera such as galvanism, magnetism, electricity, insects in the air, animalcules in the water or deleterious substances in food. Simpson insisted that there were only three possible causes of epidemic disease:

1. A peculiar influence, property or miasma existing in the air.
2. An influence existing in or emanating from the earth.
3. A contagious influence or effluvium generated in the human body while labouring under the disease and capable of exciting the same specific

disease in such predisposed individuals as are exposed to its action by direct or indirect intercourse with the infected.

He claimed that it was impossible to suppose that a disease so erratic and diffuse in its spread as cholera could be attributed to such local factors as 'the effluvium from sewers, the malaria of stagnant water'. He therefore discounted any cause other than direct specific contagion.

He was aware that those opposed to the idea of contagion held that the occurrence of several cases of cholera in the same house, the same street or the same district indicated that a local cause must be responsible. Simpson, however, argued that when a number of people resident in one place began to suffer from the disease only after they had been joined by someone who had come from some perhaps distant place where there had been an outbreak of the disease, this strongly indicated that the disease was contagious. To show that this had been the pattern of spread during the 1832 cholera epidemic, he first described the spread of the disease to Bathgate as reported to him by a local surgeon, Mr W. Gilchrist.

On 25 April 1832, three female beggars, who had been living in a part of Edinburgh where cholera was rife, walked in the direction of Glasgow as far as Newbridge, a village halfway between Edinburgh and Bathgate, in which cholera was 'perhaps more prevalent and fatal proportionally to the number of inhabitants than any other locality in Scotland'. They spent that night at a nearby farm, but next day they were unwell and found that they were unable to walk further than Broxburn, only two miles away. There they said nothing of their symptoms and were admitted to a lodging house. Next morning they could no longer disguise their illness and they were ejected by the lodging-house keeper. After lying for some time in the street, they were taken, in an open cart, the seven miles to Bathgate, where they were confined to jail. Three nurses, all residents of Bathgate, were sent by the local authority to look after them. The oldest of the beggars died on the morning of their second day in Bathgate, and her niece twenty-four hours later; the last of the three, a young woman of twenty, died on the fourth day. That same day one of the nurses became unwell; she died within eighteen hours. Simpson carefully pointed out that the parish minister and all four of the town's surgeons had visited the cholera patients but had not become infected. And, apart from the nurse, who had been in close contact with the three patients, none of the town's 3,000 residents had contracted the disease. He went on:

If we deny the contagious propagation of cholera and endeavour to explain the circumstances of such cases upon the doctrine of disease arising from a morbid influence either terrestrial or atmospheric, we cannot avoid involving ourselves in inextricable difficulties. For if this supposed influence, whether terrestrial or atmospheric, was generally diffuse over the soil or air of the town, how did it happen that it exactly attacked persons, and the persons only, of those that were attendant upon the imported sick? Were the two unfortunate nurses, who were better fed *etc* than many other poor of the place, the only individuals out of the 3,000 inhabitants of the village and out of the whole surrounding populous district of the county that were predisposed to in such a manner as to be affected with this diffuse agency? And it is perhaps important to observe that both women were between 40 and 50 and apparently of healthy constitution. They were both volunteers in the service so that we cannot ascribe the appearance of the disease in any of them to any degree of fear; their duties as nurses were neither long continued nor severe. They were each allowed soup out of the common stock provided at the general soup kitchen for the poor of the village. And had, in addition, a daily quantity of more solid and generous diet allotted to them. Indeed if we do not admit in their cases the doctrine of contagion it will be impossible to point out any cause whatever explanatory, at the same time, of their unfortunate fate and the escape of the villagers in general.

Simpson then presented no fewer than twenty-six other reports he had obtained of outbreaks of cholera in Scotland, England, Ireland, France, Germany, Russia and America during the epidemic of 1831–2. These case histories showed that, while the circumstances might vary from case to case, they could all be interpreted in the same way, and that interpretation pointed to contagion as the mode of spread of cholera. The few case histories selected from those presented by Simpson and recounted below are of outbreaks of the disease that occurred in very different locations and very different circumstances. They not only illustrate the patterns of spread of the disease but also give vivid glimpses of the distress and physical suffering that had to be endured during the epidemic of 1832.

Dollar

(Summary of a personal communication from Dr Walker to Simpson, published by Simpson in the *Edinburgh Medical and Surgical Journal*, 1838)

On 12th May 1832, a Miss Campbell, who lived and worked at the Devon Iron Works in Clackmannanshire, began to feel unwell. Cholera had been raging in the district for several weeks and, fearing that she would be committed to the local Cholera Hospital she walked the five miles to Dollar where her mother lived by herself in a cottage in the middle of the village. Neighbours noticed her arrival and next morning members of the local Health Board were called to see her. They found her in the collapsed stage of cholera. When this became known there was an immediate public disturbance in the village. She was loaded onto a cart and sent back to the Cholera Hospital at the Devon Iron Works where she died later that day.

Her mother meanwhile had been taken from her cottage and quarantined in a house half a mile outside Dollar; a friend who had visited the cottage earlier that day was sent to the same place of quarantine. The cottage and all its contents were then burnt.

Next day, old Mrs Campbell began to have the acute symptoms of cholera and fourteen hours later she died. No one in the village was ready to help with her interment. The undertaker left her empty coffin by the roadside near the house where she had died. It was left to the local surgeons to lift her into her coffin, screw it down and drive the cart that carried it to a grave outside the village. Even the horse that drew the cart had to be hired 'at exorbitant expense' from another village.

There were no other cases in Dollar. In a village of over 1,500 inhabitants only the young woman who had been suffering from cholera before arriving in the village and her mother who had shared a bed with her had died.

Doura

(Letter to the editor, the *Lancet*, 1832, p. 182)

On 20th February 1832 a young woman left Glasgow with her husband to travel on foot to Kilwinning in Ayrshire. Cholera was rampant in Glasgow at the time and after she had walked twenty miles she began to suffer vomiting and diarrhoea. She was then near the tiny village of Doura and she and her husband decided to rest up there at the house of an old acquaintance. Next day she was seen by the local surgeon who had served in India and immediately recognised the signs of cholera. Two sisters from the village were engaged to 'rubb her etc' [she was presumably in a state of collapse and already very cold to the touch] but she died that evening. No quarantine restrictions were ordered. On 24th February one of the sisters who had nursed the young woman died. Thereafter, in a little over two weeks, a further 20 died out of a total population of 37 families and 170 inhabitants.

Berlin

(Dr Becker, Letter on the Cholera in Prussia, selected and summarised by Simpson, and reprinted in *Edinburgh Medical and Surgical Journal*, February 1832)

By the early autumn of 1831, the epidemic of cholera had reached Berlin. On the 5th of September, the public dissection of a victim of the disease was performed in one of the streets near the river. Four young physicians who were present 'not satisfied with the information derived from sight, touch and smell, thought proper to ascertain the properties of the blood and the contents of the intestines by tasting these fluids'. Next morning, one of these young men, who had been having mild diarrhoea for some days, had all the signs and symptoms of cholera and within a few hours he died. His landlord had been away from home for that day but, when he returned, he too was affected and two days later he and two of his children were dead. The landlord's widow and remaining children were taken into quarantine. Thereafter there were no further cases of cholera in that house or in that street.

North Shields

(Personal communication to Simpson from Dr Edward Greenhow, North Shields)

The first person to suffer cholera in North Shields was a pauper called M'Gwin. He had been begging in Sunderland for some four months after the epidemic had first broken out there. On 8th December 1831, he had slept in a common lodging house where several of the residents were suffering all the symptoms of cholera. Next day he returned to 'his own hovel' in North Shields and by that evening he was also 'labouring under decided cholera'. He eventually recovered but on the 13th his wife had shown the first signs of cholera; she died twenty-three hours later. 'A remarkably stout healthy woman who had been sent from the workhouse for the purpose of nursing M'Gwin and his wife was seized with the disease and died within thirty hours.' Thereafter, the disease 'extended itself in the immediate vicinity of those persons' dwelling'. No arrangement for quarantine had been made.

The *Amelia*

(Professor Dickson, *American Journal of Medical Science*, No. xxvi.)

On 19th October 1832, the Brig *Amelia* left New York to sail to New Orleans. Cholera had broken out some time earlier in New York and a number of the 105 passengers on the *Amelia* had the disease before embarking. Twenty-four of those on board had already died when, on 31st October, the *Amelia* ran aground on a small sandy island twenty miles from Charlestown. There were only four residents on the island and very few dwellings but everyone from the *Amelia* was able to find some shelter. A party of wreckers from Charlestown soon arrived to recover the cargo. They soon abandoned the recovery and returned to Charlestown where one of them died. The other wreckers were ordered to return to quarantine on the island; three medical officers and a clergyman were sent to care for the sick left on the island and a lieutenant and eighteen men of the Charlestown's city guard were dispatched to prevent anyone from leaving the island. Some 150 people were confined on the island and of these 23 died. In Charlestown the sick member of the wrecking crew who had been allowed to return from the island was the only person to die of cholera.

From twenty-seven such reports from Britain, Continental Europe and North America, Simpson was able to give details of the spread of forty-one outbreaks of cholera, including many in which spread had been local, others in which spread had been from one part of a large city to another, a few (in Russia) in which transmission had occurred over many miles, and two in which the cholera outbreak had been within the closed community of a ship. In the great majority of these outbreaks he was able to show that there had been direct contact between established cases of cholera and later victims, although in a few other instances there had been apparently no such direct contact. And in several instances it appeared that efforts to quarantine those affected had been effective. Simpson claimed that the cases he cited:

> afford us sufficient precise and ample data from which to draw the conclusion that malignant cholera *can* spread by contagion. That the disease does spread in *all* cases in this manner is what the evidence by no means empowers us to assert; occasionally it has shown such anomalies as sudden and simultaneous explosions at different points in the same locality either at its first introduction and unexpected and inexplicable recurrences in places which it had visited months

or years previously . . . However, if we once do admit the evidence for contagion to be complete in some instances . . . any evidence we may thereafter adduce of its not spreading by contagion in other instances [may] be merely from the circumstance of our not being able to trace a chain of communication, either direct or indirect, between persons newly attacked and those previously attacked.

He added that, though arguing for the contagious propagation of cholera, he did not intend

to maintain that the communication of the disease from individuals to individuals is not intimately determined, and in many cases extensively promoted, by the collateral influence of other agencies operating at the same time upon those exposed individuals and by the existing degree of susceptibility of their bodies to the receipt and action of the contagious virus according as that susceptibility is modified, both by these external agencies and by the particular internal conditions of their own economies.

At that time there were many respected authorities who still insisted that ailments such as cholera were caused by miasma carried in the air or rising from the earth. This was a concept that Simpson could not accept. In his most robustly scornful style, he presented his arguments against miasma having played any part in the spread of cholera:

The whole history of malignant cholera certainly proves that no variations in the external meteorological and physical agencies to which the human system has happened to be exposed have been able to exert an influence sufficient at any time to suspend altogether the gradual progression in propagation and onward march of the disease from India over various inhabited regions of the world. The disease has shown itself in almost every kind of situation in which the body itself seems capable of existing; in every variety of geological formation that is to be found upon the face of the globe; in every kind of soil, from marshy jungles and dry deserts of the East to the most cultivated and fertile spots in Europe; it has prevailed thousands of miles inland and along the shore; on continents and in infected ships; in crowded cities and in isolated hamlets; under the extreme heat of the Indian sun and the extreme cold of a Russian winter. It has been observed to march forward in the very teeth of monsoons and has remained stationary while the atmosphere was passing over the seat of its devastations with almost the velocity of a hurricane. It stretched up the Nepal and Himalaya mountains to places 4,000 or even 5,000 feet above the level of the ocean; and it raged severely along the banks of the Caspian Sea, which are nearly 300 feet below that level. It has accompanied human intercourse from house to house, from city to city, from country to country and from continent to continent. It has travelled with man over seas, from seaport to seaport, from island to island and has even followed him across the breadth of the Indian and Atlantic oceans.

Simpson went on to elaborate on these arguments at greater length and in greater detail. But his arguments did not win the approval of the editors of the *Edinburgh Medical and Surgical Journal*. In the form of a 'Note' inserted at the end of his article, they added a long and crushing riposte. The first three paragraphs read:

In the insertion of the foregoing paper, the Editors beg leave to observe, in order to prevent any misconception on the subject of which the paper treats, that they do not by any act of insertion become responsible either for the accuracy of the statements made, or for the validity and conclusiveness of the inferences deduced.

The paper of Dr. Simpson is, it must be admitted, an able exploration of the facts and arguments which may be adduced in support of the opinion, that under certain circumstances, cholera appears to affect successively different individuals in the manner of a disease which is propagated by contagion; and in this point of view it constitutes a useful collection of facts and arguments, which deserves the attentive perusal of all those who wish to understand thoroughly the two sides of this difficult and obscure question. It must, on the other hand, however be observed, that the view here given embraces but a small portion of the inquiry relative to the etiology of cholera, and the mode or modes in which it may be propagated. It overlooks entirely the important fact, that no quarantine regulations, no measures of seclusion, non-intercourse or segregation have been capable of preventing the appearance of the distemper in the different cities and countries of Europe, or resisting its progress when it has once appeared. It overlooks also the fact that the distemper, when once developed in any community, did by no means prevail among the inhabitants in the ratio of exposure to the sick, but almost always in a ratio between which and the degree of exposure it was totally impossible to trace any connection. Again it overlooks another fact, that the disease, after expending its virulence on a certain part of the population, in all instances which came to our knowledge, gradually became extinct, or as it were, died a natural death, neither accelerated nor retarded, neither aided nor opposed by the various agents and measures which the doctrines of contagious propagation suggested.

Upon the method of investigation pursued by Dr. Simpson in his inquiry, and in establishing the point for which he appears an advocate, it would lead the Editors into too lengthened a notice to make those remarks which the subjects undoubtedly demands. This only it may be proper at present to say that, though the fact of succession in attacks may be established, it does not follow that the succession indicates the relation of cause and effect. It must be a principle more necessary in medical reasoning than in any other species of inquiry that though in establishing the relation of cause and effect, we do no more than indicate the circumstances of the latter event having followed the former, yet we are not entitled to infer the constancy of the converse proposition, *viz.* that when we establish the fact of succession between two events, we thereby establish the relationship of causation. Succession in medical facts, in short, is very similar to coincidence.

Simpson was a young man with no great reputation as a physician and no personal experience of cholera. As the recently appointed deputy to the Professor of General Pathology, he had also strayed beyond the recognised limits of his area of competence. The arrogance, even scorn, that he had shown in dismissing the belief in miasma as a cause of disease – a belief shared by the most eminent and senior physicians in Britain[11] – had evidently offended the editors. In their Note, occupying three full pages of their *Journal*, they had effectively undermined the case that Simpson had so rationally, but perhaps too robustly, presented. For some time, he did not pursue his interest in cholera.

The epidemic of cholera subsided in the autumn of 1832, but minor sporadic outbreaks continued, especially among the ill-fed poor[12] of Britain's industrial towns and villages. Then, in 1849, there was a second severe epidemic of cholera in Britain. John Snow, a surgeon in general practice in Soho in London, who had already had some experience of cholera in 1832,[13] renewed his studies of its spread. He published his thoughts in a pamphlet, *On the Mode of Communication of Cholera*.[14] He wrote that it was generally assumed that, if it was contagious, 'it must be contagious in the same way that the eruptive fevers are considered to be, *viz.*, by emanations from the sick person into the surrounding air, which enter the system of others by being inhaled, and absorbed by the blood passing through the lungs'.

However:

> Reasoning by analogy from what is known of other diseases, we ought not to conclude that cholera is propagated by an effluvium [miasma]. In all known cases in which the blood is poisoned in the first instance, general symptoms, such as rigors, headache and quickened pulse, precede the local symptoms; but it has always appeared from what the writer could observe, that in cholera the alimentary canal is first affected and all the symptoms referable to that part are consecutive and apparently the result of the local affection . . .

> . . . Having rejected effluvia and the poisoning of the blood in the first instance, and being led to the conclusion that the disease is communicated by something that acts directly on the alimentary canal, the excretions of the sick at once suggest themselves as containing some material which, being accidentally swallowed, might attach itself to the mucous membrane of the small intestines and there multiply itself by the appropriation of surrounding matter, in virtue of molecular changes going on within it, capable of going on, as soon as it is placed in congenial circumstances.

Snow suggested want of personal cleanliness as a factor in the spread and fatality of cholera; he recalled that, in the epidemic of 1832, cholera first appeared in the courts and alleyways where vagrants found shelter for the night, and that it lingered there for some time before spreading to the 'more cleanly part of the people'. But the main cause of outbreaks of the disease was 'the emptying of sewers into the drinking water of the community'. His researches had shown that in the towns which suffered most severely, the drinking water was contaminated in this way. He offered Dumfries as his first example. In the most recent outbreak there, out of a population of 14,000, 431 had died of cholera; the town's water supply was drawn from the Nith, 'a river into which the sewers empted themselves, their contents floating afterwards to and fro with the tide'.

After a lapse of seventeen years, Snow's pamphlet revived Simpson's interest in the spread of cholera. When an epidemic of the disease spread across central Scotland in 1853, Simpson asked for reports on the sanitary conditions and the state of the water supply in each of the most severely affected towns and villages in Linlithgowshire. But before he had acquired any worthwhile information he was pre-empted by John Snow.

In an outbreak in south London that year there were 286 fatal cases of cholera. The water in that part of London was provided by either the Southwark and Vauxhall Water company, which drew its supply from the faecally contaminated waters of the River Thames, or by the Lambeth company, which drew its supply from uncontaminated water much higher up the river. Snow was able to show that fatal cases of cholera had been over fourteen times more likely to occur in houses supplied by the Southwark and Vauxhall company than in those supplied by the Lambeth company. Then, in September 1854, Snow made his case even more dramatically. A particularly severe outbreak of cholera in the neighbourhood of Golden Square had caused over 500 deaths. Snow saw that these deaths occurred principally in an area within 250 yards of the pump at the corner of Broad Street and Cambridge Street. He persuaded a meeting of the vestrymen of St James' to have the handle of the pump removed; when this was done the outbreak was immediately contained.

John Snow published his final proof of the *Mode of Communication of Cholera* as a second and extended version of his pamphlet of 1849. Simpson had gone some way towards reaching the same conclusion in his pamphlet *On the Evidence of the Occasional Propagation of Malignant Cholera* in 1838, but that had been based on reports from many sources and on his study of the medical literature. Lacking John Snow's long and immediate personal experience of cholera, he had been unable to bring his investigations to an entirely successful conclusion. However, he had added strength to the arguments against the view of Evangelical physicians, such as Thomas Watson, that cholera was a dispensation from God for the correction of sin. He had also added evidence against the popular notion that the disease was caused by miasma, an invisible noxious vapour rising from the ground.

NINE

Ether

I do think you might spare her and neither heaven nor man grieve at the measure.

Shakespeare

On 16 October 1846, staff and students at Massachusetts General Hospital in Boston gathered to witness an operation which, it had been claimed, would be quite unlike any that had ever been carried out before. Operating theatres, even at the most prestigious teaching hospitals, had always been dreadful places. For generations, it had been quite usual for surgeons to appear in coats stained with the gore of long-past operations: they had removed limbs in seconds, letting the blood flow onto floors on which sawdust had been generously scattered to receive it; the place had reeked with the smell of blood, sweat and bodies. By 1846, efforts had been made to impose a more acceptable standard of decorum within the operating room and to achieve some degree of cleanliness, even if it was only by the liberal use of quantities of cold water. However, medical students watching from the gallery still had to disguise their feelings of revulsion with black humour or false displays of cold indifference as struggling patients were tied or held down on the operating table and shrieked in agony as the surgeon's knife cut through their flesh. This operation, however, promised to be different. John Collins Warren, the hospital's leading surgeon, had agreed to operate on a patient who had been given inhalations of ether. As a tumour in the neck was cut out, the patient lay perfectly still and unprotesting, and when the operation was over he reported that he had felt no pain. Oliver Wendell Holmes[1] later suggested that the state of insensibility that ether had induced in the patient should be called 'anaesthesia'.

The news of this operation in Boston changed Simpson's life. He at once recognised the full significance of what had been done. While he continued to justify his place as one of the greatest obstetricians in Britain, he worked to perfect and promote the use of general anaesthesia. His name became forever associated with what was the most immediately and most widely welcomed invention of the nineteenth century, and is still remembered as one of the greatest advances in the history of medicine.

It was always Simpson's practice to make a scholarly study of the history of any subject in which he took up an interest. In one of his earliest essays on anaesthesia he reviewed the earliest means that had been used to produce sleep and insensibility. The myrrhed wine offered to Christ before his crucifixion was a preparation of hashish, the same preparation as 'the wine of the condemned' mentioned 700 years earlier by Amos in the Old Testament. Dioscorides had been particularly successful in using mandragora to 'cause insensibility in those who are to be cut or cauterised, for being thrown into a deep sleep they do not perceive pain'. Pliny had later added henbane.[2] In Greek and Roman times Galen and Aretaeus had used decoctions or tinctures of mandragora[3] in a variety of combinations. In the thirteenth century Hugo of Lucca and Theodoric had used a mixture of mandragora and opium. In the eighth book of his *Natural Magic* in 1608, Batista Porta still recommended a 'sleeping apple' made with mandragora and opium: 'When you hold it to a sleeping man's nostrils whose breath will suck up this subtle essence which will so besiege the castle of his senses that he will be overwhelmed with a most profound sleep not to be shook off without much labour.'

How widely these various substances had been used in the distant past and how effective they had been is unknown, and Simpson did not offer any possible explanation of why they had fallen out of use. Others have suggested that these ancient recipes for the relief of surgery-related pain had quietly and gradually been omitted from pharmacopoeias after Paracelsus publically burned the ancient works of Galen and Avicenna and insisted that medicines should be used only if their virtues could be validated by observation and experience. Thereafter, alcohol or opium, or even both, might be given to dull the fears of patients about to undergo surgery, but during the operation patients could only look to the dexterity and speed of the surgeon to limit their agonies.

The notion of administering medicaments by inhalations was revived in more modern times by Thomas Beddoes at the Pneumatic Medical Institute that he had founded in Bristol in 1799. Bristol was then a favourite resort for patients suffering from pulmonary tuberculosis, asthma and other respiratory complaints, and Beddoes thought it possible that these patients might be helped by the inhalation of one or other of the gases that had been isolated and identified by Joseph Priestley in the early 1770s. As his assistant, Beddoes had appointed the nineteen-year-old Humphry

Davy and given him the task of investigating the properties of nitrous oxide. On inhaling the gas Davy soon discovered both its exhilarating and its analgesic effects. In his *Researches, Chemical and Philosophical, Chiefly Concerning Nitrous Oxide* in 1800, Humphry Davy suggested that inhalations of nitrous oxide might be used to relieve the pain of surgical operations 'in which no great effusion of blood takes place'. But he gave nitrous oxide the name 'laughing gas', and it was as laughing gas that it became best known, and as laughing gas that, for the next forty years and more, it was inhaled by the daring and fashionable as an after-dinner amusement.

Interest in the medicinal use of nitrous oxide revived in December 1844, when Horace Wells, a dentist in Hartford, Connecticut, attempted to demonstrate its analgesic properties before a specially invited audience at the Massachusetts General Hospital. Unfortunately, the patient groaned volubly and protested furiously as his tooth was prised out; the demonstration was judged a failure and Wells was humiliated.

Two years later, William T. G. Morton, who had once been Wells' partner in dental practice, thought he might succeed where Wells had failed. But first he had to find a supply of nitrous oxide. He approached Charles Jackson, who had been one of his teachers during his dental training and was now in private practice as an analytical chemist in Boston. Jackson, who was too busy on his own projects to spend time making nitrous oxide for Morton, advised him that he should instead try ether, another of the gases that Thomas Beddoes had used to treat patients at his Pneumatic Medical Institute. Ether was easily available; from the early 1830s, the inhalation of ether had been a very common amusement 'for thousands of people'[4] in Boston, Philadelphia and other cities in the eastern United States. After a number of unfortunate accidents, the recreational use of ether had become less fashionable, but in 1846 Jackson was still busily engaged in his laboratory studies of its properties and he had come to believe that it might prove to be more useful than nitrous oxide as an anaesthetic.[5] Jackson may also have been aware that Crawford Long, who had become familiar with ether as a recreational drug while he was a medical student in Philadelphia, had been using it as a general anaesthetic for minor operations since he set up in practice in Georgia in 1842. Long's effective use of ether had attracted patients and had helped build his practice but he had not revealed the source of his success in the medical press.[6]

Morton eagerly took Jackson's advice and agreed to make a few preliminary trials of ether. First he administered ether to a patient who was having a tooth extracted; afterwards the patient, Eban Frost, signed a statement verifying that he had felt no pain. Morton then persuaded Henry Bigelow, one of the younger surgeons at the Massachusetts General, to act as a witness while he performed several more dental extractions under ether. Impressed by what he had seen, Henry Bigelow agreed to ask John Collins Warren to conduct a public trial of the effectiveness of ether at the Massachusetts General Hospital. With some hesitation Warren agreed. He had been present in 1844 when Horace Wells had so conspicuously failed in his attempt to convince his audience of the anaesthetic powers of nitrous oxide. But this public trial of ether as a general anaesthetic was a complete success. Warren announced to the incredulous witnesses: 'Gentlemen, this is no humbug.'

Morton was triumphant. He was confident that he could now make his fortune. During all his trials and his public demonstrations he had disguised his ether by adding a few harmless substances to change its appearance and smell, and had called his creation 'Letheon'. Warren's public trial at Massachusetts General had successfully advertised its powers. He now planned to patent it, and to charge surgeons half the fee of all operations in which they used Letheon and the apparatus he had designed for its administration.[7] But his plan was soon frustrated. After his first public trial, Warren steadfastly refused to make any further use of Letheon until its composition was made public.[8] Morton capitulated and, on 7 November 1846, Warren used undisguised and unadulterated ether as a general anaesthetic when performing a mid-thigh amputation. A month later Henry Bigelow published a straightforward account of all the operations in which ether had been administered at the Massachusetts General by the end of 1846.[9] The news of a gas that could abolish the pain of surgery quickly spread across the United States and was carried to Britain and Europe by the new, fast transatlantic steamships.

One of the first surgeons in Britain to use ether was Robert Liston, who had been Simpson's teacher at Edinburgh between 1826 and 1828 and was now Professor of Clinical Surgery at London University. On Monday 21 December 1846, before a large audience in the theatre of University College Hospital, Liston amputated the leg of an anaesthetised man at the level of the mid-thigh. This, the most traumatic and life threatening of all the surgical operations routinely performed at that time, was quietly and successfully completed without untoward incident. When he recovered consciousness, the patient, a Harley Street butler in his thirties, asked when the operation was going to start.

Simpson was at once aware of the immense significance of what had been witnessed. As a new and unseasoned medical student at Edinburgh, he had been appalled as he watched the agonies suffered by a poor Highland woman as her cancerous breast was dissected away. Charles Darwin, Simpson's contemporary at Edinburgh, had abandoned his medical studies, in part because of a very similar experience at Edinburgh Royal Infirmary. Simpson and Darwin were not alone. Medical students had always been subjected to this same distressing initiation, and every successful surgeon had had to learn to harden his heart. When Simpson first read that the patients' agonies could be totally abolished by the administration of ether, he at once recognised that, no matter how reluctant the medical profession might prove to be towards changing the way in which surgery had been conducted for centuries, the patients would insist on having the relief of general anaesthesia, and their wishes would prevail. He meant to be at the forefront of a revolution in the practice of surgery, a revolution that he saw as now inevitable and inevitably successful. He decided he must quickly learn everything there was to know about ether. He therefore travelled to London to spend Christmas with Robert Liston and explore with him ideas on how and when the powers of ether could be used.

Not everyone in the medical profession shared this early enthusiasm for anaesthesia. From the beginning opinion among military surgeons was firmly opposed to the use of ether. The United States had been at war with Mexico since May 1846, but when ether came into use at the end of that year, the surgeon-general, Thomas Lawson, decided that the equipment necessary for its administration was so cumbersome and fragile, and the gas itself so inflammable, that ether was not suitable for military use. But other senior and influential army surgeons did not oppose the use of ether for such mundane reasons. They insisted that pain was a very powerful stimulant and a necessary aid to recovery after surgery. Even Sir George Ballingall, Regius Professor of Military Surgery at Edinburgh and veteran of campaigns in India and the East Indies, had nothing to say in support of abolishing surgical pain.

Although few surgeons in civil life in Britain took this very positive view of the value of pain, many feared that the calming effect of ether might go too far. Writing to Simpson in August 1847, a Dr Newnham reported that the initial impression of surgeons in Newcastle had been that ether had an undesirable depressing effect on the nervous and vascular systems, and for that reason its use had been discontinued; they would, however, 'rejoice to find that they had drawn too hasty a conclusion'.

Other surgeons simply feared that to use a new and untried method to abolish the patient's pain was to add a further risk to an already risky operation. To answer such fears Simpson conducted a statistical survey of the results of anaesthesia in amputations of the thigh, the leg, the arms and the forearm. In April 1848, he published his results in *Anaesthesia in Surgery: Does it Increase or Decrease the Mortality Attendant upon Surgical Operations?*, a pamphlet he arranged to have distributed widely in Britain and America.[10] In it, he compared the mortality suffered in 2,713 amputations carried out without general anaesthesia in Paris, Glasgow, Edinburgh and London with the mortality from 302 amputations performed under ether in hospitals in the same cities. The results for all four types of amputation showed the same trend, but Simpson gave particular stress to the results in the most hazardous of the operations, the mid-thigh amputation of the leg. He was able to show that when this operation had been carried out without anaesthesia, the mortality in hospitals in Glasgow had been 36 per cent; in London 44 per cent; in Edinburgh 49 per cent; and in Paris 62 per cent. As he admitted, the number of mid-thigh operations in which anaesthesia had been used in British hospitals was still very small – only 145 – but the mortality in these cases was 25 per cent. Simpson claimed his evidence suggested that it was the endurance of pain that was so depressing and destructive of the patients' vitality, and that the relief of their pain preserved not only their vitality but saved them from all 'the shock of the operation and its consequences'; his statistics clearly proved that, far from adding to the hazards of surgery, general anaesthesia led to a very significant saving of lives. However, by April 1848, when his statistical evidence of the benefits of ether was published, it had become almost irrelevant. General anaesthesia by ether was already coming into widespread use throughout Britain, Europe, the United States and beyond.

Surgeons were delighted that their patients no longer needed to be physically restrained, and that they could operate calmly on patients who remained still and unprotesting throughout. Under such conditions it was possible for them to contemplate expanding the scope of surgery and performing new operations that could be completed in more than the few seconds or minutes that conscious patients could endure. And every medical practitioner could hope that they would no longer be called on to treat patients who, because of their dread of pain, delayed or even refused operations that were clearly necessary. In a letter to his friend J. B. Fleming at Secunderabad in India, Simpson wrote: 'All here use ether in surgical operations and no doubt, in a few years, its employment will be general over the civilised world.'

The general public was even more enthusiastic. To them, the benefits of ether seemed almost miraculous. To be able to agree to surgical treatment, whenever and for whatever reason it was recommended, without carefully weighing the potential benefits against the certainty of almost unendurable pain, was something they had never thought possible. A correspondent to the *Medical Times* wrote that in all the revolutions that had ever taken place in the practice of medicine, nothing so remarkable had ever been known. The advent of anaesthesia had been hailed with such enthusiasm that 'a second Eden seemed to be dawning'. The people of Britain took to etherisation[11] as they had taken to other great innovations of the nineteenth century. There were perhaps risks. One of Her Majesty's ministers had been crushed and killed by one of the first steam trains,[12] and many feared that the human body would be unable to withstand the effects of travelling at twenty miles an hour; but all that had not dampened popular enthusiasm for the railways. Deaths during etherisation had been reported in the newspapers, and the medical profession still had some fears about its use, but this did not diminish the general public's welcome for ether. Soon it seemed that pharmacies everywhere were laying in stocks of ether, and doctors everywhere were designing apparatus for its administration.

Ether could even be fun. Sniffing ether became a popular amusement in Edinburgh in the 1840s, just as it had been in Philadelphia in the 1830s. Simpson himself greatly enjoyed the exhilarating pleasure of inhaling ether and offered it to, even pressed it on, his guests at dinner parties at 52 Queen Street. At one such dinner party on 17 August 1847, Simpson's guests included Hans Christian Andersen, the novelist Catherine Crowe, the banker C. J. Hambro and his wife, and the obstetrician John Moir. Hans Andersen recorded in his diary that he had 'thought it distasteful, especially to see ladies in this dreamy intoxication; they laughed with open, lifeless eyes; there was something unpleasant about it and I said so, recognising at the same time that it was a wonderful and blessed invention to use in painful operations but not to play with. It was wrong to do it. It was almost like tempting God. One worthy old gentleman took my part and said the same.'[13] Simpson was not offended, but neither was he deterred from enjoying ether or offering it to guests at his social gatherings.

By the summer of 1847 ether had become a familiar and valued drug, but its proper place as a general anaesthetic in surgical and obstetric practice was still uncertain. Robert Liston had been delighted by his first experience of operating on a patient anaesthetised by the inhalation of ether. But he had performed that operation in only 38 seconds, and he made it clear to Simpson that he did not intend to take advantage of the insensibility of the patient under ether to operate more slowly and more cautiously. Nor did he intend to make use of ether to undertake new, more complicated and more time-consuming procedures. Liston believed it would prove to be unsafe for ether to be administered for periods longer than a very few minutes. Simpson did not agree. He was confident he could show that ether could be used for much longer periods and, in particular, that it could be administered long enough to be invaluable in the management of difficult obstetric deliveries. For that he had to show not only that ether could be administered safely to the mother for long and uncertain periods, but also that the ether would not have a damaging effect on the child. There was also the possibility that the administration of ether, rather than being helpful, might add to difficulties of labour by inhibiting the contractions of the uterus.[14] It was therefore with considerable courage and daring that Simpson conducted his first obstetric delivery under ether on 19 January 1847.

The mother had a severely deformed and contracted pelvis. Her first pregnancy had led to a prolonged and painful labour lasting four days, during which it had proved impossible to deliver her by forceps. Even after craniotomy had been performed to reduce the size of the child's skull, it had still been difficult to deliver the dead child through her deformed pelvis. She was therefore advised of the hazards of risking a second pregnancy; but when she was next seen by her doctor she was at the end of the ninth month of pregnancy and already in labour. After a further four hours she was anaesthetised by ether, and twenty minutes later the child was delivered by forceps; the head had been severely compressed as it passed through the contracted pelvic brim and the child did not survive. However, the mother had been spared the prolonged suffering she had experienced during her previous labour, and she soon returned to normal health. Simpson was both relieved and jubilant. In a letter to his brother he wrote: 'I have delivered a woman *without* any pain. I can think of nothing else.'

He reported the success of this first case in the February edition of the *Monthly Journal of Medical Science*. In the following four weeks, with the assistance of Dr John Moir, Dr Graham Weir, Dr George Keith and Dr Ziegler, he administered ether during the labours of several of his patients,[15] including a number suffering long and difficult deliveries, and others whose labour was perfectly normal. In March he published his 'Notes on the

Inhalation of Sulphuric Ether in the Practice of Midwifery' in the March edition of *Monthly Journal of Medical Science*.

He was able to report that none of the mothers or infants had suffered any ill effect from the ether, even when it had been administered for periods upwards of half an hour. And in every case, uterine contractions had continued satisfactorily while the mother was in a 'state of anaesthesia'. In a few cases, while the apparatus for administering the ether was being adjusted, the mother became nervous and her fear seemed to diminish her contractions. But this effect quickly passed off and Simpson had 'seen no instance in which the pains were sensibly diminished in intensity or frequency after the ether had fairly begun to act. Indeed, in some cases, they have appeared to have become increased as the consciousness of the patients diminished.'[16]

At the end of his report, he added that since his first trials had shown that ether could be used effectively in controlling the pain of complicated deliveries, he had been repeatedly asked whether 'we will ever be justified in using the vapour of ether to assuage the pains of natural labour'. His answer was that if further experience continued to show that ether could be administered safely, the question would need to be changed. It would no longer be a question of whether 'we shall be "justified" in using this agent' but a question of whether, 'on any grounds, moral or medical, a professional man could deem himself "justified" in withholding and not using any such safe means as we at present pre-suppose this to be'.

In March 1847, Simpson had his report in the *Monthly Journal of Medical Science* reissued as a pamphlet, *Notes on the Inhalation of Sulphuric Ether in the Practice of Midwifery*. The pamphlet was offered for sale to the public in Edinburgh and London. He also sent many copies to members of the medical profession in Britain and overseas.

No voices were raised against the use of ether during long traumatic deliveries, or when surgical or difficult instrumental intervention was required. But there was no such consensus on the use of ether to relieve the pain of normal labour. Not every mother felt it necessary or desirable to have ether and be less than fully conscious during the eagerly awaited delivery of her child; and not every obstetrician agreed that it should be offered. Although many of his colleagues in Britain and the United States to whom Simpson sent copies of his *Notes* offered messages of congratulation, a number of influential obstetricians raised objections or reservations. Professor Charles Meigs of Jefferson Medical College in Philadelphia believed that the pains suffered during normal labour were 'a most desirable, salutary and conservative manifestation of the life force'. Professor Magnus Retzius, Head of Obstetrics and Gynaecology at the Karolinska Instituet in Sweden, had not ventured to use ether, because he thought it probable that its administration would interfere with the mother's ability to co-operate with the obstetrician during her delivery. Others were more ready to contemplate the use of ether but were deterred by the lack of any clear understanding of the nature of the unconsciousness induced by ether. If it resembled the unconsciousness of apoplexy or asphyxia, was there a risk that prolonged administration of ether might cause similar residual long-term brain damage? Even if that were to occur in only one in a thousand cases, it would clearly be unethical to administer ether in the management of a perfectly normal labour. Professor Meigs believed that the anaesthesia induced by ether was no different from the drunken stupor caused by alcohol. But did that, as Meigs suggested, leave lasting damage to the brain or the body? In the hope of finding an answer, Simpson consulted Edinburgh's police surgeon. His reply was unhelpful. He had been in office for five years, and in that time 28,357 'individuals in a state of intoxication' had been taken into custody. Of these, only three had died and in none of these cases had alcohol been the main cause of death; each year he had found it necessary to provide any form of active treatment in only eighteen or twenty cases. His conclusion was that 'altogether whisky must be the most harmless of all poisons.' Whether ether would prove to be an equally harmless poison remained uncertain.

Some objections to the use of ether were based on the obstetricians' very early and tentative experience. Charles Locock, Physician-Accoucheur to the Queen, reported that in London and in Paris, people 'are getting frightened about it [ether], as the arterial blood becomes black under its influence'.[17] There had even been a few deaths. This problem was discussed at length by Dr James Pickford in a letter published in *Aris's Gazette* on 28 May 1847. He claimed that the insensibility induced by ether was caused by vital chemical alterations in the blood. The most important of these was the damage caused to the blood corpuscles. They were first deprived of their capacity to carry oxygen; the blood then became black as myriad corpuscles were destroyed, releasing their haemoglobin into solution in the blood fluids. This led to damage of a different kind. The released haemoglobin caused depreciation in the quantity and quality of the fibrin in the blood, creating a risk of haemorrhage. Pickford was adamant that the effect of ether had nothing in common with asphyxia or apoplexy except the state of insensibility; it was something far more alarming and dangerous than any

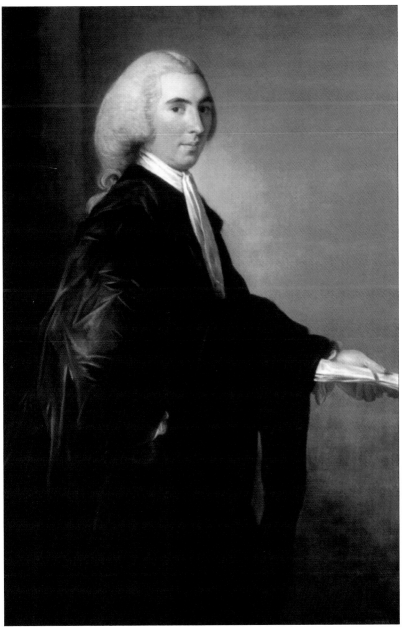

Henry Dundas (Viscount Melville), Lord Advocate, in 1775. Later War Secretary, First Lord of the Admiralty and manager of government business in Scotland during his friend William Pitt's years as Prime Minister.

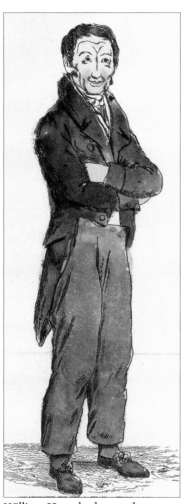

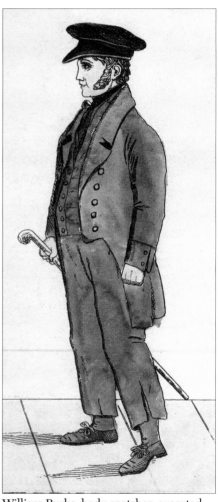

William Hare, body-snatcher, released after giving evidence against William Burke.

William Burke, body-snatcher, executed on 28 January 1829.

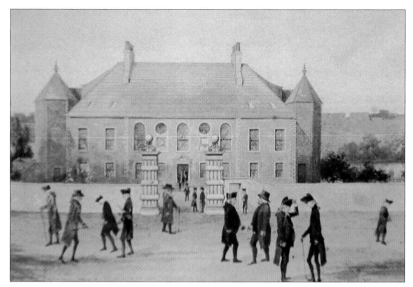

Surgeons' Hall when Simpson became a licentiate of the Royal College of Surgeons in 1830.

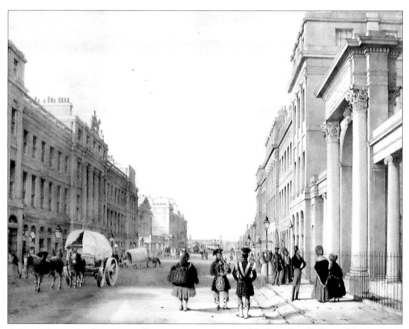

Princes Street in the 1840s when Simpson was establishing his fashionable medical practice in Edinburgh's New Town.

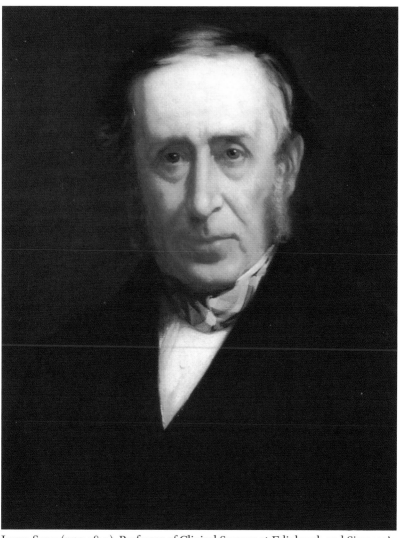
James Syme (1799–1870), Professor of Clinical Surgery at Edinburgh and Simpson's long-standing adversary.

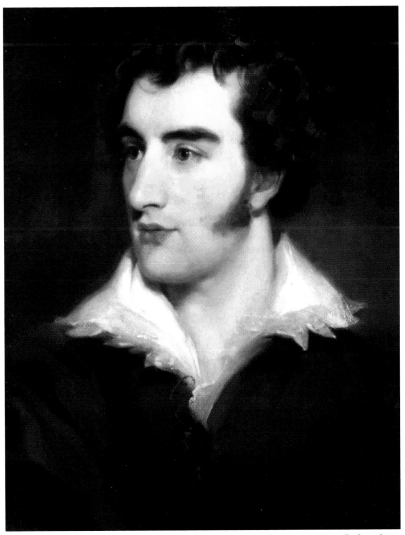

Robert Liston (1794–1847), Simpson's extra-mural tutor on surgery in Edinburgh before becoming Professor of Surgery at the new University of London. One of the first surgeons in Britain to use ether as a general anaesthetic.

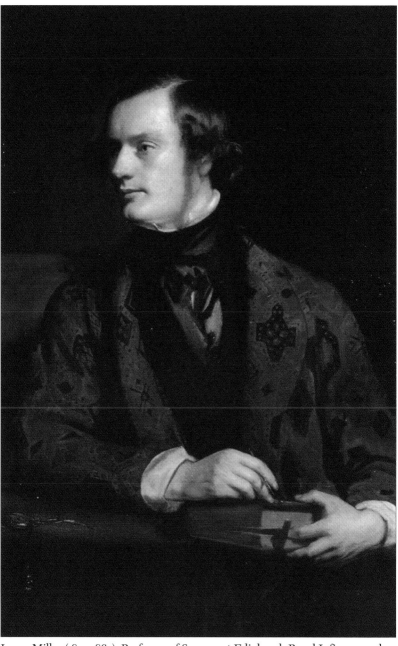

James Miller (1812–1864), Professor of Surgery at Edinburgh Royal Infirmary, who assisted Simpson by making the initial clinical trials of chloroform anaesthesia.

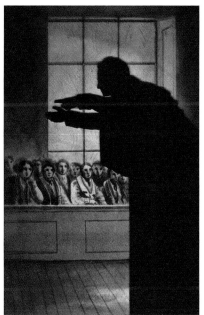

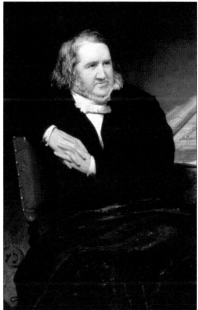

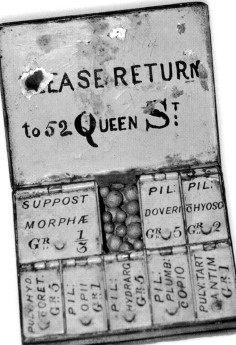

ABOVE LEFT. Rev. Thomas Chalmers. Evangelical and leader in the creation of the Free Church of Scotland in 1843.

ABOVE RIGHT. Sir James Y. Simpson, Bart., in 1866.

LEFT. Simpson's Pill Box.

RIGHT. The Coat of Arms of James Y. Simpson, mysteriously matriculated some weeks before he was created a baronet.

BELOW. St Columba's Cell (c.AD 567) discovered by Simpson in 1857 among the ruins of the ancient abbey on Inchcolm in the Firth of Forth.

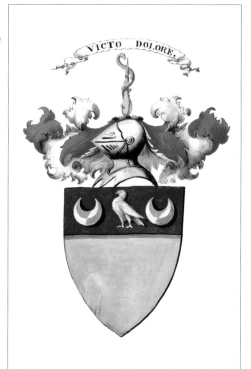

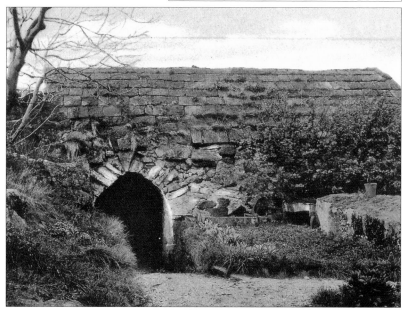

or all of these conditions taken severally or collectively. He declared that no agent which produced such a violent effect could be safely employed in the management of normal childbirth.

Months after the publication of Simpson's *Notes on the Inhalation of Sulphuric Ether in the Practice of Midwifery* the great majority of obstetricians were still not administering ether to relieve the pain of normal deliveries. Those who did not object on principle to the use of anaesthesia in normal deliveries feared that the risks in using ether might possibly outweigh the benefits. The extent and the nature of the risks was still uncertain; when mishaps occurred it was unclear whether the fault lay in the innate properties of the ether or in the technique of its administration. Although Simpson rejected the moral and ethical objections to the use of ether and attributed all the mishaps that had occurred to inexperience or incompetence in its administration, he nevertheless accepted that ether was not ideal for his purposes. As he explained to a meeting of the Medico-Chirurgical Society of Edinburgh in November 1847, he hoped to 'avoid if possible its disagreeable and persistent smell, its occasional tendency to cause irritation of the bronchi during its first inspirations'.[18] But more important were its 'inconveniences'. Simpson believed that anaesthesia should be available as an option in the management of all normal deliveries, and most normal deliveries were conducted in the patient's home. Ether needed a cumbersome administration apparatus and, in protracted cases of labour, large quantities of liquid ether, contained in large and awkward bottles, might be needed. Simpson hoped to find an alternative to ether, equally powerful but more convenient for the general practitioner to carry, and much simpler for him to administer. By the autumn of 1847 his search had already begun.

Although it had not proved to be as successful in obstetric practice as Simpson had hoped, his trials of ether in the management of prolonged and difficult labour had been of great importance in the development of general surgery. They had shown that Liston was wrong in supposing it would never be possible to use general anaesthesia to abolish the pain of operations lasting for longer than a very few minutes. Simpson had administered ether for periods of half an hour and more, and his obstetric patients had suffered no ill effects. As general surgeons discovered that their patients could be kept free of pain for ever longer periods, the need for speed became less pressing, and lightning manual dexterity ceased to be the essential skill of a successful surgeon. Surgeons could now begin to contemplate the possibility of new and ambitious operations that would have been dismissed as impossible before the introduction of ether and general anaesthesia.

For those who had first thought of ether as an anaesthetic, the outcome was less than happy. In December 1846, disappointed by the failure of his scheme to make himself rich by patenting ether as 'Letheon', Morton applied to Congress for a grant of $100,000 in recognition of his contribution to surgery by introducing ether as a general anaesthetic. His application was frustrated by the counter-claims of Charles Jackson, who claimed he had been the first to discover the anaesthetic powers of ether and that, without his work, Morton's achievements would have been impossible. Morton made further unsuccessful applications to Congress in 1849, 1851 and again in 1853. When all had failed, he made a futile attempt to sue the United States government. In pursuing his various claims he had neglected his practice and made himself bankrupt. At the age of forty-nine, while driving his buggy in Central Park in New York, he suffered a stroke and died later in hospital.

During his career, Charles Jackson made claim to priority in a number of important discoveries – guncotton, the telegraph, gastric acid, copper deposits at Lake Superior – as well as ether. All his claims were fiercely and effectively disputed. Embittered, he became an alcoholic and, at the age of seventy-five, he died in a mental asylum in Somerville, Massachusetts.

Horace Wells, after his humiliation at Massachusetts General in 1844, gave up his dental practice and made a precarious living as a travelling salesman. In 1846 he emigrated to France, hoping to become prosperous as European agent for his former partner, William Morton, selling his patented 'Letheon' products across Europe. When that project failed almost before it had begun, Wells returned to New York, where he became addicted to chloroform. In January 1848, while 'high' on chloroform, he attacked two prostitutes and was committed to a term in prison. Later, in despair, he committed suicide by slitting an artery after inhaling chloroform.

TEN

Chloroform

I esteem it the office of a physician, not only to restore health but to mitigate pain and dolours.

Bacon

In the summer of 1847, Simpson and his assistants, George Keith and James Matthews Duncan, began their search for a new inhalable anaesthetic. They hoped to find one that patients would find more agreeable than ether and that their doctors would find more convenient to administer. With the permission and co-operation of Robert Christison, the Professor of Materia Medica, and William Gregory, the Professor of Chemistry, they explored the shelves of the university's laboratories and took for testing samples of every volatile liquid that was to be found. Friends and colleagues suggested substances that they thought might possibly be the answer, and Edinburgh's leading firm of druggists, Duncan, Flockhart and Co., submitted several preparations that they had made up specially in the hope that one of them would prove to be the ideal anaesthetic, capable of dominating what promised to be a large and lucrative market.

To test these various chemicals and mixtures of chemicals, Simpson chose a procedure that was foolhardy and even potentially lethal. Early in the morning or late in the evening Simpson, Matthews Duncan and Keith would meet in the dining room of 52 Queen Street, pour the substances to be tested into saucers or tumblers, inhale their vapours and scribble notes on their effects. James Miller, the Professor of Surgery, Simpson's next-door neighbour at 53 Queen Street, called in from time to time to check on the continued wellbeing, even the survival, of the investigators and on the progress of their search.

The search had produced only headaches, nausea, ringing in the ears, dizziness and disappointment when, in October, Simpson received a visit from an old friend, David Waldie. Like Simpson, Waldie was a native of Linlithgowshire. They had been contemporaries as medical students at Edinburgh and, again like Simpson, Waldie had taken the diploma of the

Royal College of Surgeons of Edinburgh. However, he had then chosen
to make his career not as a surgeon but as a chemist. It was Waldie who
suggested to Simpson that the anaesthetic he was searching for was
chloroform.

Waldie had come to know of chloroform soon after succeeding Dr
Bett as chemist at Apothecaries Hall in Liverpool. At some time in the
early 1830s, Dr Bett had been asked by an American patient to make up
a prescription for 'chloric ether', a cordial then unknown in Britain but
popular in Massachusetts. On consulting the United States Dispensatory,
Bett discovered the cordial's composition and something of its history.
Chloric ether, or Dutch Liquid as it was also known, was a heavy, pleasant
smelling and sweet tasting liquid first produced in 1796 in Holland
by mixing ethylene with chlorine. It was a product of philosophical
chemistry; the scientists who produced it had been studying the nature
of the interaction of the two gases rather than attempting to create a new
substance to serve some specific purpose. However, for almost forty years,
physicians in Holland and America had explored its potential as a medicament. Benjamin Silliman, Professor of Chemistry at Yale, had found that
by dissolving it in alcohol, it could be recommended as an agreeable and
soothing cordial[1] helpful in the management of respiratory complaints. In
1830, in his textbook *Elements of Chemistry*[2] Silliman had described how it
could be prepared. However, Samuel Guthrie, an eccentric doctor, farmer
and amateur chemist at Sackets Harbour in Massachusetts, decided that
the method Silliman described – mixing the two difficult and unpleasant
gases, ethylene and chlorine, and dissolving the product in alcohol – was
technically difficult and unnecessarily expensive. He saw commercial
possibilities in producing it cheaply and conveniently. The method he
devised began with the mixing of three pounds of the chloride of lime,
which he used to kill the smell in his henhouses, in two gallons of rye
whiskey; his end product, as he had intended, had the physical character-
istics and the soothing properties of Silliman's cordial. But it soon became
evident that the cordial produced by Guthrie's method had even more of
the stimulating and intoxicating properties that made Silliman's cordial
popular. Silliman switched to making his cordial by Guthrie's method;
but Guthrie found that he could make more money by selling it not as
a medicament, but as 'Sweet Whiskey'.[3] It was some years before it was
discovered that the special ingredient in Guthrie's whiskey, and in Silliman's 'chloric ether cordial' prepared by Guthrie's method, was not chloric
ether (Dutch Liquid) but chloroform.

After first making it up for his American patient, Dr Bett had continued to prepare the 'chloric ether cordial', as a number of general practitioners in Liverpool had found that it was useful in the management of asthma attacks and in the relief of chronic cough. When Waldie was appointed as chemist at Apothecaries Hall he discovered that Bett had continued to prepare the cordial by Guthrie's method and, produced in that way, the mixture not only contained impurities, it also varied greatly from batch to batch in the proportion of chloroform that it contained. Waldie also heard that, in Liverpool, the vapour of this so called 'chloric ether cordial' had been tried more than once as a general anaesthetic.[4] It had proved unsatisfactory but, as Waldie later wrote, that was not surprising since the amount of chloroform in the mixture was often so small that the patient was, in effect, breathing only the vapour of alcohol.[5] Waldie introduced his own method of producing the mixture, extracting pure chloroform from the crude solution[6] and dissolving it, in a constant proportion, in rectified spirit. It was this improved product that general practitioners in Liverpool had continued to prescribe for their patients, but it was the purified chloroform that Waldie suggested to Simpson as an anaesthetic.

Unfortunately his laboratory at Apothecaries Hall in Liverpool had recent been badly damaged by fire and Waldie could not immediately provide the required sample of his pure chloroform.[7] Professor Gregory was able to produce pure chloroform in his laboratory, but not in the quantity that Simpson required. Simpson therefore ordered several ounces of pure chloroform from Duncan, Flockhart and Co. When it was delivered, Simpson thought the liquid much too heavy even to be considered. He set it aside. A few weeks later, on 4 November 1847, Simpson, Duncan and Keith had finally dismissed the last of the samples that had been assembled for testing that evening. They had been joined in the dining room by Simpson's wife Jessie, her sister Williamina, her brother-in-law Captain Petrie and Petrie's daughter, Agnes, when Simpson remembered the sample of chloroform. It was found on a side table, buried under a collection of papers. George Keith was the first to inhale its vapour from the sample in his tumbler. When Simpson and Matthew Duncan saw his reaction, they immediately tried it for themselves. All three became bright eyed and happy and, in the brief interval before they crashed to the floor, their conversation was of 'unusual intelligence and quite charmed the listeners'.[8] Simpson was the first to regain consciousness. While still on the floor he was heard to say that 'this is far stronger and better than ether'. As he looked round, Matthew Duncan was lying quite still and snoring under a chair, while George Keith was on his back kicking the supper table with 'maniacal and unrestrainable destructiveness'. Having recovered from this first inhalation of chloroform, all three repeated the experience several times. They were then certain that they had found the substitute for ether that they had been searching for. Jessie and Williamina recovered from their initial alarm; the sixteen-year-old Agnes, having demanded to try just one whiff of chloroform, immediately called out in apparent ecstasy: 'I'm an angel, oh, an angel', before sliding quietly to the floor.[9] The other members of the family then happily sampled the exhilarating vapour. The only one to resist was Williamina; Simpson, who was in the habit of teasing his sister-in-law, chased her merrily around the house with a tumbler of chloroform in his hand while she squealed in protest. Everyone except Williamina went on to enjoy the exhilarating effects of chloroform until the supply was exhausted. The celebrations continued until 3 a.m.

A few days later, on 10 November, Simpson announced his discovery to a meeting of Edinburgh's Medico-Chirurgical Society. It had been arranged that at the meeting there would be presentations by James Syme and by James Y. Simpson. It was recorded that no one could 'remember having seen a more crowded meeting of the Society'. It may have been that many had come to witness two such eminent adversaries brought together in public; it is more probable that something of Simpson's experiments with chloroform had already become known. As planned, Syme gave his account of 'A Case of Tumour of the Neck simulating Aneurism of the Carotid Artery', a remarkably frank description of a case in which he had examined the patient in keeping with the highest standards of the time but had reached a wrong diagnosis; his patient had died. He presented the case, as he said, to 'discharge the duty which devolves on every member of the profession who is so unfortunate as to commit a serious error by faithfully stating the circumstances which misled him, so that they be rendered less likely to cause similar mistakes in future'. Simpson duly presented a detailed and scholarly account of his 'Historical Researches Regarding the Superinduction of Insensibility'. It was only then that he made his 'Announcement of a New Anaesthetic Agent'. In it he discussed chloroform's chemical composition and the history of how it first came to be produced in the 1830s. He gave brief outlines of three quite different methods by which it could be prepared and described its physical and chemical properties. He listed its advantages over ether as an anaesthetic:

1. A greatly less quantity of chloroform is required.
2. Its action is much more rapid, more perfect, and generally more persistent.
3. Its exciting or exhilarating stage is far shorter, insensibility commonly supervening in a minute or two or less.
4. The time of the surgeon is saved.
5. The inhalation and influence of it are more agreeable and pleasant.
6. Its odor is evanescent.
7. No special instrument is required for its employment.[10]

He then added his recommendations on how it should be administered.

Although it was only six days since he had discovered the anaesthetic properties of chloroform, he had already used it as an analgesic to relieve the pain of dysmenorrhoea and of neuralgia. He had also used it in minor procedures, such as opening abscesses and draining ovarian cysts, and as a general anaesthetic in midwifery, 'tooth drawing' and general surgery. In all, he had used it in some fifty cases, 'all with entire success'.

The first time he used it in obstetrics was on 8 November 1847. His patient was Jane Carstairs, a doctor's wife, who had recently returned from India to live in Fife; but, as she had been warned that she might expect to have a difficult delivery, she had come to stay in Edinburgh until the baby was born.[11] Simpson wrote:

> The lady had been previously delivered in the country by perforation of the head of the infant after a labour of three days duration. In this, her second confinement, her pains supervened a fortnight before the full time. Three hours and a half after they commenced and ere the first stage of the labour was completed, I placed her under the influence of chloroform by moistening, with half a tea-spoonful of the liquid, a pocket handkerchief rolled up into a funnel shape and with the broad or open end of the funnel placed over her mouth and nostrils. In consequence of the rapid evaporation of the fluid it was once more renewed in about ten or twelve minutes. The child was expelled in about twenty five minutes after the inhalation had begun. The mother subsequently remained longer soporose than commonly happens with ether. The squalling of the child did not, as usual, rouse her; and some minutes elapsed after the placenta was expelled and after the child was removed by the nurse into another room before the patient woke. She then turned round and observed to me that she had 'enjoyed a very comfortable sleep and indeed had required it

as she was so tired but would now be more able for the work before her.' I evaded entering into conversation with her believing that the most complete possible quietude forms one of the principal secrets for the successful employment of either ether or chloroform. In a little time she again remarked that her 'sleep had stopped the pains'. Shortly afterwards, her infant was brought in by the nurse from the adjoining room and it was a matter of no small difficulty to convince the astonished mother that the labour was entirely over and that the child presented to her was really her 'own living baby'.[12]

The first patient to be given chloroform for the extraction of a tooth was a dentist's apprentice, T. D. Morrison. After agreeing to the trial he wrote a letter to Simpson freeing him from all blame should anything go wrong. The procedure was carried out to everyone's satisfaction at 52 Queen Street on the morning of 10 November.

Then, later that day, Simpson administered chloroform for three surgical operations performed by James Miller and Matthew Duncan in the presence of an invited gathering of medical men and students at Edinburgh Royal Infirmary. The first patient was a little boy of four or five who was to have a necrotic bone removed from his forearm.The boy spoke only Gaelic and there had been no means of explaining to him what he was required to do. On holding the handkerchief on which the chloroform had been sprinkled to his face he became frightened and wrestled to escape. However, Simpson held him gently but firmly and made him inhale. After half a dozen inspirations, he stopped crying and fell into a sound sleep. A deep incision was made down to the diseased bone, and by the use of forceps nearly the whole of the radius was extracted. During the operation, and the subsequent probing of the wound and the remaining parts of the bone, he gave not the slightest evidence of feeling pain. Still sleeping soundly he was carried back to his ward. Half an hour later, he was found in bed like any child newly awakened from a refreshing sleep. Questioned by a Gaelic-speaking student, he replied that he had felt no pain. On being shown his wounded arm, he looked surprised but not in the least distressed.

Simpson, after the experience of only a few days and small numbers of cases, was already fully confident that general anaesthesia by the inhalation of chloroform would prove to be one of the greatest innovations in the history of medicine. And he meant to be its champion. He therefore made quite extraordinary efforts to publicise his discovery as widely and as quickly as possible. His presentation to Edinburgh's Medico-Chirurgical

Society on 10 November was published in full in the December edition of the *Monthly Journal of Medical Science*, the journal of which he was both a proprietor and an editor. He had already submitted a full account to the *Lancet* on 12 November;[13] 'Cases of the Employment of Chloroform in Midwifery' in the *Lancet* on 21 November; and on 1 December he published yet another report in the *Provincial Medical and Surgical Journal* (forerunner of the British Medical Journal). These many communications were intended to persuade the medical profession of the virtues and safety of chloroform.

However, Simpson thought it more than probable that, in spite of making his case in the medical journals, many members of his profession would be hesitant before venturing to use an even less familiar agent than ether in the new and still somewhat mysterious business of anaesthesia. But he was confident that, if the general public could be made aware of the previously unimagined benefits that chloroform now offered, they would be his most powerful allies in overcoming whatever resistance might be offered by the medical profession. He therefore published a pamphlet entitled *Account of a New Anaesthetic Agent as a Substitute for Sulphuric Ether in Surgery and Midwifery*. Although he sent copies to the Royal Society in London and to scientists and to medical men everywhere, it was aimed chiefly at the lay public. It provided almost all the information that he had included in his articles in the medical journals, but set out in language suitable for the general reader. He assured his readers that chloroform was 'infinitely more efficacious' than ether. All that was required was 'a little liquid diffused upon a pocket handkerchief'. No strange 'kind of inhaler or instrument was required for its exhibition'. Chloroform avoided 'the inconveniences and objections pertaining to sulphuric ether – particularly its disagreeable and very persistent smell'. Since only a small quantity of liquid chloroform was required, its use was not expensive. And, above all, chloroform was safe. 'I tried it on myself.'

The *Account of a New Anaesthetic Agent as a Substitute for Sulphuric Ether in Surgery and Midwifery* was published, price 6d, on 15 November, by Sutherland and Knox in Edinburgh; that morning it was advertised on the front page of the *Scotsman*, Edinburgh's leading newspaper, and by the afternoon every copy of the first printing of 1,000 copies had been sold. The pamphlet was also published in Fleet Street in London, by Samuel Highley, and in the weeks that followed further print runs, each of a thousand copies, had to be repeated again and again in both Edinburgh and London. Simpson's report of the benefits of chloroform and the ease and safety with which it could be administered was then carried by newspapers and popular journals to an even wider public in Britain, Europe and North America.

Within weeks, his pamphlet had achieved his aim. The general public had been fully alerted to his discovery of a new anaesthetic that was even better than ether; and, as he had predicted, patients were already demanding that their doctors should have it available. Some members of the public were even buying a supply of chloroform to have ready at home. By the end of the year, established manufacturers were finding it difficult to satisfy the demand for chloroform, and new firms were being set up to produce it.

As had been the case with ether, some very influential military surgeons disapproved of the use of chloroform, and their patients, unlike patients in civilian practice, were not in a position to insist. In 1846, Thomas Lawson, surgeon-general in the United States, had decreed that ether was unsuitable for military use. Now, in 1848, he ordered chloroform for issue to all military hospitals and casualty stations serving the United States armies fighting in Mexico. However, at the military hospital at Vera Cruz, the main centre for the treatment of casualties, the surgeon in charge, John Porter, still refused to use it. He claimed, without offering his evidence, that chloroform increased the risks of haemorrhage, blood poisoning and gangrene.

During the Second Sikh War in 1848–9, the most senior British military surgeons still believed that, since pain was 'one of the most powerful, one of the most salutary stimulants known', the administration of chloroform would severely diminish the patient's chances of recovery from surgery. As late as 1854, John Hall, the surgeon in charge of the hospital services deployed for the war in the Crimea, continued to take the same view. He issued a directive cautioning medical officers against the use of chloroform, since the 'smart of the knife is a powerful stimulant and it is much better to hear a man bawl lustily than to see him sink silently into the grave'. However surgeons serving in the makeshift operating theatres close to the scene of battle were able to see for themselves that this was far from the case. The mortality from even straightforward amputations carried out without anaesthesia was appalling, and the screams of the men undergoing surgery had a demoralising effect on the badly injured casualties, lying on the ground or in the bullock carts that had brought them, as they awaited the same fate. From Edinburgh, James Syme wrote to the *Times*[14] stating that Hall was quite wrong; 'pain instead of being a powerful stimulant, most injuriously exhausts the nervous energy of a weak patient', and chloroform was 'useful directly in proportion to the severity of the injury or disease and the degree of shock'. Next day Hall replied in the *Times*, insisting that Professor Syme's opinion was 'in direct opposition to the general opinion of the profession'. But Richard Mackenzie,[15] and several other surgeons who had been students of both Simpson and Syme, had carried their own supplies of chloroform with them to the Crimea and they chose to ignore the directives of Dr Hall.

There were some early and quite different problems in civilian practice. In his various publications Simpson had given little guidance on how chloroform should be made; he had written only that 'it can be procured by various processes, as by making milk of lime or an aqueous solution of caustic alkali act upon chloral; by distilling alcohol, pyroxylic spirit or acetone with chloride of lime; or by leading a stream of chlorine gas into a solution of caustic potash etc.'. In the rush to satisfy demand, the production of chloroform by ill-informed, and often sadly inexperienced, manufacturers had unfortunate consequences. In Massachusetts the early trials of chloroform ended in disaster. Its effects proved to be wildly and dangerously unpredictable, and there were several deaths. At the Massachusetts General Hospital, early experience was so bad that chloroform was banned. Inevitably this decision, by such a prestigious body, influenced surgeons throughout the north-eastern states of America, and almost all chose to abandon their trials of chloroform and continue using ether. In December 1852, in a letter to Simpson, Dr Todd of Anderson County, Kentucky suggested that the unsatisfactory results first at the Massachusetts General, and since then at other medical centres in the United States, were due to serious faults in the way that their chloroform was made. Five years later, these suspicions were confirmed when the *American Medical Monthly* made an investigation into the quality of the chloroform being supplied from all the various sources in the United States; in July 1857 Dr Barker of Bellevue Hospital in New York wrote to Simpson: 'I suppose it will bring down on my devoted head the anathema of the manufacturers and druggists when the *American Medical Monthly* reports that the only specimen of pure chloroform they could find is that produced by Squib and myself.' When the results of the *American Medical Monthly* investigation were published, drug firms in the United States immediately sent to Duncan, Flockhart & Co. in Edinburgh for samples of their chloroform. Thereafter the quality of chloroform available in the United States improved, but by then the damage to chloroform's reputation had already been done, and in Boston and the north-eastern states it never recovered.

There were also problems in the south of England. When surgeons there made their first trials of chloroform, again many were disappointed. They complained that chloroform was much too irritant, making administration difficult because of the patient's coughing, and causing bronchitis serious enough to delay the patient's recovery. Simpson tested a sample from one of the relevant London manufacturers and found it to be acid, emitting fumes that Simpson identified as hydrochloric acid. It later became more widely understood by English manufacturers that chloroform was unstable in sunlight, producing chlorine, hydrochloric acid and phosgene.[16] In Edinburgh, Duncan, Flockhart & Co. had always taken the precaution of stabilising their chloroform by adding 1 per cent alcohol. Less experienced English manufacturers of chloroform, unaware that a stabiliser was necessary, had tried to produce chloroform of the highest possible standard of purity, with unfortunate results. Even Duncan, Flockhart's product was not stable under all conditions. In 1851, a sample of their chloroform was displayed at the Great Exhibition at the Crystal Palace; in the bright sunlight there, the chloroform turned green and had to be withdrawn.

One London doctor informed Simpson that, in England, the reason for the difficulties that so many general practitioners experienced in making proper use of chloroform was that they were not medical graduates but apothecaries, 'so as a set they are men destitute of a liberal education, the majority of them having no education at all beyond a provincial school until they went to walk the wards of a hospital. They care nothing for science. Chloroform will make its own way but it will be through the patients not the apothecaries.'[17]

In Aberdeen, chloroform had only been tried tentatively in three operations when an accident halted further trials. A druggist's shop boy, who had very quickly become addicted to chloroform, inhaled yet another generous dose and fell deeply unconscious with his head on the shop counter, his nose and mouth still in contact with the cloth onto which his large dose of chloroform had been poured. Fifteen minutes later he was dead. The accident was reported sensationally in the local press. For this and other similar tragedies, Dr Wardell of Kensington blamed Simpson. He insisted that, when informing the general public about its merits, Simpson had misled 'non-professional people' into believing that chloroform could be inhaled with complete safety; disasters had been inevitable.

Several doctors wrote to Simpson to complain that he should not have presented his discoveries and views on the use of chloroform so quickly and directly to the public. Had he addressed himself first to the medical profession, doctors would have been better prepared to meet their patients' immediate and pressing demands.

However, in spite of these difficulties and mishaps, Simpson's direct approach to the public had been successful. Had the discovery of chloroform and its advantages over ether been reported in the normal way in the medical press, surgeons would have tried it and, in time, many would have adopted it as their anaesthetic of choice. But the whole concept of general anaesthesia was new, and to use chloroform was to take a further step into the unknown. Most surgeons would have preferred a period of cautious appraisal before making free use of such a new and untried drug. But Simpson's early and vigorous advocacy created a patient demand that few surgeons found possible to resist.

Simpson was not so successful in introducing chloroform into obstetric practice. Obstetricians needed little persuasion to use chloroform in prolonged and difficult deliveries, especially when instruments were to be used. However, many objected to Simpson's insistence that chloroform should be used to alleviate the pains of normal childbirth. One wrote that pain during labour was natural and that any 'unnecessary interference with the providentially arranged process of healthy progression is due sooner or later to be followed by injurious and fatal consequences'. Impatient, as always, with opposition, Simpson replied: 'If you refuse to interfere with a natural function because it is natural – why do you ride, my dear Doctor? You ought to walk, in order to be consistent. Chloroform does nothing but *save pain*, you allege. A carriage does nothing but save fatigue. Which is the more important to be done away with? *Your* fatigue or your patient's screams and tortures? I rejoice at such bitter personal attacks and absurd misrepresentations as you indulge in for one reason. It looked as if no one were going to attack the practice [of anaesthesia in midwifery] in the way that historic fools opposed vaccination and as I predicted *would* occur. I have no such fears now.'

Simpson was equally crushing in his reply to Dr George Gream of Queen Charlotte's Lying-in Hospital in London (later Physician-Accoucheur to Queen Victoria). Gream was greatly distressed by the possibility that the administration of chloroform during childbirth might cause unseemly sexual excitement. It had been reported in the *Lancet* that a young woman, giving birth to her second child under chloroform, had dreamt that she was having intercourse with her husband. Gream protested that 'to the women of this country the bare possibility of having feelings of such a kind excited and manifested in outward uncontrollable actions would be more shocking even to anticipate than endurance of the last extremity of physical pain'. It was further reported that the young woman had offered to kiss a male attendant. Gream declared that if women were aware that this might happen under chloroform 'they would undergo even the most excruciating torture or suffer death itself before they would subject themselves to the shadow of a chance of exhibitions as have been recorded'. In gathering evidence in support of his case, Dr Gream wrote to Simpson asking for information on the incidence of lascivious dreams or indications of sexual excitement from the use of chloroform in cases under his care.[18]

Simpson replied that neither he nor any of his colleagues had ever seen behaviour such as Gream described. Further allegations of such behaviour had been 'gloated over by those who have propounded it in a way which forms, apparently unconsciously on their own part, the severest self-inflicted censure upon the sensuality of their own thoughts'. Gream, he wrote, 'was not entitled to imagine that his own lewd thoughts are typified by the thoughts or actions of his patients'. Unabashed, Gream continued to bring his concern about the sexually exciting properties of chloroform to meetings of the Westminster Medical Society until defeated by the restrained but persistent ridicule of his fellow members.

For Simpson, these criticisms by members of the medical profession were irritating but trivial. Although he had neither expected nor prepared for them, they were easily dismissed. However, he had expected another and much more powerful objection, and since he had expected that it would come from patients as well as doctors, he had prepared for it very carefully. Following the publication of his *Notes on the Inhalation of Sulphuric Ether in the Practice of Midwifery* in 1847, a number of his professional colleagues and patients objected to the use of anaesthesia during labour on the grounds that such immunity from pain during parturition was contrary to religion and the express commands of Scripture. He had expected that this objection would be repeated after the publication of his *Account* in 1848, and also that it would be put forward more forcefully. The Evangelical movement was now at its height in Britain. In 1848, the Church of England had appointed its first evangelical Archbishop of Canterbury.[19] The Church of Scotland had, some years earlier, appointed its first Evangelical moderator of the General Assembly.[20] In 1843, the Evangelical Thomas Chalmers had led over a third of the Church of Scotland's ministers and half its lay membership out of the established church to form a Free Church of Scotland in which church services consisted only of prayer, preaching of the word of God and the unaccompanied singing of the Psalms. Evangelicalism was a religion of the Word. It depended utterly on a belief in God as revealed in the words of the Bible. Simpson was a prominent member of the new, Evangelical Free Church of Scotland, and he could not lightly dismiss those who might use their reading of the words of the Bible against him.

He had prepared a carefully argued answer to the torrent of protest that he thought must surely come. To his surprise there was no such torrent. One clergyman wrote that chloroform was a 'decoy of Satan, apparently offering itself to bless women; but in the end it will harden society and rob God of the deep earnest cries which rise in time of trouble for help'. There were reports that some deeply religious women had doubts. Some consulted their ministers before agreeing to accept the benefits of chloroform during childbirth. One woman, who had gratefully sought the relief of anaesthesia during her labour, later asked for absolution for her sin. Another, Simpson was informed, had always maintained that the administration of anaesthesia in labour was an unholy work, but as her own time drew near she was most anxious to know if it could be administered by 'a plain country doctor' or by her nurse. It seemed to Simpson that although the great majority of women would gratefully accept the use of chloroform to relieve the pains of childbirth if they became severe, many would do so very uneasily because of their religious scruples. To argue against such scruples, in December 1848, he published his *Answer to the Religious Objections Advanced Against the Employment of Anaesthetic Agents in Midwifery and Surgery*.

Simpson first identified the precise Biblical source of the objections. They rested on a few verses in Genesis. These verses recorded that after the serpent and the woman had brought sin into the Garden of Eden, God had cursed both them and Adam who had allowed them to sin. The relevant passages in God's curse were:

1. Unto the woman he said, I will greatly multiply thy sorrow and thy conception; in sorrow thou shalt bring forth children . . . Genesis 3:16.
2. Unto Adam he said . . . cursed is the ground for thy sake. In sorrow shalt thou eat of it all the days of your life. Thorns also and thistles shall it bring forth to thee . . . Genesis 3:17 and 18.
3. In the sweat of thy face shalt thou eat bread . . . Genesis 3:19.

Simpson argued that the agriculturalist who now pulls up and destroys the thorns and thistles which the earth was doomed to bear is never looked upon as erring and sinning in doing so. Man was doomed to till by the sweat of his brow but now, instead of his own sweat and personal exertions, he employs the horse and the ox, water and steam power, sowing, reaping and grinding machines to do this work for him and elaborate the bread which he eats. If the first part of the curse must be read literally and acted on literally, why not the second and third? Further, in Genesis it is also written that man was told that out of dust 'wast thou taken, for dust thou art, and unto dust shalt thou return'. If man is so doomed to die, why should those physicians who feel conscientiously constrained from relieving the agonies of woman in childbirth use their skills to prevent man from dying?

Later in his pamphlet Simpson claimed that curses imposed for sins committed in the Garden of Eden had, in any case, been rendered void, since 'Christ is everywhere declared to be an all-sufficient sacrifice for all the sins and crimes of man'. Bringing together various passages in Matthew 9 and 12, he wrote: 'Christ the man of sorrow, who hath given himself up as an offering and a sacrifice to God, surely hath borne our griefs and carried our sorrows for he saw the travail of his soul and was satisfied.'

He then went on to show that, even if the curse had still been valid, the meaning of the word 'sorrow' had been misunderstood. In Genesis 3:16, the Hebrew word translated as 'sorrow' was *etzebb*. In Genesis 3:17 the Hebrew word translated as 'sorrow' was *itztzabbon*. Both these Hebrew words were derived from the same root, *atzabb*, which (according to Tregelle's translation of *Gesenius's Hebrew and Chaldee Lexicon*) could mean both a) to labour or to fashion, and b) to toil with pain, to suffer or to be grieved. Simpson quoted several places in the Bible where *etzebb* and *itztzabbon* had been used in passages where their sense was clearly 'to labour' or 'to toil'. He then instanced several other passages where the sense was clearly 'pain' or 'agony'; there the word used had been *hhil* or *hhebhel*. He concluded that the English version of God's curse, 'in sorrow thou shalt bring forth children', should have read 'by labour thou shalt bring forth children'. 'Labour' was not only the correct translation, it was peculiarly apt in describing human parturition. 'The greatest characteristic in human parturition as compared with parturition in the lower animals is the enormous amount of muscular action and effort (labour) provided for and usually required for its consummation. The erect position of the human body renders a series of peculiar mechanisms, arrangements and obstructions necessary in the human pelvis for the prevention of abortion and premature labour and for the well-being of the mother during pregnancy. But these same mechanical arrangements all render at last the ultimate expulsion of the infant in labour a far more difficult and more prolonged process than in the quadruped. The human mother is provided with a uterus immensely more muscular and energetic than that of any of the lower animals. The uterus is many times stronger and more powerful than the uterus, for example, of the cow. The great characteristic of human parturition is the vastly greater amount of muscular effort toil or labour required for its accomplishment.'

As always, Simpson embellished and dignified his writing with references to both ancient and modern literature. The authors he quoted included Luther, Calvin, Aquila, Rosenmuller, Dathe, Bishop Patrick, and Sir Walter Scott. But toward the end of his defence of anaesthesia during childbirth, he again quoted from the Bible. 'And the Lord God caused a deep sleep to fall upon Adam; and he slept; and he took one of his ribs and closed up the flesh thereof.' He offered this passage as affording evidence that our Creator himself used means to save poor human nature from the unnecessary endurance of physical pain.

Simpson's *Answer* was published in Edinburgh and London, and thousands of copies were sold. Theologians and leaders of the Church of Scotland, the Free Church of Scotland[21] and the Episcopal Church in Scotland all wrote to congratulate him. Some of the most exalted dignitaries of the Church of England expressed their approval of what he had written. The powerful opposition that he had anticipated failed to appear. In July 1848, Simpson wrote to his friend Protheroe Smith in London that 'the religious opposition to chloroform have ceased among us'.

Within a year of Simpson's introduction of chloroform, surgeons and their patients had become secure about their confidence in the benefits and advantages of chloroform. For general surgery, chloroform had become the anaesthetic of choice in Britain, the south and west of the United States, France, Germany, Austria, Italy, Russia and India. However, Simpson had been less successful in promoting the use of chloroform in midwifery. In October 1848, he reported that he had delivered 150 patients under anaesthesia by chloroform. One child, already known to be dead three weeks before the mother went into labour, was born in a 'putrid state' at an estimated gestational age of seven months; one mother had died of puerperal convulsions two weeks after delivery; another had died of acute endocarditis three weeks after delivery; but there had been no death or mishap that could be attributed to the use of chloroform.

No series of a similar size had been carried out elsewhere, and the reports from obstetricians that Simpson received in the first weeks and months were disappointing. One obstetrician wrote that 'there is a strong prejudice in England against chloroform in midwifery but chloroform

will make its own way. But it will be through the patients not the apothecaries.'[22] In Ireland, early experience had not been encouraging. In Dublin,
Professor Evory Kennedy's first patient suffered a convulsion while chloroform was being induced; Dr Churchill had administered chloroform to
Lady Drysdale during her delivery but 'without success'; Dr Coombe had
used chloroform a number of times but was still afraid of it; at his first
trial of chloroform, Dr Tyler had given too much and 'labour was retarded'.
On the second occasion he had given too little and 'could not say that
labour went uninterruptedly and without pain'; after a year, obstetricians
in Dublin were still reluctant to use chloroform because of their 'dread of
bad consequences'. [23] In Aberdeen, because of the early difficulties that had
occurred during its use in general surgery, chloroform had not even been
tried in midwifery.

However, in spite of early hesitations and difficulties, obstetricians soon
became very ready to administer chloroform when operative or instrumental intervention was necessary in order to save the life of the mother or
child. Simpson's persistent difficulty was in promoting the use of chloroform during normal deliveries. He took the view that the proper indication for the use of chloroform was not the nature of the problem or the
need to use instruments but the intensity of the pain and degree of distress
being suffered by the mother. Even the pain of what would be generally
considered a normal delivery might, on occasion, be beyond the tolerance
of the mother. Whether or not the use of chloroform was indicated should
therefore depend on the circumstances of the case and the judgement of
the obstetrician. This was a view that Professor Meigs of Philadelphia could
not accept. He considered it to be unethical. He wrote: 'Should I exhibit to
a thousand patients merely to prevent physiological pain and for no other
reason and should I destroy only one of them I should feel disposed to
clothe me in sackcloth and cast ashes upon my head for the remainder of
my days.' Simpson respected Meigs' case and the two continued to correspond in an entirely friendly way. Simpson was confident that the case
Meigs made would fall when it was shown that in normal labour it was
not necessary to have the patient completely unconscious; the patient need
only be given the small and entirely safe dose of chloroform necessary to
alleviate her pain. Meigs, and many others, were equally certain that the
administration of general anaesthetic could never be made completely safe.

Meigs' case had been strengthened by a major problem first reported in
January 1848. There had been a sudden unexplained death under chloroform in Newcastle upon Tyne. The patient was Hannah Greener, an illegit-

imate girl of fifteen whose mother had died when she was born. Hannah was noticeably underweight but otherwise well grown and in good health, apart from the pain from her in-growing toenails. In 1847, she had the nail of her left great toe removed under ether. After the operation she had been unwell and much upset by her short stay in hospital. When it became clear that she should have the same toenail on her right foot removed, it was decided that the operation should be done at home and under chloroform. On the morning of the operation she was nervous and fretful, and when the surgeon and his assistant arrived in the afternoon she burst into tears. She was seated in an armchair near the fire and told, perhaps rather briskly, to stop crying. About a teaspoonful of chloroform was put onto a cloth, which was then held closely over her mouth and nostrils. After two breaths she tried to pull the cloth away but was ordered to put her hands on her knees. After about half a minute, her eyes were closed, she was breathing normally and seemed to be at the required level of anaesthesia. However, when the first incision was made, she seemed to jerk in reaction, and more chloroform was quickly administered. She then suddenly blanched and, after a few feeble and rapid breaths, stopped breathing completely. Water was dashed on her face and brandy was poured into her mouth in the hope that she might swallow it. When these efforts failed, she was laid on the floor and the surgeon tried to bleed her, first from her arm and then from her neck. Barely a trickle of blood flowed from her veins and it was clear that she was dead. It was estimated that no more than two minutes had passed between her first whiff of chloroform and her death. At post-mortem her lungs were thought to be 'in a very high state of congestion', but no other possible cause of death was discovered. Sir John Fife, the Newcastle surgeon who carried out the post-mortem, attributed the death to congestion of the lungs due to inhalation of chloroform. The jury accepted his verdict.

Simpson had promoted chloroform as a safe anaesthetic and it had been administered to Hannah Greener exactly as he had recommended in the *Lancet* of 21 November 1847. As always, Simpson refused to retreat from a position he had taken in public. He insisted that Hannah Greener had been suffocated by the brandy forced into her mouth when she was already too deeply unconscious to swallow; he also pointed out that the measures taken to resuscitate her had been sadly inappropriate.

However, a second death followed in February 1848 in Cincinnati. The patient, Mrs Simmons, was thirty-five years old and in good health; she was to have a number of 'stumps' of teeth removed. She was anaesthetised by inhaling chloroform from a glass globe containing a sponge completely saturated with liquid chloroform. After an estimated twelve breaths she seemed to be insensible and the operation began. She was already pale and, as the last root was drawn, her arms and body suddenly became rigid. Her breathing had stopped and no pulse could be felt. Artificial respiration was tried. Electric shocks caused the muscles of her limbs to contract, but they had no effect on her heart. Mrs Simmons, like Hannah Greener, died within two minutes of taking the first inhalation of chloroform.

A few more such deaths followed. They occurred randomly as isolated incidents and almost anywhere that chloroform was used. But even Sir John Fife, the surgeon who had performed the autopsy on the victim of the first of these incidents, continued to use chloroform. He did not believe that chloroform was a toxic substance, but rather that Hannah Greener had shown an abnormality, an idiosyncrasy, in her reaction to it. Soon idiosyncrasy was offered as the explanation for any sudden death in the first minutes of induction of anaesthesia by chloroform, and the phenomenon became known as chloroform syncope. Reports of chloroform syncope did not deter Simpson. He continued to advocate the use of chloroform, comfortable in the knowledge that, in Edinburgh, it had been administered to large numbers of patients and there had been no deaths or other serious mishaps. Properly administered by his method, chloroform was safe.

In London, John Snow[24] was sure that the position taken by Simpson was untenable. After setting up in general practice in Soho in 1838, Snow had become interested in the problems of breathing, asphyxia and resuscitation. By the 1840s, for use in his experiments, he had designed a number of pumps and instruments for the measurement of the flow of gases. When the inhalation of ether came into use in 1847, he was therefore well prepared to become one of the first to practise as an anaesthetist and, within a year, he had become the leading anaesthetist in London. In his view, Simpson had been reckless both in the way he had introduced first ether and later chloroform into obstetric practice. Simpson had administered ether to a woman in labour without having any proper experimental evidence of its effects and dangers. When introducing chloroform Simpson had either ignored or not known of the studies of the French physiologist Marie Jean Pierre Flourens.

In 1847, Flourens had shown that the inhalation of chloroform induced insensibility in experimental animals, but he had concluded that chloroform was 'wonderful but terrible' and much too dangerous for use in humans. Since then, Snow had taken Flourens' work a stage further by addressing the question of why deaths occurred during the induction of anaesthesia by the inhalation of chloroform but not by the inhalation of ether. These careful and complex studies he reported to meetings of the Westminster Medical Society, and his conclusions were reprinted in the *Edinburgh Medical and Surgical Journal* in March 1849.[25] He confirmed that the actions of ether and chloroform were similar. Both could produce a desirable degree of anaesthesia. At a higher dosage both caused paralysis of the nervous mechanism that drives respiration; if the dosage was increased still further, both could cause paralysis of the action of the heart. But, in practice, there were important differences. His experiments on animals had shown that when air saturated with ether was inhaled at sufficiently high dosage, first respiration would stop and then, after an interval, the heart would stop – not due to the direct action of ether but simply due to the lack of oxygen. As a result, if the administration of ether was immediately withdrawn when breathing stopped, but before the heart stopped, the patient could be easily revived by any of the well known and well practised forms of artificial respiration. However, by Snow's calculations, chloroform was at least three times more powerful than ether. When air saturated with chloroform was inhaled it produced insensibility more quickly than ether and went on to paralyse breathing more quickly. By that time, even if the administration of chloroform was immediately withdrawn on the cessation of breathing, there was already enough of this very powerful gas in the lungs so that, when absorbed, it could directly poison and paralyse the action of the heart even before the heart had begun to suffer from the lack of oxygen. The patient was then effectively dead and could not be revived by artificial respiration or by any other means.

Snow acknowledged that chloroform was an excellent anaesthetic; indeed, it was his own anaesthetic of choice. But he condemned the way in which Simpson recommended that it should be administered. When a measure of liquid chloroform was dropped onto a pocket handkerchief held over the patient's mouth and nostrils, it could never be known how much of the vapour from that measure was inhaled by the patient and how much was dissipated into the surrounding atmosphere. He particularly deplored Simpson's early assertion that anaesthesia was best induced by 'giving a large, full and rapid dose of it at once'. That, he believed, was highly dangerous. His experiments had convinced him that chloroform was safe only if it made up no more than 5 per cent of the mixture with air being breathed by the patient. Chloroform should therefore only be administered by equipment capable of delivering it at a controlled concentration and at a controlled rate.

Simpson did not agree. He had indeed advised that anaesthesia should be induced by administering one initial large powerful dose of anaesthetic gas when the gas was ether. During the period of some minutes required for ether to bring about the loss of consciousness, the patient often became excited and difficult to manage; an initial, large powerful dose of ether had the effect of abolishing or shortening that difficult period. Chloroform induced loss of consciousness quickly without any significant period of excitement; there was therefore no reason to administer a large initial dose. As he had advised in his *Notes*, in midwifery cases it was only necessary to sprinkle a few drops of the liquid chloroform onto a pocket handkerchief and hold it over the nose and mouth for a minute or two; for surgical cases chloroform was best given on a handkerchief folded into a cup form, with the open end placed over the patient's nose and mouth. For the first few seconds, it should be held at a distance of half an inch or so from the face and then gradually more and more closely. Only in very unusual circumstances should a larger quantity of chloroform be poured onto a handkerchief and immediately held close to the face of the patient. Simpson also recognised that the victims of chloroform syncope were not the elderly, the sick and the feeble but the young, active, alert and anxious patients presenting for minor surgery. These were patients who were most likely, either in their eagerness to co-operate or more probably in their anxiety, to take large sudden deep inhalations of chloroform during induction. He had always insisted that, before and during induction, the patient should be kept as quiet and calm as possible. He later made a change in his administration of the anaesthetic; he placed a thin piece of fabric loosely over the patient's nose and mouth, leaving generous space for air, and applied the chloroform, drop by drop, to the fabric. A manufacturer adapted this method by producing a wire frame to hold the fabric over the patient's nose and mouth; the wire frame could be folded and contained in a leather box that could be conveniently carried in the doctor's hat.

Simpson's method had the support of the public and the majority of the medical profession. The public welcomed chloroform anaesthesia as the blessing of the age, and looked to have it quickly and conveniently available whenever and wherever it was needed; they had no wish to see its use restricted by some ill-understood need to have elaborate special equipment. Medical practitioners naturally wished to respond to the expectations of their patients and they found that chloroform could be administered conveniently, cheaply and apparently safely, as Simpson instructed. At Edinburgh, medical students were obliged to attend a lecture on the principles of anaesthesia and, before graduating, to take their turn in administering chloroform to patients at Edinburgh Royal Infirmary according to the strict rules laid down by Professor Simpson.

Elsewhere, the studies published by John Snow caused some to lose faith in Simpson's technique of administration. In hospitals in London, chloroform continued to be used, but it was administered by special equipment in the strictly controlled way advocated by John Snow. The administration of chloroform was left to those with special experience and training; hospitals appointed their own specialist anaesthetist; and the principles and practice of anaesthetics was not taught to medical undergraduates. However, general practitioners everywhere continued to rely on Simpson's methods as most suitable for their purposes. By whichever method it was administered, chloroform, the anaesthetic that Simpson had introduced in 1847, continued to be the anaesthetic of choice for general surgeons in Britain, the British Empire, Europe and the southern United States for over fifty years. But for these fifty years the question of how it should best be administered remained unsettled. So too did the questions of whether and when chloroform should be used to relieve the agony of natural childbirth.

ELEVEN

Fortune, Family and Fame

There is a tide in the affairs of men.
Shakespeare

In 1847, when Simpson began his very public and costly campaign to promote the use of his new anaesthetic, he had only recently freed himself from years of debt. In 1839, his brother Sandy, who had lent him financial support during the lean times of his first years in practice, had lent him a further £500 to help meet the cost of his election as Professor of Midwifery. In 1840, Simpson had repaid his brother in full but immediately borrowed £1,200 (at 4 per cent interest) from his father-in-law, Walter Grindlay. He used that loan to support his family in a life style in keeping with his newly acquired status in Edinburgh society, while he built up the large, fashionable and lucrative private practice that would, in time, earn him financial independence. For three years, his father-in-law had not pressed for the return of any of the capital or even for payment of the interest, but in 1843 the Grindlay shipping business was in financial difficulty.

Walter Grindlay, now aged eighty-five, blamed Sir Robert Peel for his troubles.[1] It was on the advice of a Parliamentary committee of enquiry chaired by Peel that British banks returned to the gold standard in 1823. The gold standard had been abandoned by the government in 1797 as a device to make credit to help meet the vast expense of the war with France; banks were relieved of the obligation to pay gold in return for the notes they had issued. In the twenty-six years that followed, this policy of easy money made it possible for Grindlay to build up a prosperous business. Easy credit allowed him to buy his ships and fit them out on the voyages that made him wealthy. The bonanza of the sugar trade with the West Indies was past its peak, but it was still highly profitable, and the killing of a single bull sperm whale in the South Seas could yield 12 tons (3,024 gallons) of sperm oil worth £80 a ton. Those of Grindlay's ships that were engaged in the sugar trade could normally be expected to return with a substantial profit within a relatively short time, but his ships hunting sperm whales in the South Seas could be at sea for many months before they brought home any return for his investment. While the banks allowed him easy credit he had prospered, but after Britain returned to the gold standard, extended credit became hard to find and his business was no longer so profitable. In April 1843, when one of his ships was long overdue and he had been refused help by his banks, Grindlay appealed to Simpson. Simpson did not reply but left it to his wife to come to some arrangement with her brother Richard, now the managing partner in his father's business. In her letter to Richard, Jessie explained that after paying all the New Year accounts and buying various 'indispensables', there was only enough left in the bank to pay the servants' wages. However, she expected that by the end of the month, the fees received by 'the doctor' would be more than enough to cover her household expenses, in which case she would be able to let Robert have £40 or £50.

The immediate crisis passed, but Simpson decided he should begin to repay to his father-in-law a debt that now amounted to £1,365 15s. The whole sum had been repaid when, in May 1847, the banks once more refused to allow the Grindlays credit. Again the Grindlays saw Sir Robert Peel, now the Prime Minister, as the villain. In spite of increasing poverty in Britain throughout the 1840s the government refused to heed calls to repeal the Corn Laws, which imposed high duties on imported wheat and made bread expensive. However, the great famine that began in Ireland in 1845 forced Peel not only to repeal the Corn Laws but also to allow gold to leave the country, in order to pay for the importation of grain. In 1847 the importation of grain increased sevenfold, and the outflow of gold forced the bank of England to increase its interest rate to 10 per cent. In a letter to his sister Jessie, Richard Grindlay wrote that if she had been reading the money articles in the papers she would know 'of Sir Robert Peel's absurd act obliging the banks to curtail their issue of notes in proportion as the gold leaves the country instead of, as common sense would dictate, increasing the issue of notes to fill the vacuum caused by the abstraction of gold to pay the Yankees for their bread stuff. We are in a queer state. Bank of England notes are not to be had.' The Grindlays were temporarily embarrassed. Two of their ships, the *Champion* and the *Envoy*, were on their way home from the United States with some £6,000 worth of freight, but they had made long passages out and were not expected for two or four weeks. Richard was afraid they would not be in time to meet certain payments that 'must be met to the day'; he therefore asked Jessie to approach Simpson for a loan of £200 or, if possible, £300 until his ships arrived.

After a few days Jessie was able to send the money. Richard's reply to Jessie on 13 May provides the first evidence of Simpson having offended his brother-in-law. Richard wrote: 'I have yours of the 10th only this morning with enclosures. I began to fear my letter had miscarried. Brothers and sisters may take some liberties with each other but I had hardly expected there to be any dubiety about my honesty. I was perhaps too intimate with James at one time but it was before he showed himself in his true colours. I avoid him now as much as I can without positively cutting him. His ways are not my ways. If they were I would be greatly unfit for my present position where I have to act for others to the extent of thousands.' There is no further reference to the quarrel in Simpson's correspondence and the cause is therefore obscure, but it probably relates to Simpson's idiosyncratic and inconstant attitude to money. Although he and Richard continued to do business together they never communicated directly, only through Jessie.

Simpson continued to make further small financial contributions to the Grindlay shipping business when help was required but, after the death of Walter Grindlay in 1851, he made no further loans; instead he bought a third share in a number of the family shipping ventures. Within a few years, in partnership with Elisabeth, his mother-in-law, and Richard, his brother-in law, he had a share in four trading vessels: the *Nepaul*, the *British Queen*, the *Falkland* and the *Kate Kearny*. One unusually profitable ship's voyage brought Simpson £2,900 but, in most years, his share in the Grindlay shipping business brought him an annual income of some £4,000.[2]

Other investments that he made on his own account were not always so successful. He bought the *Araminta* for £4,500 in a very unlikely and very unsuccessful venture to ship guano from the New Hebrides to Ireland. He lost £600 on a scheme to extract oil from Irish peat bogs. And he showed a certain naivety in the arrangement he made to invest in sugar plantations in Tobago. In 1859, he agreed to buy from a Mr O'Neil a half share in two estates, Whin and Auchenskioch, for £2,500 and £3,000. He accepted O'Neil's undertakings first to remain on the island to manage the estates and, second, to return Simpson's money if the estates failed to make a profit. Between 1860 and 1866 Simpson advanced a further £3,400 to meet the cost of laying in new crops. But, after making the deal, O'Neil promptly returned to Britain, leaving the estates in the care of overseers. Most of the sugar cane that they raised over the next seven years was used to produce rum, which they sold locally; only a small proportion of the estates' product was exported for profit in the sugar market in Britain.

When, in July 1867, Simpson sold his interests in Tobago, he recovered only £2,000 of his total investment of £8,900.

Among his profitable personal business ventures was his investment in shale oil production in West Lothian. In 1860 he invested £5,800 as one of the founding partners of the Mid Calder Oil Company, which later grew to become the Oakbank Oil Company, one of the most successful and long surviving shale oil companies in Scotland; he also bought a large block of shares in Young's Paraffin Light and Mineral Oil Company. He invested in gold mining in South Africa with shares in De Beers Mining Company Limited and Gold Fields of South Africa Limited.

Over the years other investment schemes – some apparently sound, some adventurous and some bizarre – were proposed to Simpson and, if the idea behind them intrigued him, he was happy to invest. When they failed he did not grieve over them; he could well afford the loss. Even in the early 1850s, his private practice was already one of the most lucrative in Britain. His pamphlets, and the reviews and discussions of his pamphlets in popular journals and newspapers, had broadcast his fame across Europe as the foremost obstetrician and gynaecologist of his time. Patients were attracted not only by the news of his almost legendary skills, but also by his readiness to break with convention. He insisted that mothers should no longer be made to suffer the worst agonies of childbirth. He made it clear in his writings that he believed the treatment women received should not be dictated by the customs and attitudes of a male-dominated society; women should be encouraged to make decisions on matters that affected their health according to their own convictions and in response to their own needs. In the 1850s this was not a commonly held view, even among women. Few women thought of asserting their equality with men or of challenging the prevailing legal doctrine which held that all of a wife's possessions and earnings were vested in her husband. It was usually only wealthy fathers who could use the costly legal devices necessary to draw up marriage settlements for their daughters that ensured they could hold property and have private incomes which gave them a degree of independence from their husbands. It was over half a century since Mary Wollstonecraft had published *A Vindication of the Rights of Woman*, but feminism as we now understand it had not yet been born. Nevertheless, there were already some numbers of well informed, and often wealthy, women who were attracted by Simpson's advanced views, and they now looked to him not only as an obstetrician and gynaecologist, but also as a general physician. They came to Edinburgh from every part of Europe to see him. It was said that, in the 1850s and

1860s, the docks at Leith were kept busy unloading 'cargoes of ladies from Rotterdam, Le Havre and Copenhagen.'[3] In 1860 the Empress Eugenie came from Paris to consult him, taking up residence in the Douglas Hotel in St Andrew Square. Colonel Ewart marked the occasion by parading the 79th Regiment (Ross-shire Buffs) past her windows, while the regimental band played 'Parlant pour la Syrie'.

It was not only women of advanced views who consulted him. In the 1850s and 1860s Simpson had many stoutly conventional ladies as patients in what was by far the busiest practice in Scotland. An American obstetrician who spent some time as Simpson's guest at 52 Queen Street wrote that the house seemed to him to be a private hospital rather than a home. It had been a large house when Simpson bought it in 1845, but it was enlarged in 1846, and later alterations and extensions doubled its original size. Apart from the accommodation for his family and his two assistants, there were rooms for visiting doctors from England, Ireland, Europe or America who came to discuss his ideas and study his methods, as well as for those patients who travelled long distances to see him, or needed to rest or recover from their operative treatments before returning home. On the first floor there was a consulting room for Simpson and, on the floor below, consulting rooms for his two assistants.

In his first years at Queen Street, Simpson did not keep an appointment system. Patients began to arrive as early as 7 a.m. to make certain of seeing him. At the door they were met by Jarvis, who combined the offices of Simpson's butler and his factotum. Jarvis showed those patients who were distinguished by their rank or position in society to the right and upstairs to wait in the drawing room. He directed the others through the hall to a large room towards the rear of the house, where they waited to be seen by one of Simpson's assistants; patients who could not find a chair sat on the stairs or wherever there was space. To achieve some degree of order, patients were asked to draw a number on arrival, and they were called in to be seen in that order. But every day, often before every patient had been seen, it was necessary for Simpson to leave Queen Street to lecture at the university, or to visit patients in the Royal Maternity Hospital or at their homes. At 5.30 p.m. he returned home to have what he called a 'west country tea' of bread and ham, fish and custard pudding before rushing out to make more calls in the city. Many patients left Queen Street without having been seen, even after hours of waiting. Simpson received many letters of complaint and after a time he adopted a more regular routine, which he followed for the rest of his life.

In the morning, he rose at 6 a.m. – or as early as 2 or 3 a.m. if he was in the mood to write on the project most occupying him at the time. He then prepared his lectures or wrote letters. At precisely 7.30 a.m. the *Scotsman*, the *Courant* and the *Daily Review* were delivered to him in his room; later they were thrown over the banisters as he descended, his arms full of books, for prayers in the dining room at 8.15 a.m. Prayers were attended by the family, the butler, the cook and six maids, and any guests then living in the house. Simpson read the lesson and his children led the singing of the psalm.

At breakfast he was never alone. It was his practice to immediately invite any interesting and distinguished visitor to Edinburgh that he might happen to meet – writer, politician, painter, actress, academic – to join him at 52 Queen Street for breakfast or lunch on any day they might find convenient. In addition to such chance visitors he might also be joined by obstetricians, physicians or surgeons who had come to Edinburgh specifically to meet and talk with him, or by archaeologists and scientists with news of their researches. As they arrived they were usually welcomed by his sister-in-law, Williamina, who seated them as seemed appropriate at his table.

At 9.30 a.m. he left in his brougham, drawn by a dashing pair of greys, to visit patients in their hotels or homes. Always he wore a black coat of the same cut, black trousers, a white choker with a carefully tied neck-cloth and a brightly coloured waistcoat. Outdoors in the winter, he wore a long sealskin overcoat and, winter and summer, he always had a distinctive round black hat with a narrow brim, which he either carried in his hand or wore tilted back on his head. He was accompanied in his carriage, and even into the patient's bedroom, by one of a succession of large, friendly coach dogs. While with his patient, he never allowed himself to appear hurried, and he always took time to talk to and amuse any children who made an appearance during his visit. But between visits his coachman was instructed always to drive as fast as possible, since time was short and not a moment was to be wasted. Simpson liked speed. Whenever possible he enjoyed travelling on the newest and fastest steam trains. The favourite phrase forever on his lips was 'come away, come away' as he urged others to keep up with him.

Between 11 a.m. and noon he lectured to his class at the university. Then lunch at home followed the same pattern as breakfast, taken in the company of people he knew well and people he had never met, and the conversation was never idle or trivial. His first patients arrived at 1.30 p.m.;

as always they were shown either upstairs to the drawing room or to the waiting area on the ground floor. Those in the drawing room might find themselves sharing the room with writers and poets hoping for Simpson's endorsement of their work, artists hoping to draw or paint him or sculptors planning to make his bust in plaster or marble. But whatever the bustle in the drawing room or the inconvenience of their long waits, his patients were always charmed by the attention and care he gave to their complaints and their anxieties. When an assistant called him to the ground floor to see a patient of particular interest or difficulty, that patient experienced the same charm and careful attention. All necessary operations were carried out immediately. No bills were presented, since Simpson expected all fees to be paid when the patients were seen and treated. When the patient was attended to by one of his assistants, the customary guinea usually passed from one palm to the other during the handshake at the end of the consultation. Patients seen by Simpson were left to decide for themselves the size of the fee appropriate to their own assessments of their positions in society, and in keeping with the value they put on the services they had received. For the most part, the fees that Simpson collected at 52 Queen Street varied from £30 to £300; the fee presented by a particularly eminent and wealthy patient could be very much greater but, on the other hand, no payment was ever accepted from a member of a clergyman's family. When the patient had been seen, her treatment completed and her fees paid, Jarvis whistled for a cab from those waiting patiently on the special rank near Simpson's house.

In the late afternoon, when the last patient had left, Simpson set off once again in his brougham to see patients in hospital or at their homes. He was usually able to return home for tea with his family and a hour or so of talking or playing games with his children. He was then off again at 7.30 on his round of visits, returning home often at 11 p.m. or later to have supper of a boiled egg, an hour with his books and then to bed. Simpson seldom dined out, and he did not smoke and drank only water. However, when he entertained at home he did not allow his own abstemious habits to limit the generosity of his hospitality; he dined at 6.30 – on one occasion with as many as twenty-six guests – and he was an excellent host. Conversation at the table was always lively, intelligent and enlightened. Dinner might be followed by coffee and an erudite or amusing lecture given by one of his guests. But Simpson's preferred after-dinner entertainment was the portrayal of great names of history or fiction in colourful and faithfully costumed *tableaux vivants*, the audience further enlivened in some cases by short whiffs of chloroform. But no matter how he had spent his evening Simpson was always easily roused by the night bell at the door of his house summoning him at any hour to a patient in labour in any part of the city.

Oddities continued in the way that Simpson conducted his practice. He kept no diary of his appointments, relying entirely on his memory. Inevitably appointments were forgotten or passed over in favour of more urgent or more interesting cases. This problem was made worse by his frequent absences from Edinburgh and the fits of depression,[4] headaches, body pains and palpitations[5] that confined him to bed for three or four days at times of particular stress. His failures to keep appointments caused disappointment for his patients and inconvenience for his obstetric colleagues who had to be hurriedly called for in his absence. Unfortunately, he rarely felt it necessary to apologise. His friend Argyll Robertson felt compelled to write to him a quite remarkable letter from a physician to such a prominent and successful colleague:

> Reports are everywhere current of your inattention to patients who place themselves under your care; that you neglect one set of patients for the sake of an other; that you make appointments, keep patients in their beds waiting for you day after day; that letters remain unanswered; and that patients are often left in ignorance whether to alter, continue, or give up remedies you have prescribed; and in short it is said by some that a patient cannot with safety intrust [sic] herself to your care from these causes . . . If even a slight foundation be given for a continuance of these reports in the public mind, no talents however great will ultimately bear up against them.
>
> Now such instances of inattention must result from one of two causes; either that you have more practice than any single individual is equal to, or that there is want of due arrangement. If the former, in my opinion you should decline taking charge of a portion of your patients to whom you feel you cannot do justice. If the latter, let your arrangements be changed. Whenever on leaving a patient you fix a day for again visiting her, enter it at the moment in your visit-book. Let it be at all times most correctly kept. If there be any which you find you cannot accomplish let a note be immediately sent to the patients intimating the circumstance and fixing when you will call. If sent for unexpectedly to a case in which you are likely to be detained let a message be sent to those expecting you. I am certain if you were to adopt some such method you would do away with many

of the current reports. If in the same manner you have not time to answer letters of consultation fully at the time they are expected, let a short note be written mentioning the circumstances. Excuse me for stating the absolute necessity of some change being made. Your present mode must be injurious to your patients and will ultimately be much more so to yourself.

Simpson was not offended. He delegated a greater share of his work to his assistants, but made no other noticeable change in the somewhat disordered management of his time.

Also, he never felt it necessary to include an accounting system in the financial management of his practice. The income received from Simpson's practice was only discovered at the end of each day when Jarvis emptied his master's pockets. But that could only be an estimate: Simpson might well have used a folded £10 note to stop a window from rattling in the wind, or he might have paid a street trader with a £5 note and been in too much of a hurry to wait for change. Simpson was not greatly interested in money. One patient persistently offered him £1,000 to visit her, but since he believed her complaint to be imaginary he just as persistently refused. It is probable that Simpson had no more than a vague idea of how much he earned, but an experienced visiting obstetrician who spent some weeks in his company estimated that his annual income from his city practice alone was at least £10,000.

Almost until he died, Simpson continued travelling to manage the births of children in the great houses of Scotland and England. His fees were vast. And, every day, gifts varying from game to elaborate and heavy pieces of fine silver were delivered to his house.

Even before his practice had reached its height, his house in Queen Street was overcrowded each day with people of all ranks of society, and filled with the clatter and bustle of a small hospital. Order was only maintained by the presence and loud, gruff voice of Jarvis, Simpson's general factotum. As a retreat from this constant hurly-burly, Simpson bought a house on the coast at Trinity, near the fishing village of Newhaven. Viewbank[6] was a square stone house facing west over the Firth of Forth. In the garden he planted groups of lilac, laburnum and apple trees, as well as beds of white roses. He improved and extended the lawn until it was possible to play bowls. Occasionally in the evening he brought visitors for a game and to enjoy the peace but, whenever possible, he preferred to come by himself to do some gentle gardening and read in peace. And Viewbank was a convenient base for his occasional archaeological explorations of the island and ruined abbey of Inchcolm.

When at Viewbank on a Sunday, Simpson attended Newhaven Free Church. He became friendly with the minister, Mr Fairbairn, and involved himself in the minister's schemes to improve the living standards of his parishioners and reduce their alarming consumption of alcohol. As a basis for Mr Fairbairn's reforms, Simpson prepared a statistical account of the parish, recording the number of houses, the number of inhabitants in each house, the number of places licensed for the sale of alcohol, and the quantity of alcohol consumed by the inhabitants; he also made a survey of the sanitary conditions in the village. He attended the fishermen's wives and contributed to the building of a new church.

However, Viewbank had been bought primarily for his children. Two of his daughters had already died: his first child, Maggie, had died at the age of four in 1844 of bronchopneumonia following an attack of measles; and Mary, aged two, had died of scarlet fever in the winter of 1847. Two of his later children were semi-invalids. From infancy, James had suffered a progressive skin disease and partial blindness; although Simpson consulted the recognised experts of the time, no diagnosis was ever established. Jessie had reacted badly to vaccination in infancy and was severely afflicted by cow-pox; she seemed to be a happy child but was never completely well, probably the victim of vaccinia encephalitis. For all but the winter months, Simpson kept his wife Jessie and the children – David, Walter, William, Magnus, Eve, James and Jessie – at Viewbank, while he lived, as he said, 'as a bachelor' at 52 Queen Street.

From 1847, the structure of the household gradually changed. Simpson's wife seemed never to recover from the deaths of Maggie and Mary. She gradually withdrew to her room and the consolation of her religious pamphlets and her increasingly frequent inhalations of chloroform. Her central role in Simpson's household came to be occupied by her sister Williamina. And much of her part as a parent to her children was assumed by her husband. Simpson was a fond, careful and attentive father. He had suffered agonies of grief when Maggie and Mary died; he was to suffer again when James died at the age of fifteen and Jessie at seventeen. He was always close to all of his children. When he was at home he found time to spend an hour or more with them every day. When they were apart he wrote to them regularly, usually late at night, and he looked for prompt reports in reply. One September, when the children were on holiday at Port St Mary House, Captain Petrie's home on the Isle of Man, Simpson wrote to his daughter: 'My dearest Eve, of course there is no ink in that barbarous isle or you would have written me long ere this. Try pencil – it will do quite well – and tell me how the first of women is doing.' After a light-hearted report on the activities and accomplishments of the family dogs, his letter ends: 'But my paper is done, and I must stop. Love to Mamma and all. Ask Magnus what murders he has committed with his gun and tell Willie that I was greatly pleased with his letter. Your affectionate papa, JYS.'

Simpson supervised the children's education, taking care to provide what he believed had been wanting in his own. He had been taught Latin and Greek, but he had become convinced that it would have been more to his advantage to have learned modern languages; he sent his sons abroad to acquire a mastery of French and German. Later, Walter was sent to explore the great archaeological sites in Spain and Egypt. David, when he became a medical student, spent a summer visiting museums and sitting in on classes at the leading medical schools in Europe; he wrote to his sister, Eve, of his astonishment that their father was known and honoured everywhere he went. To his children, Simpson was their father who, as they discovered, was also a great man, rather than a great man whom they knew to be their father.

The part that he had played in the introduction and development of anaesthesia brought Simpson many honours. He was elected an Associate of the Academy of Medicine in Paris and a member of prestigious medical societies almost everywhere at home and abroad. He received the Order of St Olaf from the King of Sweden, and was awarded the Monthyon Prize of the French Academy of Science and the degree of DCL by Oxford University. In 1848, he was invited to take the chair of Midwifery at St Bartholomew's Hospital in London. To one of those who had pressed him to accept, he replied that since the Queen came regularly to Scotland there could be no reason for him to move to London; London had nothing to offer him that he did not have in Edinburgh. In Edinburgh he was master of the Royal Maternity Hospital. He had his clinic and busy private practice in Queen Street. He was free to practise as he chose, and to pursue whatever line of research attracted him.

His position in Edinburgh was enhanced in 1850 by his appointment as Physician to Edinburgh Royal Infirmary, by his election as President of the Royal College of Physicians, and later by his election as President of the Medico-Chirurgical Society of Edinburgh. These offices were conferred on him in recognition of his international reputation as medical scientist and practitioner. That Simpson accepted them was not as an indication that he was willing to conform to the ethos and outlook of Edinburgh's medical establishment. His inaugural address to the Medico-Chirurgical Society was a masterly review of the progress of medicine and surgery since the beginning of the century, but he took the opportunity to make clear his position as President of the Society. He promised that while every freedom would be given to professional debate, he would ensure that, 'if possible', nothing would be said that might 'unnecessarily' hurt the feelings of any member, present or absent. Nevertheless, he insisted that the science of medicine could only be promoted 'by the stimulus of mind upon mind, like the friction of iron upon iron'.[7] As a student he had come to believe that he could only succeed in his profession by battling against a complacent and self-serving medical establishment. That his career had, until now, been spectacularly successful did not suggest to Simpson that his battle was over.

TWELVE

Homoeopathy, Mesmerism and Blackmail

*Men often swallow falsities for truths, dubiosities for certainties,
feasibilities for possibilities and things impossible as possibilities
themselves.*

Thomas Browne

In February 1850, Simpson was summoned to London for a meeting with
Prince Albert at Buckingham Palace. As President of the Royal Society of
Arts, the prince was then acting as patron and master planner of a Great
Exhibition of the Works of Industry of all Nations at which, in 1851, the
world was to be shown the best that Britain had contributed towards the
progress of mankind. It had been decided that chloroform must be one of
the exhibits, and the prince looked to Simpson for his thoughts on how it
should be presented. The meeting passed off very well. The prince was 'very
kind and gentlemanly', taking Simpson on a tour of the palace, showing him
his library and introducing him to the Prince of Wales and the younger
children.

Before returning to Edinburgh, Simpson spent some time exploring the
Roman antiquities at the British Museum. But while in London, he suffered
an injured and poisoned finger, and during his long and cold journey north
he began to feel unwell. When he reached home, he already had a large and
painful abscess under his arm. He was now very ill. At first he refused to
have the services of a surgeon, but his assistants and his wife were together
able to persuade him that his life was in danger, and James Syme was sent
for. The abscess was opened and drained and thereafter Simpson made a
slow but, in the end, satisfactory recovery. After a period of convalescence
at home, he travelled abroad to make a leisurely tour of some of the leading
medical schools and medical museums of France, Belgium, Holland and
Germany.

By the summer, he was well enough to return to his busy practice. But his
illness had brought an end to his brief period of harmony with James Miller.
They had both been pupils of Robert Liston in Edinburgh and they had

been good friends until, in 1842, the Chair of Surgery became vacant. James Miller applied for the post and at first Simpson gave him every possible support. But when Simpson discovered that his enemy, James Syme, was also canvassing for Miller, Simpson dramatically changed sides and gave his support to Miller's rival, Robert Lizar. In public, Simpson tried unsuccessfully to explain his sudden loss of confidence in Miller by referring to a case in which one of Miller's surgical patients had died unexpectedly and tragically soon after the operation. Simpson's late and unscrupulous opposition did not affect the outcome of the election. Miller was appointed to the chair, but he felt wounded that Simpson had so casually and unjustly tried to damage his reputation and career.

However, four years later Miller let that pass when he found himself in a position to assist in Simpson's first crucial trials of ether and chloroform. As we have seen (Chapter 10), his ready and unselfish assistance proved to be invaluable. Yet only months later when, as Simpson's next-door neighbour, he was immediately available and more than capable of performing the necessary operation, he had been sidelined. It added to the slight that Simpson had apparently thought it necessary to set aside years of open hostility and call in his long-standing enemy, James Syme.

Simpson was unrepentant, and two years later he again attempted to damage Miller's reputation. Simpson had been called to see Mrs Johnstone, a neighbour living at 34 Queen Street. It was an unusually difficult gynaecological case and his efforts were unsuccessful. He decided that it had become necessary to have the specialist services of an experienced surgeon. Miller was called in and, although the patient's condition had already become critical, he immediately agreed to operate. Unfortunately the patient died. Miller claimed that the death was due to 'peritoneal infection' resulting from Simpson's earlier interventions. Simpson, however, claimed that Miller had cut an artery by mistake and that the patient had died from blood loss. Miller was the first to publish a pamphlet in his defence, but Simpson quickly replied in kind. Both attracted supporters among the medical profession in Edinburgh and thereafter a very public and undignified dispute was conducted in the local press. The affair was also reported in the *Lancet* and other medical journals, and in them the prevailing opinion was that any surgeon suddenly 'put in the position of Miller ought to receive the sympathy and not the reproach of his brother practitioners'. Simpson, never able to accept defeat or contradiction, retrieved Mrs Johnstone's mattress in order to demonstrate that the blood that it had absorbed was compatible with a major haemorrhage. The dispute continued for two months and only came to an end when the leading physicians and surgeons in Edinburgh joined together to draw up a document that, without expressing an opinion as to the relative amount of blame attributable to the two disputants, required both to take the earliest opportunity to express their regret for the damage that their unseemly public wrangle had done to the profession. There was some lingering sympathy for James Miller; for Simpson, however, the incident only added to his growing reputation as someone who attracted twice the practice and conducted three times the productive research of any other medical man in Edinburgh but made ten times the number of enemies within his profession.

When a very young man, without influential friends or political patronage, he had been quick to assume that every member of Edinburgh's medical establishment, both in the university's Medical Faculty and in the College of Physicians, must be his enemy. When a number of these long-established members of the medical profession openly opposed his election to the Chair of Midwifery, they became his enemies for life. When he himself had become established as Professor of Midwifery at Edinburgh and gone on to achieve international fame by his contributions to obstetrics and surgery, he acquired new enemies. These included everyone who attempted to detract from the merit and significance of his achievements. Among them were those who attempted to deny him his prime place in the development of general anaesthesia, and his part in the discovery of chloroform.

First there was Dr Glover, a physician in Newcastle. In a letter to Simpson in November 1847, he wrote that he had just read Simpson's pamphlet on chloroform and could hardly believe his eyes when he found that Simpson had not taken the least notice of his own laborious researches on chloroform. He claimed to have published the results of animal experiments in which he had demonstrated chloroform's power of producing 'narcotism and, in one experiment, even the insensibility of the animal to pain'. Simpson did not conceal his rage. In his long and dismissive reply he wrote: 'I was most ignorant of your ever having written one word on chloroform or aught allied to it. I find, on talking over your letter with some professed therapeutists and chemists here, that they were just as ignorant of your paper as I was. If I had known of your paper, I am not at all sure that I would have quoted it. Altogether you poisoned and half poisoned several animals by injecting chloroform into their blood vessels, stomach and peritoneum. Surely this has nothing to do with the anaesthetic effects of chloroform as inhaled by the lungs.'

Such attempts to deny Simpson his place in the advancement of general anaesthesia continued until the end of his life. In January 1870, in a letter in the *Boston Medical and Surgical Journal*, Dr Henry Bigelow bitterly objected to Simpson being honoured as the inventor of chloroform, 'one of the greatest medical discoveries of modern times'.[1] Simpson wrote to Bigelow giving a full and accurate account of his part in the discovery and introduction of chloroform, but three months later he had cause to write to Bigelow again:

'Towards the beginning of the present year, I sent in reply to your groundless accusation, an answer in the form of a letter to yourself; and subsequently I received from you a written note in which you stated you were not disposed to pursue the subject further. In consequence I dismissed the matter entirely from my mind; and I deeply regret, both for your own sake and for the peace and character of our honourable profession, that you did not adhere to your resolution. For I have just received a slip of printed statement, unaccompanied by one word of writing but drawn up in the form of a letter from you to me, in which you continue the subject in terms more bitter and personal than before. On first perusing it, my impression was that it was too querulous in tone and temper to deserve an answer.' However, he did answer in a long and erudite history of the development of anaesthesia since Greek, Roman and mediaeval times and making clear his part in that history. He received no reply.

Simpson had also offered fierce rebuttals to those who attacked him for his use of chloroform in midwifery. One of the first to do so, in March 1847, was Samuel Ashwell, physician and lecturer in midwifery at Guy's Hospital in London. Simpson replied: 'A few hours ago I received the *Lancet*. Your strange paper in it has done me good. I have seen the time when such a scurrilous attack as yours would have irritated me. Now-a-days such things produce the very reverse so that I fancy I am getting quite hardened. Great abuse and great praise sound to me now very much alike. For I feel the greater good I can ever accomplish for my profession and for humanity, the greater will always be the temporary blame attempted to be heaped upon me by bigoted members of the profession. Of course you are aware that it would be quite *infra dig* in me to reply publicly to such a personal attack as you have chosen to send to the *Lancet*, [but] I will readily convince you how utterly wrong you are in error of all points. In our profession duties of omission and commission amount to the same crime in principle. To prolong your medical prejudices, you argue that you and your brethren are entitled to perpetrate medical cruelties and torture to poor women who commit themselves to your care. To confess to you the truth, my blood feels chilled by the cruel inhumanity and deliberate cruelty which you and some members of the profession openly avow. And I know that you will, in a few years, look back with horror at your present resolution of refusing to relieve your patients merely because you have not yet had time to get rid of some old professional caprices and nonsensical thought to the subject.'

Even towards distinguished members of his profession with whom he had been on friendly terms for some time, Simpson was crushingly forthright if they ventured to disagree with him. Robert Collins, an eminent obstetrician in Dublin and a former Master of the Rotunda, questioned the statistics in one of Simpson's articles in the *Provincial Medical Journal*. Simpson replied: 'I have often stated that your work is a most admirable collection of obstetric cases and data. Your data are, I believe, exceedingly accurate and valuable but your own deductions from these extensive data are equally, in most cases, extremely inaccurate and valueless.'

Simpson was equally belligerent toward his critics in the medical profession in Edinburgh. Nevertheless, on 5 December 1850, he was elected President of the Royal College of Physicians of Edinburgh. Since first being made a Fellow, he had taken little part in the business of the college, been fined many times for his absence from its meetings and made no effort to make himself popular. However, he was now clearly the most distinguished member of the college and it was in recognition of his eminent place in the profession that he was elected. Apart from its routine business, in 1850 the college was engaged in four major issues – medical reform; public health in towns and cities; medical services in the Highlands and Islands; and the place of homoeopathy in medical practice. The college's part in the negotiations on medical reform was being very capably led by Robert Renton; W. P. Alison had been, for some years, the college's chief advocate of public health measures for towns; and the investigation into medical services in the Highlands and Islands was being ably conducted by Charles Darwin's friend, John Coldstream. As President of the Royal College, Simpson gave his formal support but played no more active part in the college's campaigns on these three important issues. But he was more than ready to take the lead in countering the infiltration of homoeopathy into medical practice, not only in Edinburgh but in Britain. It was an issue that had been causing him concern for some years.

In 1842, when John Thomson resigned as Professor of Pathology at Edinburgh, a majority of the members of the university's Faculty of Medicine had moved to have the chair abolished. However, Simpson had persuaded the patrons of the university to retain the chair, and later he had been successful in securing the appointment for William Henderson. For almost ten years, Henderson had been a very successful extramural lecturer on the Practice of Physic; he had published several important works on the diseases of the heart and had become recognised as an expert in histopathology. But to Simpson's intense embarrassment, soon after his appointment to the Medical Faculty of Edinburgh University as Professor of Pathology, he revealed himself as a convert to homoeopathy. He joined the staff of the Homoeopathic Dispensary that had been established in Stockbridge in Edinburgh in 1841; in 1845, he published his *Enquiry into the Homoeopathic Practice of Medicine*; and since then he had been attempting to introduce homoeopathic treatments in his ward at Edinburgh Royal Infirmary. Simpson, feeling directly responsible for his appointment, was now determined that Henderson should be deprived of his chair and prevented from teaching and practising at Edinburgh Royal Infirmary. But not only Henderson; he was determined that homoeopathy should be completely disassociated from established medical practice throughout Britain.

The founder of homoeopathy, Samuel Hahnemann, was born in 1755. He studied medicine at Leipzig and Vienna, but when he took his degree he was already disillusioned. The medicine that he had been taught at these long-established and greatly respected medical schools had offered him no single universal principle according to which all cases of all diseases could be treated. Without such a single guiding principle he had felt unable to practise, and he had made his living as a translator of texts. But he had continued to theorise and he eventually formulated a principle based on two counter-intuitive ideas. The first was that a disease should be treated by administering a substance that, if administered to a healthy person, would produce the same symptoms as the disease; the second, that the effectiveness of such a substance would be increased not by increasing the dose, but by diminishing it. Armed with this principle he took up medical practice. His ideas attracted some support among the many, both doctors and patients, who were dissatisfied with the widespread practice of polypharmacy: when one elaborate and possibly expensive medicament failed it was usual for another to be added and, when that too failed, yet another was added, followed possibly by a fourth. In Edinburgh, the former President of the Royal College of Physicians, W. P. Alison, was well known as a very liberal polypharmacist; Professor Syme, on the other hand, had little faith in any of the commonly used medicaments and prescribed only preparations of rhubarb for his patients. It was generally recognised that there existed very wide differences and very great problems in the drug treatment of disease, but Simpson insisted that, as an answer, Hahnemann's homoeopathy was 'absurd and negative'. After Hahnemann's death it had become even more absurd. By the 1840s, it had become accepted by even the most committed homoeopathic practitioners that Hahnemann's principles should not be strictly observed in cases 'when life seems almost extinguished', 'in cases of poisoning', 'in all cases of external injury', 'in severe and prolonged consti- pation' and 'in cases of syphilis'.[2] In such cases effective conventional treat- ment must be used. Homoeopathy had become not a science but a faith. In the United States candidates for admission as members of one homoeo- pathic institute were required to swear: 'By our Saviour Jesus Christ, who suffered and died for us, redeeming our sins by his precious blood . . . not to treat patients but by medicaments whose effects have been well proved, which are in the domain of pure homoeopathy as I have acknowledged and declared in my profession of faith.' The candidate had also to swear 'to propagate the knowledge of the principles of Pure Homoeopathy by all lawful means in [his] power'.[3] Simpson was particularly incensed that homoeopathists should seek to enjoy the status and privileges conferred by Fellowship of the Royal College of Physicians of Edinburgh (or member- ship of any other established medical corporation in Britain) yet be intent on undermining the principles on which that status and those privileges were based.

Simpson proposed that homoeopathists should follow the example of the many clergymen in Scotland who, in 1843, had 'as an act of common honesty, withdrawn themselves from those corporations and communions whose principles they could no longer hold'. They had voluntarily left the Established Church to form their own Free Church. The homoeopathist should do likewise and voluntarily leave the established medical institu- tions and create institutions of their own.

On 2 May 1851, only a few months after Simpson became its presi- dent, a meeting of the Royal College of Physicians of Edinburgh formally agreed four resolutions. In summary, these were: a) that the college should continue to decline to admit homoeopathic practitioners as Fellows; b) that Fellows who endangered the reputation of the college by becoming homoeopathic practitioners should withdraw and sever their connection with the college; c) that no Fellow of the college should meet practitioners of homoeopathy in consultation or co-operation; d) that although the college had not thought it expedient to take active steps for disclaiming those Fellows who had become homoeopathic practitioners or co-operated with homoeopathic practitioners, it had the power to do so and would use that power summarily should it prove necessary.

The full text of these resolutions was sent to the Royal College of Surgeons of Edinburgh, the Royal Faculty of Physicians and Surgeons of Glasgow and the Provincial Medical and Surgical Association (the British Medical Association from 1854), and all three bodies adopted them in formulating their own policies on homoeopathy. Simpson's resolutions were particularly effective in curbing the practice of homoeopathy in Edinburgh, since only Fellows of the colleges of Physicians or Surgeons were eligible to practise and teach medical students at Edinburgh Royal Infirmary. Deprived of his Fellowship of the Royal College of Physicians, Henderson was obliged to resign from his position as a clinical teacher. Since, as Professor of Pathology, he was not required to teach therapeutics, he was allowed to continue to lecture to medical students at the university until he retired in 1859. Even so, Simpson continued to fulminate against him. He had made another enemy.

Although Simpson could not have been more forthright in his rejection of homoeopathy or more active in persuading others to follow his lead, only four months after his resolutions had been made public, he was accused, in a letter published in the *Lancet*,[4] of 'fostering the dangerous error' of homoeopathy. Even by the standards of the time it was a letter of unusual virulence. The author, 'Isaac Irons', declared it was regrettable that the patrons of Edinburgh University had tolerated for so long the 'leprosy' that had 'infected' Professor Simpson, and extraordinary that they had not dismissed him from the chair that he was 'polluting'. 'Isaac Irons' also claimed that Simpson was not only meeting in consultation with homoeopathists, but was also 'throwing his house open to mesmeric *soirees*'; thus, in private, countenancing the quackery that he denounced in public. But for the 'inconsistent conduct' of Simpson as President of the Royal College of Physicians, it was 'impossible to believe that the rampant quackery in the university and among the population of Edinburgh could ever have reached the present disgraceful position'. The letter went on:

'But it is not the homoeopathy and mesmerism only which Dr. Simpson has fostered, it is to him that we chiefly owe that infinitely more dangerous and disgusting quackery in midwifery which rages like pestilence in London and in every town and village throughout the Empire and in some of our most distant colonies. To Dr Simpson we owe the invention of the dangerous weapon called the uterine sound or poker; pessaries which have justly been designated as infernal and impaling uterine machines to cure retroversions which never existed; instruments for pumping the uterus to excite menstruation. To him we owe the hysterotome for slitting open the os uterus to cure sterility; and to Dr. Simpson we owe the attempt to revive the brutal practice of turning in cases of distortion of the pelvis; of attempting to substitute the Caesarean operation for the induction of premature labour. To him we owe the attempt to subvert the established practice in placental presentation by extraordinary statistical tables. And lastly we owe to the genius of the Professor of Midwifery in the University of Edinburgh the baby sucker.'

The letter was wildly malevolent. As President of Royal College of Physicians, Simpson had made it clear that he regarded the theory of homoeopathy as irrational and its practice reprehensible. He had not 'fostered homoeopathy': he had taken strong action to suppress it. Nor had he 'fostered mesmerism'.

The craze of mesmerism (or animal magnetism) had its origins in the concepts of Franz Anton Mesmer, an Austrian physician practising in the 1790s. It had later been taken up in Paris and was introduced to Britain by Professor John Elliotson of London University in 1837. At a series of meetings at University College Hospital, Elliotson demonstrated his ability to influence his subject's nervous system by making certain hand movements and causing the warmth of his body to penetrate the subject's body in the form of a ubiquitous but invisible magnetic fluid.[5] Elliotson's demonstrations were later exposed as fraudulent and he was forced to resign from his chair. Nevertheless, a few unorthodox surgeons found that, in some cases, mesmerism (alternatively 'animal magnetism' or 'hypnotism') seemed to be capable of inducing a degree of anaesthesia sufficient for minor operations.

Mesmerism had not been taken up by the medical profession in Edinburgh. It was true, however, that William Gregory, the Professor of Chemistry at Edinburgh University, was an enthusiast for both phrenology and mesmerism. But Gregory took no part in the teaching of therapeutics or in the practice of medicine. There could therefore be no reason for Simpson, as President of the Royal College of Physicians, to act against Gregory as he had acted against Henderson. In any case, Simpson regarded mesmerism as harmless. In the same issue of the *Lancet* that carried the 'Isaac Irons' letter, Simpson had written: 'I do not believe and never did believe in animal magnetism. During the last ten or fifteen years I have seen experiments made in the subject and have repeatedly made them myself.

In the course of them I have witnessed very interesting physiological and psychological results, such as the production of sleep and perversions of sense but I have no belief whatever that these effects are the effects of any power, force, agency or entity, such as is understood by the term animal magnetism, passing from the so called mesmeriser to the so called mesmerised. On the contrary, these experiments have convinced me that these and other phenomena of the like kind are merely effects produced by the mind of the mesmerised upon his or her own economy; they are only self-mental acts as independent of any mesmeric influence as the phenomena of common sleep or common dreaming.'[67]

In his letter, 'Isaac Irons' had condemned almost every one of Simpson's innovations in obstetrics and gynaecology as quackery. But they had all been openly presented at meetings of the Edinburgh Obstetrics Society, and all had later been described in full in the medical press. Nothing had been kept secret and none of his innovations had been exploited for personal gain. All but one had found a respected place in obstetric or gynaecological practice. The exception was his 'baby sucker'. This had been introduced by Simpson as a possible 'substitute for the forceps in tedious labours'. Whereas forceps grasped the sides of the head as the infant was pulled forth, in Simpson's invention the head was held by a rubber cup attached by suction to the infant's scalp, while the infant was extracted by at least as much pulling power as could be safely achieved by forceps. After trying several changes in the designs of the suction caps and the pumps needed to create suction by extracting the air from the cap, Simpson had presented his 'Air Tractor' to a meeting of the Edinburgh Obstetric Society in December 1848. This early version, scorned by 'Isaac Irons' as a quackery, did prove to be unsatisfactory in practice but, when synthetic materials more suitable for the purpose became available a century later, the concept was shown to be sound by the production of the very successful Ventouse Vacuum Extractor.

The 'Isaac Irons' letter was both offensive and libellous, and several of Simpson's colleagues urged him to take both the author and the editor of the *Lancet* to court. Others argued that the letter was so obviously outrageous that it could not possibly do damage to Simpson's reputation. However, Simpson had recognised at once that the author of such an offensive letter could only be his former opponent and more recent antagonist, the lecturer on midwifery at St George's Hospital in London, Robert Lee.

Robert Lee, born in Melrose in 1793, had studied medicine at Edinburgh and taken his MD degree in 1814. He then served as assistant to

James Hamilton, the Professor of Midwifery and Diseases of Women and Children at Edinburgh, for three years until he moved to London to take charge of the epileptic son of the Honourable William Lamb (afterwards the Prime Minister, Lord Melbourne). He later studied in Paris for a year, but then suffered a long and serious illness. On his recovery, in 1824, he was offered the appointment as physician to the governor-general of the Crimea. After his return to London, in 1827 he was appointed physician to the British Lying-in Hospital and began to lecture on midwifery at the Webb Street School of Anatomy and Medicine. He published numerous papers on obstetric pathology and in 1830 was elected Fellow of the Royal Society. Five years later he was given the prestigious appointment as lecturer on midwifery at St George's Hospital. When James Hamilton died in 1839, Lee applied to succeed him as Professor of Midwifery and the Diseases of Women and Children at Edinburgh.

He was a formidable candidate. He had been Hamilton's assistant; he had more than twenty years of clinical experience of midwifery and the diseases of children; he had been teaching midwifery for a decade; he had written many scientific papers; he was a Fellow of the Royal Society. Yet the appointment was given to Simpson, who was only twenty-eight years old; a doctor of medicine for only seven years and with only three years' clinical experience of midwifery; the author of only four scientific papers; and almost unknown outside Edinburgh. Lee was deeply humiliated. His resentment was still evident more than five years later.

In March 1845, Simpson published a 'Memoir on the Spontaneous Expulsion and Artificial Expulsion of the Placenta before the Child in Placental Presentation'.[8] He quoted the leading authorities of the time, who were agreed that of all the accidents of childbirth the one most dreaded was when the afterbirth was implanted over the opening of the mouth of the uterus so that in labour it presented before the child, causing dangerous haemorrhage. By listing the published results of fifteen respected obstetricians he was able to show that, in these cases, one in three of the mothers and two in three of the children died. Simpson claimed that mortality could be reduced if, when all conventional procedures had failed, the obstetrician turned the child so that he could grasp its feet and forcibly deliver it past the afterbirth. In his experience Simpson had found that, when the child had been pulled to safety, the collapse and contraction of the uterus quickly stopped the haemorrhage. In an article in the *Medical Gazette*,[9] Robert Lee claimed that by advocating such a manoeuvre Simpson was 'departing from the rule that has been established in the treatment of cases of placental presentations for the last two hundred years and the established rules of practice in the treatment of cases of such vital importance'. Without mentioning Lee by name, Simpson wrote to the *Lancet*[10] to make it clear that he was not suggesting that his manoeuvre should replace conventional treatment, but that it should be used when conventional treatment had failed. Lee now changed tack; in a piece in the *Lancet*, mysteriously signed A.B.,[11] he claimed that there were contradictions in Simpson's statistics and demanded that he should 'inform readers which table is correct and what he thinks the value of the two tables to be when put together'. Simpson replied by publishing his 'Notes on the Statistics of Placenta Praevia: Exposition of the Errors of Statement of Dr. Lee.'[12] This long, fully documented and carefully argued article in the *Lancet* began: 'It is well known that when the cuttlefish wishes to escape and hide itself, it empties its ink bag so as to darken the surrounding water and cover its retreat. In his last paper Dr Lee has scattered his ink upon the pages of the *Lancet* with apparently the same object.' Simpson then went on to reveal in detail fifteen 'errors of statement' in Dr Lee's various publications on placenta praevia since 1845. Lee had no answer, and made no further attacks on Simpson until he sent his 'Isaac Irons' letter to the *Lancet*.

Simpson responded to that letter in typically robust style. In a letter to the same journal he began: 'For some time I was at a loss to determine whether it was not my duty to repel, by very different measures from the present, the attack in the *Lancet* published under the assumed name of 'Isaac Irons'. Among the circumstances which have principally decided me to follow the present simpler method is the unanimous conviction which all my medical friends who have either written or spoken to me on the subject have expressed on one point *viz* that there is in the medical profession only one individual who does use, on professional subjects, language so indiscreet as that of the well known writer in question; and that, after all, this individual was scarcely legally responsible for his own outbreaks of violence ... On this as on other occasions 'Irons' strangely seems to suppose that the medical profession are weak-minded enough to mistake mere personal abuse and scurrility for argument while he evidently forgets it is, to the contrary, generally acknowledged that such weapons are seldom or never used, except in cases where all proper and legitimate arguments are actually wanting.' Simpson then went on to counter, point by point, the attack made on him by Lee in his 'Isaac Irons' letter. Lee (still as 'Isaac Irons') renewed his attack in the next edition of the *Lancet*, but Simpson decided he could now be ignored.

Simpson had been badly ruffled by these public exchanges in the medical press. He felt it necessary to respond to the explanation that had been offered by the editor of the *Lancet* for his decision to publish the scurrilous 'Isaac Irons' letter. The editor had written: 'Dr Simpson will not fail to recollect that his name is systematically published as that of one of the Editors of the *Edinburgh Monthly Journal of Medical Science,* a work that habitually contains very gross imputations on the reputation of and conduct of the hospital physicians and surgeons of this metropolis. In consequence of not having repelled such attacks we have been accused of exercising undue forbearance and even of showing culpable partiality towards Dr. Simpson and his colleagues of the northern journal.' For Simpson this attempt at justification was almost as insulting as the letter itself. He reminded the editor that, in the past, the *Lancet* had published 'various anonymous letters from "Irons" and others containing attacks and misrepresentations regarding myself and my practice nearly as unprincipled and as violent as that which has just appeared'. On the other hand, 'since becoming one of the proprietors and editors of the *Monthly Journal,* I can honestly declare that I have never written one single word of blame or imputation against any London medical man. You must excuse me, however, for adding, that after what has happened, I do not pledge myself to be equally lenient for the future.'

In spite of his differences with the editor, Simpson was confident that, by his correspondence in the columns of the *Lancet*, he had cleared himself of Lee's accusations of quackery and sympathy with homoeopathy in the eyes of the medical profession. But, as always, Simpson thought it even more important that he should make his condemnation of quackery and his total rejection of homoeopathy clear to the general public. In 1852, he published a carefully argued but damning book (21 chapters and almost 300 pages) entitled *Homoeopathy: Its Tenets and Tendencies, Theoretical, Theological and Therapeutical.*[13] It was very well received by the public; a second edition was published in 1852 and a third in 1853.

When he felt himself attacked on professional issues, Simpson's response was always immediate and aggressive. But he was much less decisive when confronted with issues that concerned his private life. In 1854, he allowed himself to become involved in a matter that later led to his becoming a target of blackmail.

From time to time, with the assistance of his wife, Simpson organised the early care of illegitimate children born to patients in his private practice. He found suitable foster parents for the child and arranged for them to receive regular payments from the father, or other supportive relative, to meet the cost of the child's continuing care. It was Jessie's task to keep in touch with the fostering family, to ensure that the payments for the child's care were being received and, when appropriate, to convey news of the child's progress to the mother. In most cases the arrangement worked well, but there were occasional difficulties. For example, one father, William Cowan, who lived in Ireland, wrote to Simpson promising to hold himself 'responsible for all the costs and charges of whatever kind that may be incurred in the caring of the child called Mary White now nursing with Mrs Alexander', one of Simpson's most reliable foster mothers. Cowan paid £15 in advance for one year's nursing care, but thereafter he made frequent specious excuses for his repeated delays and failures in making subsequent payments.

Simpson was almost always able to overcome such difficulties. However, in June 1852, he became involved in a case that was to cause him great embarrassment. A Miss Nicol, suffering from what she believed to be a rapidly growing abdominal tumour, had travelled some distance to Edinburgh to consult James Syme. Syme found her to be in an advanced stage of pregnancy and called on Simpson to take charge of her case. Simpson duly managed her delivery and arranged for the child to be cared for by Mr James and Mrs Mary Quinton. The Quintons had no children of their own and were eager to adopt the infant on condition that the natural parents would not, at any later time, seek to reclaim him. This was agreed. Mrs Quinton was paid £7.50 for the first six months' care, a nursemaid was engaged and the child was christened Rochester Quinton. Six weeks later Jessie was able to write to Miss Nicol, informing her that the child was progressing very well and was already 'a little idol' to his new parents.

After a satisfactory trial period of six months, the payments to Mrs Quinton were increased to £50 a year and James Quinton, an Oxford graduate, was employed as Simpson's secretary on an annual salary of £90. The Quintons were still living in lodgings in Edinburgh when in July 1854, a lady whom Mary Quinton had long thought of as a close friend made what seemed to be a generous offer. The lady knew that Mary Quinton had hoped, at some time, to increase the family income by taking in students as boarders. To make that possible, her friend proposed that the Quintons should take over the lease of her house in Castle Street. She also offered to leave behind in the house all her furniture, to be paid for later when the Quintons had gathered together the necessary funds. The Quintons were delighted to accept the offer, but soon after taking possession of the house they discovered that the rent was already many weeks in arrears and that the furniture left so generously for their use had never been paid for. When the creditors pressed for payment, John Quinton began to misappropriate money that he had been given by Jessie Simpson to settle her household bills. This was only discovered when warrants were issued summoning Quinton to appear at the debtors' court and the full extent of his difficulties could no longer be hidden. When Simpson was informed he immediately dismissed John Quinton from his position as his secretary and began legal proceedings to have him prosecuted for theft.

Three times Mary Quinton wrote to Simpson asking for an interview. Three times he made no reply. Then very late one evening, she called on the Rev. Thomas Guthrie, the leading figure in the Free Church in Scotland, the church to which both she and Simpson belonged. Guthrie found her in the deepest agony, plunged, as he said, into such grief that he had difficulty in informing any right notion of her sad story. She showed Guthrie a letter that she had written but had not yet sent to Simpson. In it she appealed to Simpson, as a fellow member of the same Christian church and as one with whom she had shared the same sacramental table, for his forgiveness. She reminded him that for two and three quarter years her husband had been his willing and laborious servant; night after night he had worked with him well after midnight and had often been with him before daybreak. Her husband's debts amounted to only a little over £200. 'Could he only remain in your service a few months longer instead of being cast away hopeless and uncared for, he would retrieve his position and I would have no fear of the future. Otherwise I can only view him as a lost man.' Mary Quinton asked Guthrie for his help by passing this, her fourth, letter to Simpson. This he did, calling next morning at 52 Queen Street to deliver the letter and a note in which he very gently suggested a degree of compassion, since 'the temptation into which John Quinton has fallen mingles a large share of pity with blame'. Simpson dropped his legal proceedings against John Quinton but did not re-employ him. Now deprived of both John's salary of £90 and the £50 that Mary had continued to receive every year for the care of the child even after the child had been adopted, the Quintons took refuge with Mary's sister in Notting Hill in London.

Simpson heard nothing more from them until January 1865, when the young Rochester ('Bobby') Quinton was given the opportunity to become an apprentice with an architect in London. Since the Quintons could not afford the necessary fees, Mary's sister wrote appealing to Simpson for the required £52. Simpson did not answer and the fees were paid by Mary's sister. But when Simpson was honoured by being created a baronet, Mary

Quinton resorted to blackmail. She wrote to Simpson demanding that he should arrange for Bobby's natural parents to set up a trust to provide for his education and maintenance; alternatively he should provide the necessary funds himself. She threatened that if he did not comply she would 'consult three or four clergymen'. When, yet again, Simpson did not answer, she wrote to a number of clergymen and other prominent citizens in Edinburgh claiming that Simpson was Bobby's father and that he should be made to reveal the name of the mother. And once again Thomas Guthrie was persuaded to act as her go-between with Simpson.

The accusation that he was the child's father at last stung Simpson into vigorous action. He wrote to Guthrie and sent copies of his letter to Edinburgh's two daily newspapers.

Dear Sir,

Some time ago you asked the name of the parents of the child whom Mrs Quinton took home some years ago under the sole condition that he should not be taken back from her by the parents and that he should be entirely surrendered over to her. It is unnecessary, I believe, to state to you that I would transgress most grossly the principle of professional honour if I complied with such a request. The secret could do no good to Mrs Quinton since the mother is in poverty and dependence. She may find the parentage of the child from other quarters, if she thinks fit, but she cannot possibly hope to extract the information from me.

But as you have written on the matter I venture to trouble you with it in another light. Mrs Quinton has written to Professor Syme on the matter. Mr Syme and I are not friends nor even on speaking terms but he has informed Mrs Quinton that he called me to see the mother a few days before the baby was born, she having come a long distance to be under the professional care of Mr Syme for a supposed tumour. After the child was born I had to make arrangements for it being given out to nurse and was thus led into some considerable expense on the matter.

I have heard from a number of quarters that Mrs Quinton has behaved in the matter in a way which either you must get her to rectify thoroughly at once or I shall deem it my duty to hand the subject to my lawyers. Mrs Quinton has stated that I am the father of the child. I demand that she forthwith contradict this indelicate suggestion. She well knows who the father is. Out of compassion

I refrained from allowing a most painful prosecution being instituted against a person in whom she was deeply interested. She is a villainous wicked woman. I expect her to furnish an apology to me.

Yours sincerely,

J. Y. Simpson

The threat of legal proceedings put an end to Mary Quinton's attempt at blackmail and Simpson suffered no further public accusations of having fathered an illegitimate child. But this hint of scandal was cherished by his enemies and rumours persisted. It seems possible that, had Simpson dealt with Mary Quinton's first challenge in 1854 in the same robust way in which he dealt with challenges offered by his professional colleagues, this quite unfortunate attack on his character might have been prevented. The allegations that had been made lingered in the minds of his enemies and were later revived and used against him.[14]

THIRTEEN

Influence and Power

Men in great place are thrice servants, servants of the state,
servants of fame and servants of business.

Bacon

During the first ten years of her marriage, Queen Victoria had seven children, and each one of her deliveries left her feeling 'so battered'.[1] When, in
1850, Simpson was invited to Buckingham Palace to discuss the medical
exhibits to be included in the coming Great Exhibition, Prince Albert
discussed with him the effects and potential benefits of inhaling chloroform during childbirth. Following that conversation, it was decided that
the Queen should have chloroform administered to relieve the pain of
any future deliveries. Three years later, on 7 April 1853, during the delivery
of her eighth child, the Queen found her first experience of 'that blessed
chloroform soothing and delightful beyond measure'.[2] A few days later, Sir
James Clerk, the Queen's physician, reported to Simpson that 'Her Majesty
was greatly pleased and has never had a better recovery. I know this information will please you, and I have no doubt that it will lead to a more
general use of chloroform in midwifery practice in this quarter [London]
than has hitherto prevailed.'

From the beginning, Simpson had been aware that many obstetricians, especially in London, had been opposed to the use of chloroform
during childbirth. The *Lancet*, the most widely read medical journal in
Britain, had trumpeted that 'in no case could it be justified to administer
chloroform in perfectly normal labour'. But Simpson had always been
confident that the resistance of the medical profession would, in time,
be overcome by the demands of their patients. Any fears caused in the
patients' minds by occasional reports of mysterious deaths during the
administration of chloroform were overcome by their anxiety to be free
of the agonies that so often had to be endured while giving birth. Now
in 1853, that most iconic of patients, the Queen, had insisted on taking
advantage of the relief offered by chloroform and, as Sir James Clerk had

predicted, the opposition to Simpson and his pain-free childbirth was silenced.

Honours followed. Simpson was awarded honorary membership of the most distinguished medical societies in Europe and America. He was elected a Foreign Associate of the Imperial Academy of Medicine in Paris. He received the Monthyon Prize of a gold medal and 2,000 francs by the French Academy of Sciences. These honours and the great achievements that they celebrated increased Simpson's status in the eyes of many distinguished men, several of whom had influence in the corridors of power. The most powerful of Simpson's friends was Prince Albert's close associate, the Duke of Argyll. Since the abolition of the office of Secretary of State for Scotland in 1746, the distribution of government patronage in Scotland had been left in the hands of a succession of unofficial 'managers'; in the 1850s and 1860s the manager was the Duke of Argyll. Simpson had first met the duke in 1844[3] when he had been called upon to treat his wife, and since then they had been on very friendly terms. Simpson had often been a guest at Inveraray Castle, and his wife Jessie and their children had spent several happy summer weeks at Torriesdale, another of the duke's castles at Carradale in Argyll.

Simpson enjoyed his new access to power and influence. He was delighted to demonstrate that he was in a position to come to the aid of even his long-standing enemy and former rival, James Syme. In 1849, Syme published a monograph, *On Stricture of the Urethra and Fistula in Perineo*. In it he described a new operation for what was a notoriously difficult condition to correct. Although he had performed the operation on only eleven patients and had followed them up for only a very few weeks, he claimed that his operation produced very much better results than had ever been achieved by conventional procedures. Since stricture of the urethra was a chronic condition which very often recurred after treatment, there were many surgeons who thought that his very few and very early results could not justify his claims. The controversy grumbled on until 1851 when John Lizars, one of Syme's less successful rivals in Edinburgh, published a pamphlet on the subject in which he suggested that Syme had not reported the serious complications suffered by his patients; that he had not revealed the true number of cases in which his new operation had failed completely; and that he had not published the overall mortality among the patients he had tried to treat. Syme wrote to the *Medical Times* to deny Lizars' accusation, but the editor considered his letter so vitriolic as to be actionable and refused to publish it. Syme then sent a letter to the *Monthly Journal of Medical Science* in which he stated that in making his accusations Lizars had gone 'beyond the pale of professional respect and courtesy'. Lizars brought a case of libel against Syme.

When the case came to court in July 1852, Simpson testified in Syme's favour. The jury agreed that Syme's comments had been justified and found against Lizars. However, there were many among the medical profession who had a much clearer understanding of the issues involved and were convinced that there had been a miscarriage of justice. The *Medical Times* continued to take Lizars' part and complained of 'Syme's overwhelming conceit'. At the next meeting of the Provincial Medical and Surgical Association, at Oxford in 1853, the Official Orator, Mr Hester, made disparaging comments about the unseemly dispute between two of Edinburgh's leading surgeons that had by then continued for over three years. He was particularly scathing about the part played by James Syme, and his remarks were published in full in the *Transactions* of the association. Syme protested and, when he received no immediate apology, he felt obliged to resign from the Association. Simpson now came to his rescue. Simpson addressed no fewer than five long and carefully argued letters to the President of the Association, Sir Charles Hastings. In the final and most threatening, he wrote: 'I cannot see how, by any possibility, the Council of the Association could with regard to justice and the dignity of the Association defend, as they appear to do in the last number of their journal, the professional abuse uttered by Mr Hester and so far homologate it as deliberately to refuse Mr Syme any expression of regret that such a very offensive and untrue statement should have been allowed to be published in the official organ of the Association. I state my sincere conviction that Mr Hester's abuse of Mr Syme is most unfounded and untrue; that the publication of it in your *Transactions* is, to say the very least, unfortunate; that its defence and homologation by the Council will prove most untenable. Therefore, before any ulterior steps are taken let me beg, through you, to appeal earnestly once more to the gentlemanly feeling of the members of your Council for the quiet and proper settlement of the matter.' The President and council of the Provincial Medical and Surgical Association capitulated, and the matter was settled to the complete satisfaction of Simpson and, perhaps to a lesser degree, of Syme.

In his first years in Edinburgh, Simpson had felt alienated and threatened by Old Corruption, the network of power and influence that could make, or more probably break, his career. Now some twenty years later he had the power and influence to make or break the careers of others.

The nature and extent of his powers soon became evident. In the autumn of 1853, Robert Jameson announced his retirement from the Regius Chair of Natural History at Edinburgh. A number of distinguished naturalists wrote to Simpson informing him of their intention to apply for the post and asking for his support. The most eminent of these was Edward Forbes, FRS, a former Professor of Botany at King's College, London and President of the Geological Society of London. Already on friendly terms with Simpson, he wrote:

> My Dear Simpson,
> Since I found on enquiry at the Home Office that Professor Jameson's proposed retirement is likely to prove a *bona fide* proceeding, I am taking prompt measures towards endeavouring to become his successor. After much consideration I am determined to renounce London for Edinburgh, provided I can obtain Professor Jameson's post in its entirety.
>
> An office of such importance will doubtless attract many candidates and be much intrigued for, hence I require all possible support. You are, I believe, intimate with the Duke of Argyll, to whom I have written on the matter and who will doubtless be consulted. If you would in any way back my cause with him, and more especially give him to understand that my presence in the University would be acceptable to the Professors, you would do me much service.

As it was a regius chair, the appointment of a successor to Professor Jameson was not the responsibility of the university's patrons, the Town Council. As a Crown appointment it was in the hands of Scotland's 'manager', the Duke of Argyll, who appointed Edward Forbes. However, within a year, Forbes died. Argyll, himself an eminent scientist and a Fellow of the Royal Society, at once wrote to consult Simpson on the choice of a successor: 'I heard of Edward Forbes's death with dismay. It is an irreparable loss to science. I think there can be no doubt that if we could secure adequate emoluments for both branches of a divided chair [Zoology and Geology] the division would insure the best and most adequate teaching. Agassiz[4] is a great name. But I doubt whether, with all his fame, he was equal to Forbes; nor do I think he is a great palaeontologist, except in the *fish* department. But of this I am not sure.'

It proved impossible to create separate chairs of Zoology and Geology as Argyll had hoped. After some further consultation and careful consideration, George Allman, Professor of Botany at Trinity College Dublin and a president of the Linnaean Society, was made Regius Professor of Natural History at Edinburgh.

In the years that followed, Simpson's support proved invaluable to candidates for appointments not only in Edinburgh but throughout Britain and elsewhere. However, his influence was, for once, frustrated in 1855 when W. P. Alison resigned from the chair of the Practice of Physic. This had long been regarded as the senior and most prestigious of the medical chairs at Edinburgh, and it had become almost customary for it to be filled by the promotion of the holder of one of the more 'junior' chairs, usually the Professor of the Institutes of Medicine. However, as it was not a regius chair, the successor to Alison could only be decided by the votes of the patrons of the university, the thirty-three members of Edinburgh's Town Council.

As Alison had been unwell for over two years, his resignation had long been expected and, in that time, a number of physicians had let it be known that they had ambitions to succeed him. Of these, the most likely candidates were thought to be John Hughes Bennett, the Professor of the Institutes of Medicine; Andrew Douglas, a physician at Edinburgh Royal Infirmary and a popular clinical teacher; William Gairdner, a successful lecturer on the Practice of Physic at Edinburgh's extramural medical school; and Andrew Wood, a lecturer on the Practice of Physic and greatly respected Secretary of the Royal College of Physicians of Edinburgh. In a letter to a friend explaining his reasons for intervening in the election, Simpson wrote that privately he 'wished particularly Dr Bennett to get the vacant chair in order that we might get Dr Sharpey down by this arrangement to our university'.[5]

William Sharpey had been born in Arbroath, and had graduated in Medicine at Edinburgh, since which time he had been a close friend of Charles Darwin. In 1855, he was Professor of Anatomy and Physiology and Dean of the Faculty of Medicine at University College, London, and Secretary of the Royal Society. He was already recognised as the foremost physiologist of his time in Britain.[6] Simpson was confident that, if Bennett could be successfully promoted to the chair of the Practice of Physic, he could then secure for Sharpey the resulting vacancy as Professor of the Institutes of Medicine. On this occasion Simpson's objectives were fully shared by James Syme and other members of Edinburgh's Faculty of Medicine.

The protocol for the election of a Professor of Medicine at Edinburgh was somewhat complicated. The voting was carried out in two stages, and every town councillor had a vote at each stage. It was customary for there to be an interval of approximately two months from the day the chair became vacant until the day on which the new professor was to be elected; in this case the interval was set at seven weeks. In that time each candidate was expected to have printed a 'Catalogue' of the appointments he had held, a list of his publications in the medical press, and other contributions that he may have made to medical practice or medical science; 'Testimonials' from as many medical colleagues, patients and influential patrons that he could find to support him; and at least one 'Address' to the patrons of the university to set out his intentions should he be appointed to the chair. All these documents had to be published and distributed not only to members of the Town Council but to members of the medical profession and the general public in Edinburgh so that, if they wished, they might communicate their views to town councillors. During the seven weeks, candidates had the opportunity to canvass every member of the Town Council, appealing for them to pledge their votes in both stages.

Only days before Alison resigned it seemed probable that he would be succeeded by John Hughes Bennett. Bennett had the advantage of having been Professor of the Institutes of Medicine for five years, and of having been an excellent lecturer and teacher. He also had the powerful support of both Simpson and James Syme. But he was unpopular among his colleagues. One of his rivals later wrote that: 'He had no grace of any kind, religious, moral or aesthetic. It was said that he arranged the abortions [aborted foetuses] of his mistress on his mantelshelf when he lived in Paris and exhibited them to his fellow students. He was reckless in his statements, greedy of money and fees, coarse and uncourteous in his language and conduct and much better fit for the stock exchange and society of bulls and bears than scientific men.'[7] Simpson was afraid that, because of Bennett's difficult personality, he might be defeated in the election by Andrew Wood. Wood had the support of the majority of the fellows of the College of Physicians, and he was a member of the Free Church, a church that was very well represented among the members of the Town Council. If Wood were to be elected, Simpson's scheme to find a place in Edinburgh for William Sharpey would come to nothing.

On 13 October, a physician in York, Thomas Laycock, was surprised to receive a letter from Simpson.

My Dear Dr. Laycock,
Dr Alison is to resign today or tomorrow from the chair of the Practice of Physic, his health being very bad indeed. I do not know how it will be disposed of or who will be considered for it. But

perhaps it would be a professorship for which you would consider it right to come forward. It is certainly the highest medical chair in our Scotch Universities. And consequently, I may say, in Britain. Think over it or rather *act* at once, if you have any idea of it. None of us professors can or will interfere in any way. The patronage is in the hands of the Town Council who always strive to put the right man in the right place.

Yours very truly,

J. Y. Simpson

Laycock was Physician to York County Hospital and a lecturer at York Medical School. He had received all his medical training in England but had taken his MD at Goettingen in 1839. He published his *Treatise of the Nervous Diseases of Women* in 1840, which included references to Simpson's work. Thereafter they had continued to correspond, and Laycock had visited Simpson in Edinburgh, with Simpson calling on Laycock whenever he was visiting patients in or near York. Nevertheless, Laycock was surprised and puzzled by Simpson's letter. But he was very ready to leave York which, in his experience, was 'not an improving place', and he found the unexpected suggestion that he might be a credible candidate for a chair in Edinburgh very flattering. He wrote to Simpson to reassure himself that an English physician, trained in England and with a degree from a German university, would be acceptable in Scotland. Simpson replied by telegram: 'All doctors acceptable . . . not an hour should be lost, several have already applied.' Next morning Laycock left York by the 9 a.m. train to Edinburgh. He had arranged to put up at Mackay's Hotel in Princes Street, but on his arrival Simpson pressed him to be his guest at 52 Queen Street for the duration of the contest.

Throughout his campaign, Laycock received invaluable advice and encouragement from Simpson's friend Robert Chambers, from Simpson's assistant, William Priestly, and from Simpson's cousin, the surgeon William Carmichael. But while the other candidates were assisted in their canvassing by 'committees' of supporters, Laycock conducted his canvassing by himself. In his letter inviting Laycock to become a candidate, Simpson had stated that he would 'not interfere in any way' in the election. Laycock was therefore surprised to see that Simpson was 'arranging and concocting testimonials [for every candidate] with all the enthusiasm of a busy apothecary' and openly giving support and encouragement to John Hughes Bennett.[8]

Even without Simpson's personal help Laycock conducted a skilful campaign. Many very distinguished men in England (including the Archbishop of York) wrote enthusiastically in his support; in all he was able to summit 90 testimonials; Bennett submitted 280. Calling on town councillors to solicit their votes, Laycock was calm, straightforward and courteous; when they informed him that they had pledged their first votes to Bennett or Wood, he congratulated them on the wisdom of their choice and modestly appealed for their second votes. It was a tactic that won him a large share of second votes.

As the campaign progressed, the town councillors' voting intentions were openly declared, and a week before the election was due it became clear that, for the first round of the election, Gairdner could only be sure of four votes and Douglas of only one. Both withdrew from the contest. On the evening of 1 October, with only one full day of campaigning still to go, the supporters of the three candidates reviewed the votes that had been pledged for the first and second rounds of the election. They found that, for the first round, Wood had promises of 12 first votes, Bennett 11 and Laycock 10. Bennett would therefore survive the first round, but he had so few promises of additional second votes for the final round that he could not possibly win. Laycock, on the other hand, had so many promised votes for the second round that he could easily beat either of the other candidates. However, that seemed irrelevant, since he was destined to be defeated in the first round by one vote. Wood, confident that he had already won, arranged to celebrate with a champagne lunch for his supporters on the day of the election. Bennett, although his defeat seemed inevitable, did not withdraw from the election or release the town councillors who had promised to support him from their pledges.

Simpson, as always, refused to accept defeat. His somewhat devious scheme to bring Sharpey to Edinburgh had clearly failed, but he could at least prevent his old adversary Andrew Wood from being elected to the most prestigious medical chair in Scotland. He immediately put pressure on those town councillors who had promised their votes to Bennett to abandon what had now become a lost cause and vote for Laycock instead. On the morning of the election, one switched his vote in the first round and gave it to Laycock, bringing the totals to 12 for Wood, 11 for Laycock and 10 for Bennett; Bennett was eliminated. In the second round, the number of second votes that Laycock had so carefully solicited, together with further defections from Bennett's support, brought his total to 18 against 15 for Wood. Wood was devastated, and his celebration was cancelled. It was

Simpson who was seen to celebrate. His plan to make a place for Sharpey in Edinburgh had been frustrated, but he was now determined to show that he had been the author of Laycock's success. That afternoon he left his patients to the care his assistants and drove the professor-elect triumphantly around Edinburgh in an open carriage.

Both Bennett and Sharpey were disappointed by the result, but both went on to add even greater distinction to their reputations as physiologists in the chairs they already held. At Edinburgh, Laycock was also successful as the first Professor of Medicine at Edinburgh to give special attention to mental disorders. However, he was not always happy there. Less than two years after his appointment, Simpson, with the support of others among the medical professors, tried unsuccessfully to undermine him by attempting to persuade the university's patrons to establish a chair of Clinical Medicine; had Simpson succeeded, Laycock would have lost the right to teach medical students at Edinburgh Royal Infirmary. Some years later, Laycock wrote privately that 'Simpson was a singular compound of reckless generosity and selfishness, so treacherous and so vengeful that it was difficult to say whether he was most dangerous as a friend or an enemy'.[9]

Even after his election, Laycock still had difficulty in understanding Simpson's motives in so urgently inviting him to become a candidate for the chair of the Practice of Physic at Edinburgh. For his part, Simpson later denied that he had been in any way responsible for Laycock's decision to put himself forward. In a letter to his friend Mrs Tootal, he wrote: 'I have been often very amused by the reports circulated by my professional brethren in regard to Laycock's election. If you ask Dr Noble of Manchester, you will find that it was he and another physician (I forget who) that were living at the time with Dr Laycock at the York Meeting who advised and urged him to become a candidate. When he did come down, the first thing I told him was that, along with some other professors I wished particularly Bennett to get the vacant chair in order that we might get Dr Sharpey down by this University. I am sure of one thing, when towards the end when I did begin to interest myself in the matter at all I worked harder for Bennett than I would do again for any other man.' This seems disingenuous. Simpson makes no mention of the letter he sent to Laycock on 13 August 1855 or the telegram that followed two days later. Nor does he mention the generous and vital help that Laycock received from Simpson's assistant William Priestly, his close friend Robert Chambers and his cousin William Carmichael, or the hospitality that Laycock enjoyed at 52 Queen Street throughout the campaign.

It was only after some time that Laycock came to understand the nature of Simpson's stratagem. Simpson did indeed mean to work hard for Bennett's election, but he feared that Bennett might be narrowly beaten by Andrew Wood. By running Laycock as a second credible, but nevertheless unlikely, alternative candidate, he believed he could ensure that Bennett would be elected. Laycock could be relied on to collect a respectable number of first votes, but not enough to prevent him from being eliminated at the first round of the election. Simpson was confident that he could then persuade those who had pledged their second votes to Laycock to transfer them to his prime candidate, Bennett. When, unexpectedly, it became clear that Bennett could not win, Simpson saw that he could at least defeat Wood by putting pressure on those who had pledged their second votes to Bennett to transfer them to Laycock. The move was successful and Laycock was duly grateful for the support that Simpson had given him. But five years later, Laycock wrote in his journal that he had come to believe that Simpson's 'ultimate objective' had only been to use him 'as his warming pan' in preparing a place for Sharpey at Edinburgh.

Perhaps Simpson should not be condemned for this ruthless use of his power and influence. His letter to Mrs Tootal, quoted above, indicates that he was not proud of the tactics that he had employed, but it may well be that he would have considered them fully justified had he been successful in bringing to Edinburgh such an eminent medical scientist as William Sharpey.

James Syme had supported Simpson in his efforts to elect Bennett to the chair of the Practice of Physic, and during this unusual period of harmony they had joined together in a project to provide the army with much-needed medical officers. Britain was at war. For some time the expansionist Nicholas I of Russia had been hoping to secure Britain's help in dismembering the ailing Ottoman Empire. When Britain declined to co-operate, the aging Nicholas I prepared to occupy Ottoman territories as far south as Constantinople and Jerusalem. Since such moves would threaten Britain's communications with India, British forces were deployed to bases in the Mediterranean. When in February 1852, the authorities in Jerusalem transferred custody of the Sanctuary of the Nativity from the Greek Orthodox Church to the Roman Catholic Church, the ensuing riots gave Nicholas I a pretext for intervening to protect the interests of his co-religionists; Russia gathered her forces on their borders, threatening to invade Moldavia and Wallachia, then still nominally part of the Ottoman Empire. Napoleon III of France, eager to be seen as the protector of the Roman Catholic Church, responded by sending a battle fleet through the Bosphorus into the Black Sea. Over the following months the crisis mounted. By June 1854, Russian armies had invaded Moldavia and Wallachia; a French army had been sent to Bulgaria to oppose them and restore the integrity of the Ottoman Empire; and British forces had sailed past Constantinople into the Black Sea. Leaving a depot and hospitals at Scutari on the shore of the Bosphorus, the British had then sailed north to join the French at Varna in Bulgaria.

At Varna it immediately became evident that the British army's medical services were inferior in numbers and organisation to those available to the French. However, when cholera broke out at Varna both armies suffered catastrophic losses. The French commanders, believing that the disease was caused by the foul air at Varna, evacuated their sick from the ramshackle building that served as hospital for both armies and dispersed them widely in the surrounding countryside.[10] There, separated from their efficient medical services, they died miserably in their thousands. Some of the British sick were sent to the crumbling military hospital at Varna; others were sent on the long sea journey to Scutari, where conditions were no better. In both places the orderlies who were expected to provide nursing care were poorly trained old soldiers. Since they were issued with generous rations of rum in the belief that rum was a preventative against the disease, the orderlies were persistently drunk. Few of the British sick received any form of hospital care. Most were left to themselves, and were buried by their friends. William Russell, *The Times'* correspondent, wrote that 'horrors occurred here every day. Walking on the beach one might see some straw sticking up through the sand and on scraping it away with his stick be horrified by bring to light the face of a corpse.' Many of the men who were still free of cholera 'seemed verging on insanity. They might be seen drunk in the ditches by the roadsides under the blazing sun, covered with flies.' In the outbreak of cholera the allied armies suffered the deaths of over 10,000 men, including many of the military surgeons who had been most attentive in caring for them.

The reports from Varna published in *The Times* made the British public begin to question the competence of the army's medical services. Their worst fears were confirmed by the reports published after the army's first major battle, at the Alma in the Crimea on 20 September 1854. *The Times'* diplomatic correspondent, Thomas Chenry, reported that 'the worn out pensioners who were brought out as an ambulance corps are totally useless, and not only are surgeons not to be had but there are no dressers or nurses to carry out the surgeon's directions and to attend on the sick during intervals between his visits. Here the French are greatly our superiors. Their medical arrangements are extremely good, their surgeons are numerous and they have the help of the Sisters of Charity who have accompanied the expedition in incredible numbers. These devoted women are excellent nurses.'[11]

By 13 October, only four days after the reports from the Alma had been published in London, Florence Nightingale obtained the authority of the Home Secretary, Lord Palmerston, the Foreign Secretary, Lord Clarendon and Dr Andrew Smith of the Army Medical Department to lead a party of four nurses to 'help the state of the Scutari hospital'.[12] However, the minister responsible for army administration in the field was Sydney Herbert, the Secretary at War. Herbert persuaded Miss Nightingale to accept instead the 'Office of Superintendent of the female nursing establishment in the English General Military Hospitals in Turkey'. Miss Nightingale accepted the appointment, and with a government-sponsored group of forty nurses she sailed for Scutari on 21 October. To find a way to help relieve the shortage of army medical staff at Scutari and the Crimea, Herbert, with the helpful thoughts of other cabinet members (including the Duke of Argyll), decided to send out surgeons and physicians in civilian units to be attached to the army. From London, a group led by Holmes Coote and Spenser Wells agreed to run civilian hospitals first at Smyrna and later at Renkoi. Simpson was given authority to send a second group. However, he was already convinced that hospitals, especially hospitals crowded with casualties, were unsafe places to perform surgical operations. In June 1854, Richard Mackenzie, a young surgeon at Edinburgh Royal Infirmary who had ambitions to succeed Sir George Ballingall as Professor of Military Surgery, had already gone out to join the 72nd Highlanders, and he was already showing what could be achieved by a regimental surgeon operating not in a hospital, but in the open air near to the battle.[13] With the active co-operation of James Syme, Simpson sent out more young surgeons to follow Mackenzie's lead. With the exception of Joseph Lister, who was a Quaker and opposed on principle to war, all the resident staff of Edinburgh Royal Infirmary – Heron Watson, Alexander Struthers, John Beddoe, John Kirk, George Pringle and David Christison – went out to the Crimea, where they served with great distinction.

As the conflict continued, the British public became increasingly critical of the conduct of the war. Britain's forces had been sent from Varna into the Crimea to deprive the Russians of the great Black Sea naval and military base at Sevastopol, but after almost four months Sevastopol had still not been taken, and Britain's inadequately equipped and badly led army had lost large numbers of its men in battle and even larger numbers to disease and neglect. In January the government was forced to resign. The civilian surgeons sent to the Crimea by Simpson had not cured the deficiencies of the army's medical services but, by their presence, their high level of skill, and their liberal use of chloroform, they had made the treatment of military casualties at least more humane. Until the end of the war in 1856, Simpson continued to correspond regularly with the new Prime Minister, Lord Palmerston, the new Secretary of State for War, Lord Panmure, and the Minister at War, Sidney Herbert.

Simpson's authority now extended well beyond the field of midwifery, and his influence reached beyond Scotland. In November 1856, he was invited to assist in finding an acceptable scheme for the regulation of medical practice in Britain. After many years of war, economic depression and political unrest, Britain was emerging as the world's richest nation. In this newly prospering Britain, there were many more people who could afford to pay for medical care and, in a country that was being rapidly, heedlessly and unhealthily urbanised, there were many more occasions for that aid being sought. But for prospective patients there was little to guarantee the professional competence of those who offered their services.

In the most badly served counties in Scotland – those in the Highlands and Islands – one in four of the medical practitioners in 1850 had no recognisable qualification and no licence to practise.[14] In England the situation was much worse; in one rural county it had earlier been estimated that nine out of ten practitioners were quacks[15] and, in the whole country, the *Association Medical Journal* was able to identify '21,435 persons practising without qualification'.[16]

But even among those medical practitioners who had a licence to practise from a 'legitimate and proper source', there were many who were poorly educated, inadequately trained and professionally incompetent. There were no fewer than twenty authorities in Great Britain and Ireland (Table 13.1) with the power to license medical practitioners, and each one set its own standards. In some cases, those standards were so low as to defeat the purpose of the licensing system. Confidence in the integrity and competence of the whole medical profession was inevitably undermined since 'in every one of its ranks, medical, surgical or obstetrical, numerous and melancholy examples of utter incompetence of licensed charlatans present themselves daily'.[17]

Table 13.1 Licensing Authorities for Great Britain and Ireland in 1850

The Royal College of Physicians
The Royal College of Surgeons of England
The Apothecaries Society of London
The University of Oxford
The University of Cambridge
The University of Durham
The University of London
The Royal College of Physicians of Edinburgh
The Royal College of Surgeons of Edinburgh
The Faculty of Physicians and Surgeons of Glasgow
The University of St Andrews
The University of Glasgow
The University of Aberdeen
The University of Edinburgh
The King and Queen's College of Physicians in Ireland
The Royal College of Surgeons in Ireland
The Apothecaries Hall of Ireland
The University of Dublin
The Queen's University of Belfast.
The Archbishop of Canterbury[18]

In 1853, the Home Secretary, Lord Palmerston, described the medical profession as 'a labyrinth and a chaos'.[19] From the earliest years of the century, there were a number of attempts made by individual medical practitioners to produce a scheme for the regulation of the training and practice of medical practitioners in the United Kingdom, but each one failed to attract general support within the profession. Since it appeared that the medical profession was unable to reform itself, in 1844 the Home Secretary, James Graham, drew up his own bill 'for the Better Regulation of Medical Practice throughout the United Kingdom'. Its main purpose was to create a central administrative body, largely composed of non-medical members, to supervise and co-ordinate the work of the profession's various and disparate licensing bodies. However, after almost two years the Home Secretary had been unable to secure sufficient backing for his bill to be debated in Parliament, and he was obliged to withdraw it. But the threat remained that, if the profession did not regulate itself, the government might find it necessary to impose state control. Stung into action, bills promoted by sections of the profession were tabled in Parliament in 1844,

1845, 1846, 1848, and 1854. All failed because of unresolved differences among the various sections of the profession.

Each of the many licensing bodies in the United Kingdom had its own charter, and its own, often long-established, privileges or monopolies. For example, early in the sixteenth century the Royal College of Physicians of London had been given the right to grant licences to practise medicine in London and within seven miles of London; much later the college's licentiates were also allowed to practise elsewhere in England. Since 1599, the Royal Faculty of Physicians and Surgeons of Glasgow had possessed the sole right to grant licences to practise medicine or surgery (or both) in the area of the ancient (but now defunct) see of the Bishops of Glasgow – but only there. By an Act of 1533, the Archbishop of Canterbury still had the authority to grant licences for the practice of medicine anywhere in England. Curiously, from 1822, graduates of the new University of London were entitled to practise anywhere in England except London. To add yet a further complication, the Apothecaries Act of 1815 enabled the Apothecaries Society to license medical men not as physicians or surgeons, but as 'general practitioners', the first time this designation had been used in an official government document; unfortunately the wording of the Act did not make it clear whether the legislation applied to the United Kingdom or only to England.

Every one of the twenty licensing bodies had its own peculiarities. It was virtually impossible to achieve complete unison in expressing the views and aspirations of such a large number of disparate and competing bodies in a single reform bill. As the debates continued throughout the 1850s, the protagonists for reform tended to fall into two major groupings.

One group formed round the universities of Edinburgh and Glasgow, then by far the largest medical schools in Britain. In 1804, they had agreed that they would conform by establishing a curriculum to be completed by students proceeding to the MD degree. By 1824, the curriculum at both universities included all the subjects – including Surgery, Midwifery and Pharmacy – that would prepare their medical graduates for a career in general practice. In each of the years that followed, Edinburgh and Glasgow together produced more medical graduates than all other British universities, and more than ten times the number produced jointly by the universities of Oxford and Cambridge. Therefore, when the regulation of the medical profession again became the subject of urgent debate in the 1850s, the vast majority of medical graduates practising in Britain had been trained at Edinburgh or Glasgow. They had completed a curriculum based on the skills needed by a general practitioner, and had been carefully examined in all of those subjects before graduating.

Since almost every medical man in Britain, no matter what his ultimate ambitions were, had of necessity to begin his career in medicine or surgery as a general practitioner, there were many among those drawing up the regulatory plans who argued that it would be appropriate for everyone entering the profession in future to train first as a general practitioner. Already, for over a generation, a majority of Edinburgh or Glasgow MDs had been doing just that. It therefore seemed fitting that the degree of MD should be confirmed as the single common qualification for entry to the medical profession. This was the concept that was at the heart of the bill to regulate the medical profession drafted for presentation to Parliament by Lord Elcho.[20] He envisaged a single university-trained medical profession, including all physicians, surgeons and apothecaries, and a single medical register of all those legally entitled to practise in the United Kingdom that would record the university from which the practitioner had graduated, although not his designation as physician, surgeon or apothecary.

This was in sharp contrast to the provisions of the bill being drafted by Thomas Headlam.[21] He represented the views of an alliance of all the medical corporations of the United Kingdom, assembled and dominated by the Royal College of Physicians of London. This college was the most ancient and the most elitist of the licensing bodies in the United Kingdom, and it had great influence in political circles in Britain. It insisted that the divisions in status that existed within the medical profession should be maintained. Headlam's bill therefore called for separate registers for physicians, surgeons and apothecaries, and for all practitioners to be examined and enrolled by the appropriate royal college or corporation before being admitted to the relevant register. But, in practice, the structure that it planned to maintain existed only in the populous and wealthy metropolis of London. Outside London, all medical practitioners made the greater part or all of their income from general practice. Viewing the London scene, the Provincial Medical and Surgical Association (the precursor of the British Medical Association) found it strange 'to find first a Royal College of Physicians in possession of a charter granted by Henry VIII in the sixteenth century with which they would lord it over their brethren in the nineteenth, a charter whose basis is the paramount absurdity that physicians can alone be educated at the universities of Oxford and Cambridge, schools of no note in the annals of medicine. We find next a College of Surgeons governed by a self-perpetuating council, distinguished in all their acts by a selfish anxiety for their own interests. And we come lastly to an Apothecary's Company, the essence of whose existence is the astounding fact that persons called upon to treat disease must not use the means of doing so, must not administer those remedies in the study of which his life may have been spent."[22]

Although fully conscious of these 'absurdities', the Provincial Medical and Surgical Association was nevertheless, at first, ready to ally itself with the Royal College of Physicians of London and support Headlam's bill. The great majority of the association's members were not university graduates and they could not accept the alternative proposal, put forward by Lord Elcho, that a university degree should in future be the only qualification for entry to the medical profession.

Neither of the sharply contrasting bills being put forward by Headlam and Elcho was able to attract wholehearted support within the profession. Headlam promised a structure for the profession that was too strictly hierarchical and not in keeping with the practicalities of everyday medical practice in most parts of the country. Elcho's bill, on the other hand, was too radical and too idealistic; it was perhaps theoretically attractive to have a university educated medical profession, but the university medical schools in England were too few, too small and in the case of Oxford and Cambridge too deliberately elitist to make that possible in practice.

In the spring of 1855, Simpson drew up an alternative bill of his own.[23] In May he had a meeting with the new Home Secretary, Sir George Grey, to solicit the support of the government. However, the Home Secretary decided to put all three draft measures, Headlam's, Elcho's and Simpson's, 'on ice' until the medical profession was able to give them more careful consideration. Simpson immediately dropped his plan to put forward a measure of his own. His main objective had been to oppose the Royal College of Physicians' vision of a strictly hierarchical medical profession. His own experiences as a young man, struggling to build a career against the prejudices of an established elite, had set his mind against such a concept. Since the Home Secretary had made it clear that the government would not legislate on medical reform for some months, he decided that he could most effectively frustrate the London college's intentions by using the available time to persuade Lord Elcho to make his bill more realistic.

In the months that followed, Simpson and John Storrrer of London University became Elcho's chief advisers. Simpson visited Elcho in London, and Elcho called on Simpson whenever he was in Edinburgh; at other times they communicated by letter; and, from London, John Storrer regularly wrote to Simpson to consult him on the re-drafting of what they now privately referred to as 'their Bill'.[24]

Early in 1856, William Cowper, the President of the Board of Health, was appointed chairman of a House of Commons select committee appointed by the Home Secretary to examine and report on the measures for medical reform that had been put forward by Headlam and Lord Elcho. Cowper found both bills unsatisfactory, and in November 1856 he announced that he intended to put forward a bill of his own. For Lord Elcho, Storrer and Simpson it immediately became 'a great matter for Cowper to have at hand a man to refer to who has the confidence of the university party'.[25] It was clear that the best person to act as their go-between with Cowper was Simpson himself. Cowper's wife was his patient, and Cowper travelled with her when she came to see him in Edinburgh; when in London, Simpson was in the habit of calling on Cowper and his wife. Simpson and Cowper now also began to communicate regularly by letter. Cowper came to rely on Simpson's support. In one letter on 13 May 1857 he wrote: 'All goes swimmingly. I trust you will not fail to let me have authentic evidence that the Scottish Universities are not consenting to Headlam's Bill. Any kind of hint as to the position of the Scottish corporations will be welcome. What is the actual present position of the College of Physicians in regard to the approval of the Headlam Bill? If you have time, find me anything that may be useful.'

When the provisions of Cowper's bill became known, the British Medical Association (the Provincial Medical and Surgical Association until January 1857) found that it now offered an alternative to Headlam's bill that did not threaten to make a university degree the essential qualification for entry to the medical profession. On 3 April, Sir Charles Hastings, President of the association's council, wrote to Simpson to inform him that the Reform Committee of his association had 'agreed to support Mr Cowper's Bill with some modifications'. He added that his committee had also re-examined Lord Elcho's bill and found it acceptable, apart from its proposal that the General Council to be appointed to regulate the profession should be nominated by the Crown. 'There is really no other material difference between the Bills and as Lord Elcho has signified his willingness to alter his Bill insofar as the constitution of the Council goes, I really do not see why the two Bills should be fought over before parliament. Why should the respective supporters not join behind one good Bill. I find it most probable that the College of Physicians in London will oppose both Bills. That makes it the more important that the other professional bodies should unite forces instead of being a divided body.' When Simpson informed him of Hastings' message, Lord Elcho agreed to withdraw his bill, leaving a slightly amended version of Cowper's bill to go forward with the guarantee of government support. That bill proposed that all the existing licensing bodies (with the exception of the Archbishop of Canterbury) should continue to examine and license new entrants to the profession. It also provided for the establishment of a new body to regulate the profession, to be called 'The General Council of Medical Education and Registration of the United Kingdom' and made up of a representative of each of the licensing bodies,[26] together with six members to be nominated by the Crown.

On 6 July 1858, when Cowper's Medical Bill reached its vital committee stage, Simpson's assistant, William Priestly, was present in the House of Commons. That evening he reported to Simpson:

> The Medical Bill passed through committee, as you already know by my telegraph, by large majorities whenever there was a division . . . Headlam, when his amendments came, had no chance whatever. He was beaten 3 to 1. Mr Walpole [the Home Secretary] had not left him a leg to stand on. Mr Walpole's business view of the whole question was masterly and Lord Elcho rendered most valuable service throughout. But for Lord Elcho, a clause in addition to the Bill after it was through would have been tacked on by Headlam which would virtually have subverted the universities entirely. It was simply that crafty clause in Headlam's last Bill with that little word 'and' instead of 'or' which would have compelled all MDs to go to [be enrolled by] the College of Physicians. Lord Elcho caught it immediately but could not get Mr Walpole to see the drift. When Lord Elcho had spoken it roused Mr Secretary and he supported Lord Elcho most effectively to throw it out. Now is your time for Lord Elcho's LLD.

The next day, Cowper wrote to Simpson: 'I am glad to inform you that my Bill went through Committee without material alteration. Headlam's amendments did not meet with any favour from Walpole as I feared when I wrote to you. We are now safe unless the Colleges can bewitch the House of Lords.' The London College of Physicians did, as Cowper had suspected, attempt to 'bewitch' the Lords. At the end of July, when the text of the bill to be considered by their Lordships was published, it mysteriously contained the clause requiring medical graduates to enrol with the Royal College of Physicians that had been rejected by the House of Commons. Simpson was informed by telegram, and the same evening he set out for London. The following day, with some assistance from his powerful medical and other friends in London, in the course of a few hours he had the alterations expunged and the bill restored to its original form. When the Lords came to discuss the bill in the last week of July, the British Medical Association had gathered for its annual meeting at the Royal College of Physicians of Edinburgh. It was there that Simpson received a telegram informing him the bill had passed. When his telegram was read to the meeting by the President of the association, Sir Charles Hastings, 'the hall rang with cheers'.[27] The meeting formally acknowledged that, for this achievement, after so many years of controversy and delay, the profession was indebted principally to Professor Simpson. He had played a crucial role in the introduction of a formula for regulating the medical profession in Britain that was to continue to operate essentially unchanged into the twenty-first century.

FOURTEEN

Private Practice, Archaeology and Semmelweis

*Wearisome condition of humanity, created sick and commanded
to be sound.*

Brooke

In November 1858, in a letter to a friend, Simpson wrote that he had never begun the new academic year so unwillingly. The summer had been one of the brightest and happiest in the whole of his life. The Archaeological Institute of London had met in Edinburgh in June, and it had been an agreeable week of 'nothing but dinners and evening parties'. He had later gone abroad with Jessie for their first holiday together for three years. Then, on his return, when he became caught up in the critical last stages of shaping the legislation for medical reform, he had been delighted by the prestigious and powerful support he had been able to command in London. But now in Edinburgh for the winter term, he could only look forward to further bitter confrontations with his fellow members of the Faculty of Medicine.

As a student and a radical, Simpson had resented the political and social prejudices of a Medical Faculty that always seemed ready to exclude him from advancement in his career. Now in his maturity, and a member of that Faculty, he still saw the other members as his natural enemies, seemingly intent on setting limits to his ambitions. For their part, the senior members of Faculty had, from their earliest years in the profession, been accustomed to looking down on midwifery as an 'ignoble art' that required neither the learning of a physician nor the courage and dexterity of a surgeon. Simpson had proved to be an accomplished scholar and writer, as well as an outstanding practitioner. They might have come to accept him as a worthy and respected colleague had it not been for his arrogance in straying from his proper field of obstetrics to pontificate on matters on which other members of the Faculty were the recognised authorities. After almost two decades of persistent conflict Simpson had attracted open personal enmity and distrust. At Simpson's first Faculty meeting after his bright and happy summer, James Syme, the Professor of Surgery and his arch-antagonist, condemned his contribution to the business of the meeting as 'false and calumnious', Syme later apologised to the Principal of the University for the unfortunate expression he had used, but he did not apologise to Simpson.

American obstetricians, who had crossed the Atlantic to visit him, found that Simpson was not so revered by the medical profession in Edinburgh as he was in Boston or Philadelphia. His historic work on anaesthesia had won him international fame, and he had been proudly recognised in Edinburgh by his election as President of the Royal College of Physicians in 1850 and President of the Medico-Chirurgical Society in 1852. But in his everyday practice he had acquired the reputation of being unreliable. As every year passed, he continued to agree to see more patients than he could possibly fit in to the time available. Every day he worked many tireless hours, but he was frequently absent from Edinburgh, attending privileged patients or lecturing to learned societies in some distant part of Britain. Patients whom he could not see felt let down; and those who were passed over while he attended to some more important case felt humiliated. Simpson employed three very able assistants, and every patient received efficient and competent care. But the patients, and the general practitioners who had referred them, had been led to expect the personal attention of the great man himself. And there were those who believed that Simpson not only promised to see too many patients, but also tended to promise them too much. He was an enthusiastic pioneer of the new discipline of gynaecology but he seemed eager to the point of recklessness in attempting operations that were still largely untried. He was not a highly skilled surgeon and in difficult cases he found it necessary to call for more expert assistance; even so, operations that had promised so much had, on occasions, very disappointing results. Simpson was the best of obstetricians and an excellent physician. His work on anaesthesia had transformed surgery and relieved the suffering of millions. No one denied his genius. But there were many in the medical profession in Edinburgh who were uneasy. They feared that his genius and his ambitions were carrying him too fast and too far, and that by the late 1850s he had already over-reached himself.

This was not a view shared by his hospital patients or by his students. Every day when in Edinburgh, he visited the patients in his ward for women and children at the Royal Infirmary, and the young and usually very poor women at his lying-in hospital in the Canongate. They could be confident of receiving a standard of care that they were most unlikely to find elsewhere. Even on days when he could not be present himself, their care was delegated to medical staff who had been trained in his methods

and had received his clear and comprehensive instructions. At his classes
at the university, Simpson attracted more medical students than any other
lecturer. Their first assessments of his qualities as a teacher are recorded in
a formal address presented to him by his students at the end of the winter
session in 1848. They were surprised and delighted that, unlike their other
professors, he did not read his lectures but seemed to engage closely and
personally with his audience. They were impressed by the warmth and
fervour of his delivery, and were greatly entertained by his account of the
fictions and absurdities he had discovered in his reading of the early literature of obstetrics. His presentation of his own medical, pathological and
practical doctrines was always clear and logical. They admired his erudition
and his mastery of the current literature, which enabled him to guide them
in selecting authors on whom they could rely. They commented particularly on the value of his regular course of practical exercises on his obstetrical machines (models), and the opportunity they were given to put their
theoretical instruction to the test in practice with patients at his public
dispensary. These, they said, were only some of the benefits that had earned
their most sincere gratitude. In the years that followed, Simpson amended
his lectures to take account of advances in knowledge. As demands on
his time increased he made every effort to ensure that, as far as possible,
other engagements did not take priority over his teaching; but on the few
occasions when he could not be present he arranged that his place should
be taken by a very able young obstetrician and lecturer, Alexander Keiller.

Simpson more than fulfilled his obligations to his students, and to his
patients in the public hospitals. But his professional life centred on his
private practice. Visiting obstetricians who were allowed to observe him
at work were surprised to discover that obstetric or gynaecological cases
made up rather less than half his practice. The majority of his patients
were women and children referred to him as a very successful, modern
and greatly admired general physician always ready to try every new drug
and every new treatment.[1] Only a very small proportion of his patients
were permanent residents of Edinburgh. The city authorities calculated
that, every year, the many patients who travelled long distances to consult
him added £80,000 (or £6,000,000 at current values) to the income of
Edinburgh's hotels and boarding houses. A short stout man in a dark coat
and a round black hat on his flowing grey hair, sitting with book in hand
in an elegant brougham, Simpson was a familiar sight as he was driven by
his coachman, George Wilson, from one Edinburgh hotel to the next.[2]
His patients were always at once encouraged by his confidence and his

easy charm. Formidable at meetings of the Faculty, to his young patients watching out for his arrival he was 'dear little fat Simmy'.[3]

Years before, in 1839, Simpson had stated that his ambitions could only be fully achieved by his 'pen' as well as his 'lancet'. In the late 1850s, the demands of his practice left him only a stolen hour early in the morning or late at night for his writing. But precious stretches of useful time became available when he was called to cases in distant parts of the country. He travelled to patients in Scotland as far north as Keith and as far west as Argyll; in England from Scarborough across to Cumberland and south to Manchester, London and Brighton. Summoned, as often as not, by the new telegraph, he went by rail to the station nearest to his destination and was met there by a coach sent by the patient's family. The staff at railway stations in many parts of Britain had good cause to remember him; he was always accompanied by a great load of books and papers and, if he was to travel overnight, by a hammock-like 'bed' that had to be suspended from poles rigged up between the seats of the compartment. On his return to Edinburgh, he was always careful to thank and reward the railway staff who had given him their very necessary assistance.

His long journeys gave him time for reading, and there was more time after he reached his patient's bedside. The time required for the management of an obstetric case was always unpredictable and the family usually insisted that he should continue to be at hand during the infant's first days: at least four or five days were necessary when he was called to see a child through the early dangers of diphtheria; advising on the terminal care of a patient dying of tuberculosis would take perhaps as many days; and no family that had been anxious enough to summon him from distant Edinburgh would be satisfied if he spent less than two or three days with them. For much of these days, Simpson was free to read and draft the text of pamphlets and essays, to be dictated to his two secretaries when he returned to Edinburgh.

He wrote on archaeology as well as on medicine. As a child, Simpson had been introduced by his uncle, George Jervais, to the study of the fossils, ancient stones and monuments in the hills surrounding his home in Linlithgowshire. His interest in archaeology continued for the rest of his life and went much deeper than that of the average gentleman amateur. His house in Queen Street became a favourite meeting place for dedicated archaeologists from every part of Britain and, in November 1861, he was appointed Professor of Archaeology at the Royal Scottish Academy. During the 1850s and 1860s, Simpson wrote a number of important essays and monographs;[4]

all but two were extended versions of papers delivered to the Society of Antiquaries of Scotland or to the Royal Society of Scotland. His publications did not form a series connected by a common theme.[5] Each one was prompted by a particular experience, request, or event. His *Notes of Some Ancient Greek Medical Vases for Containing Lykion*, for example, published in Edinburgh in 1856, followed from a visit to the British Museum in 1852; his *Was the Roman Army Provided with Medical Officers?* was written as his response to a direct question from Sir George Ballingall, the Professor of Military Surgery; his masterly review, *Archaeology: Its Past and Future* marked his election as Vice-President of the Society of Antiquarians of Scotland; *On an Old Stone-Roofed Cell or Oratory in the Island of Inchcolm* was the report of a discovery made during one of his many visits to an island he could see from Viewbank, his house on the shore of the Firth of Forth.

Like all his writings on medical subjects, his major works on archaeology show evidence of many long laborious hours of research in his library. Each one begins with an exhaustive historical review of his topic; his most quoted early sources are Herodotus, Pliny, Bede and Hector Boece. His evidence is set out in meticulous detail and discussed logically and at length. Each of his publications ends with a clear statement of his conclusions. The Roman army did have medical officers, at least in the time of the Empire even if not before; the Cat-Stane at Linlithgow marked the grave of the grandfather of Hengist and Horsa; the small building being used as a pigsty on Inchcolm in 1857 was originally an oratory established by St Columba in the sixth century AD. In his *Antiquarian Notices of Syphilis in Scotland*, Simpson discounted the common notion that syphilis had spread so quickly across Europe because it did so as an epidemic contagious fever; his well documented and argued thesis was that syphilis was then, as now, a venereal disease. That it spread so rapidly in the fifteenth and sixteenth centuries was the result of the sexual practices in a civilisation which might find a cardinal with as many as fifteen children, and in which were strict rules that determined how much a bishop could take from church funds to provide dowries for his daughters. One of the specimens described in his *On Some Scottish Medical Charm-stones, or Cure-Stones* was the *Talisman* of Sir Walter Scott's novel, and it was only one of several cure-stanes in the keeping of old Scottish families.

In *Is the Great Pyramid of Gizeh a Metrological Monument?* Simpson displayed his delight at debunking the effort of scholars with whom he disagreed. In a number of presentations, including one to the Royal Society of Edinburgh in 1866, Professor Piazzi Smyth, the Astronomer

Royal for Scotland, had claimed that the Great Pyramid of Gizeh (Giza) was not built as a mausoleum but as 'a marvellous metrological monument to contain within its structure material standards as measures of length, capacity and weight for men and nations for all time'. But Simpson pointed out that the early historians from Herodotus onwards had all agreed that the pyramid was a mausoleum. Since then, many excavations had shown that the chambers and internal structure of the pyramid conformed to the general design of the chambers and crypts of burial mounds, cairns and barrows elsewhere, including those that Simpson had visited in Ireland with his archaeologist friend, Sir William Wilde. Smyth claimed that the porphyry coffer found in the King's Chamber inside the pyramid was not a sarcophagus but a divinely ordained 'standard measure of capacity and weight' with the capacity of a cauldron that would contain exactly four quarters of wheat. Simpson argued that a standard of measurement 'should be measurable'. Every surface of the coffer was uneven and, from one part to another, its sides and bottom varied widely in thickness; it had been measured at different times by twenty-six different observers and always with very different results. Simpson concluded 'that this vessel formed under alleged Divine inspiration as a measure of capacity for all men and all nations, and particularly for these latter profane times, is in truth nothing more and nothing less than an old and somewhat misshapen stone coffin'.

To Simpson's amusement, Smyth had also claimed that the standard of linear measurement was the length of the base line of the pyramid which had been divinely set to measure one Hebrew Sacred Cubit (each one ten-millionth of the earth's semi-axis of rotation) multiplied by the number of days (365.25) in the year. Here Smyth had taken it upon himself to correct Newton's estimate of the length of the ancient Sacred Cubit. Newton had taken a cubit to be equal to the normal pace of a man, that is, one third of his height. Newton had made a number of calculations of the size of the ancient cubit to allow for the differences between tall and short men and had published a mean value of 24.75 inches. Smyth assumed, wrongly, that in his calculations Newton had used the Roman foot rather than British inches; Smyth repeated Newton's calculation making allowance for the difference between the Roman and British foot, producing a measurement for the Sacred Cubit of 25.07 inches.

Simpson happily pointed out that, in his 'Dissertation upon the Sacred Cubit of the Jaws and the Cubits of the Several Nations', Newton had allowed for the difference between the Roman and British foot, and therefore his estimate of the Sacred Cubit of 24.75 inches must stand. But, in any case, the length of Newton's Sacred Cubit was completely irrelevant, since those building the pyramid in 2160 BC could not possibly have heard of Newton or his calculations. And the base of the pyramid was useless as a standard measurement. The base of the north side of the pyramid had been measured five times, and the lengths recorded had varied from 9,110 to 9,163 inches. More recently Mr Inglis from Glasgow had measured all four sides and found a difference of 18 inches between the longest and the shortest.

Simpson's final comment was that if Smyth's figures and methods were used, at least something 'very exact and marvellous' could be proved: 'If the polar axis of the earth be held as 500,000,000 inches and Sir Isaac Newton's Sacred Cubit be held as Professor Smyth calculated it to be, the long diameter of the brim of my hat is one forty-millionth of the earth's polar axis.'

Neither Simpson's interest in archaeology nor his demanding practice as obstetrician and physician was allowed to divert him from his writing as a medical scientist. By 1859, his efforts to promote the use of chloroform had come to a very successful end and his case for the use of anaesthesia in normal childbirth had been clearly and very persuasively made. He was now able to return to a subject that had first caught his attention more than a decade earlier: puerperal fever. For centuries there had been scattered cases in which mothers had died of a malignant fever only a few days after the birth of her child. But for the midwife (or the male accoucheur, should one be called in) attending the delivery in the patient's home, there seemed nothing to distinguish one fever from the many other fevers endemic in the local community at the time. It was only in the middle years of the eighteenth century, when the first lying-in hospitals were established and large numbers of poor mothers were brought together from their wretched homes to be delivered in a public ward, that this one fever was recognised as a distinct entity worthy of its own name, puerperal fever. In almost every case the mother felt well in the first day after delivery, but on the second or third day she became unwell with a high fever and, as the disease progressed, a grossly distended and painful abdomen; the pain often became as severe as the worst of her labour pains. Once puerperal fever was recognised, it became clear that it was responsible for more than half of all maternal deaths. It has been estimated that in the eighteenth century in Britain, between 6 and 9 of every 1,000 mothers delivered at home contracted puerperal fever,[6] and of these a third or more died, usually after two or three days of great suffering. In lying-in hospitals the death rate was three or four times greater, and during epidemics of puerperal fever the death rate in lying-in hospitals became more than twenty times greater.[7]

In the early eighteenth century the common notion was that puerperal fever was caused by the suppression or retention of the lochia, the uterine discharge that followed childbirth. However, the twelve epidemics of puerperal fever that occurred in England between 1760 and 1788 led to a belief that puerperal fever was spread by 'miasma', the invisible emanations from decomposing vegetable or animal matter carried in the air. However, Professor Alexander Hamilton, the father of Simpson's predecessor as Professor of Midwifery at Edinburgh, believed that the cause of puerperal fever was more specific and had something in common with the cause of erysipelas, the potentially fatal disease that was so common in surgical wards. In 1783, in his *Outlines of Midwifery*, he had written: 'In hospital practice there is no doubt but that the disease is produced by specific contagion from the air of the wards. It is particularly observed in surgical wards that there is such a state of air as produces almost in every wound, even the slightest symptoms of erysipelas and even mortification. In the Edinburgh Royal Infirmary, when the lying-in ward was there, it was observed that, when such state of the air was present, puerperal fever raged violently but at no other time.' Hamilton's ideas attracted little immediate attention outside Edinburgh, but after an epidemic of puerperal fever in Aberdeen, Alexander Gordon carried them an important stage further.

Alexander Gordon had studied medicine in Aberdeen, Leyden and Edinburgh before becoming a surgeon in the Royal Navy in 1780. Released from the navy on half-pay in 1785, he spent almost a year training in midwifery in London before returning to Scotland as Physician to the Obstetric Dispensary in Aberdeen. After a full and careful account of the epidemic of puerperal fever in 1789–92 he wrote: 'The cause of the epidemic fever was not owing to a noxious constitution of the atmosphere for, if it had been owing to that cause, it would have seized women in a more promiscuous and indiscriminate manner. But this disease seized such women only as they were visited or delivered by a practitioner or taken care of by a nurse who had previously attended patients affected with the disease.' He had begun his treatise by asserting: 'I could venture to foretell what women would be affected with the disease upon hearing by what midwife they were to be delivered or by what nurse they were to be attended during their lying-in; and almost in every instance my prediction was correct.'[8] Gordon also noted that while the epidemic of puerperal fever raged in Aberdeen there was, at the same time, an outbreak of erysipelas

ACCOUNT

OF A

NEW ANÆSTHETIC AGENT,

AS A

SUBSTITUTE FOR SULPHURIC ETHER

IN

SURGERY AND MIDWIFERY,

BY

J. Y. SIMPSON, M.D., F.R.S.E.,

PROFESSOR OF MIDWIFERY IN THE UNIVERSITY OF EDINBURGH;
PHYSICIAN-ACCOUCHEUR TO THE QUEEN IN SCOTLAND, ETC.

" I esteem it, the office of a Physician, not only to restore health, but to mitigate
pain and dolours."—BACON.

COMMUNICATED TO THE MEDICO-CHIRURGICAL SOCIETY OF EDINBURGH,
AT THEIR MEETING ON 10TH NOVEMBER 1847.

THIRD THOUSAND.

EDINBURGH:

SUTHERLAND AND KNOX, PRINCES STREET.

LONDON : SAMUEL HIGHLEY, 32 FLEET STREET.

MDCCCXLVII.

Simpson's announcement and account of his discovery of chloroform to the
general public of Britain and North America.

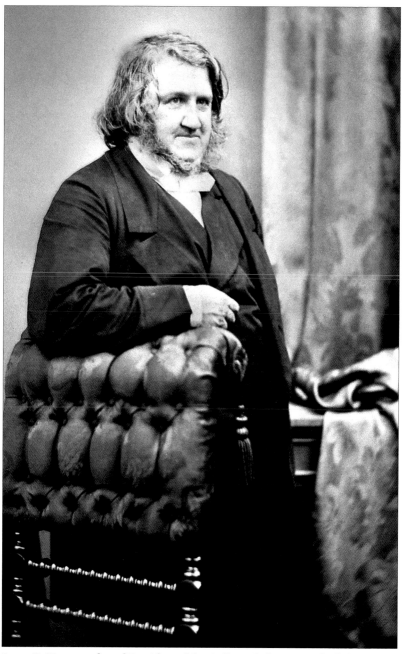

James Y. Simpson, elected President of the College of Physicians of Edinburgh in 1850.

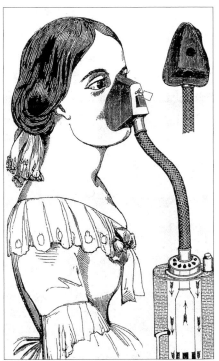

LEFT. The apparatus designed by John Snow, London's first anaesthetist, for the administration of chloroform.

BELOW. An inhaler designed for the recreational use of chloroform.

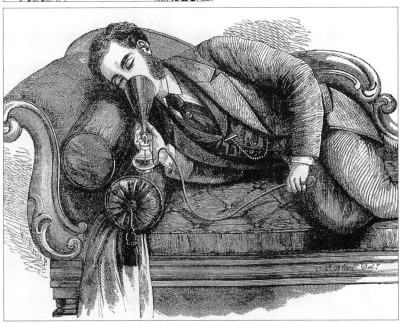

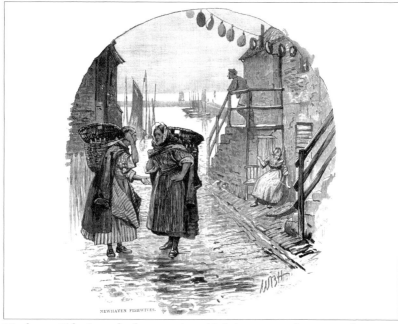

NEWHAVEN FISHWIVES.

Newhaven Fishwives who for centuries sold their wares on the streets of Edinburgh. Simpson studied the social conditions in which they lived in their home village near his house, Viewbank, at Trinity.

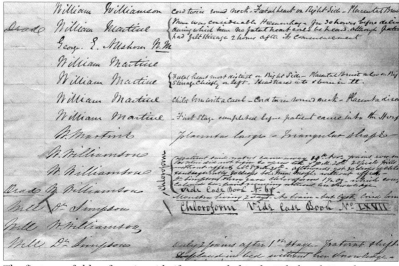

The first use of chloroform in midwifery recorded in the Edinburgh Royal Maternity Hospital Case Book.

ANSWER

TO

THE RELIGIOUS OBJECTIONS

ADVANCED AGAINST

THE EMPLOYMENT OF ANÆSTHETIC AGENTS
IN MIDWIFERY AND SURGERY.

BY

J. Y. SIMPSON, M.D., F.R.S.E.,

PROFESSOR OF MIDWIFERY IN THE UNIVERSITY OF EDINBURGH, AND PHYSICIAN-
ACCOUCHEUR TO HER MAJESTY IN SCOTLAND.

" For every creature of God is good, and nothing to be refused, if it be received with
thanksgiving."—1st Timothy iv. 4.

"Therefore to him that knoweth to do good and doeth it not, to him it is Sin."—James iv. 17.

EDINBURGH:

SUTHERLAND AND KNOX, 58, PRINCES STREET.
LONDON: SAMUEL HIGHLEY, 32, FLEET STREET.

MDCCCXLVII.

Simpson's *Answer* to the expected religious objections to the use of anaesthesia in childbirth, widely distributed to the general public in Britain and North America.

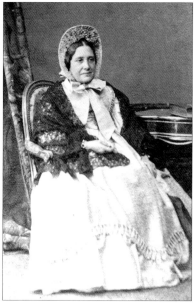

Lady Simpson.

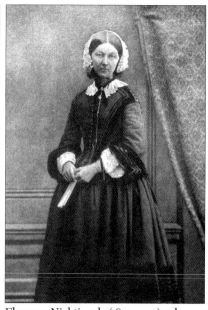

Florence Nightingale (1820–1910), who took nurses to serve in the war in the Crimea; Simpson sent surgeons.

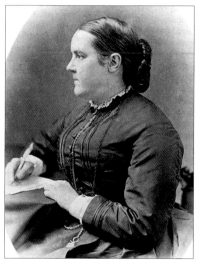

Sophia Jex-Blake (1840–1912), founder of the Edinburgh School of Medicine for Women, in 1887.

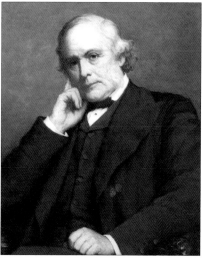

Joseph Lister (1827–1912), Professor of Surgery at Glasgow from 1860, at Edinburgh from 1869 and at London from 1877: a pioneer of antiseptic surgery.

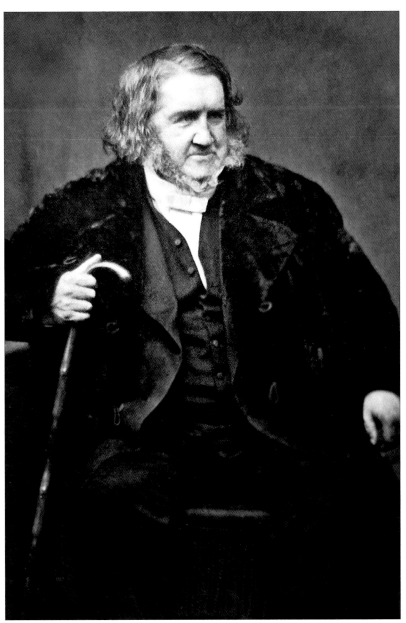
Sir James in his last years wearing his famous seal-skin coat.

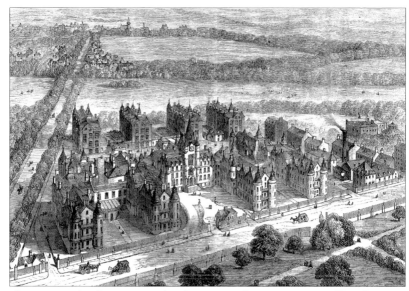

The new Royal Infirmary, completed in 1879. Built as interconnected but distinct pavilions, it shows the influence of Simpson's ideas on the control of hospital infection.

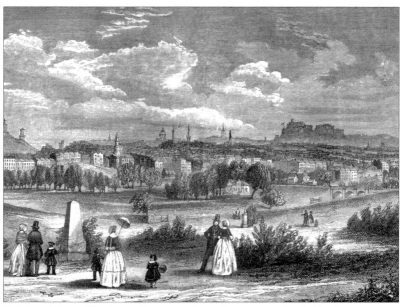

Edinburgh from Warriston Cemetery where Simpson was buried in 1870.

in the surgical wards of the city's hospital. 'I will not venture to positively assert that puerperal fever and erysipelas are precisely of the same specific nature, but that they are connected, that there is an analogy between them, and that they are concomitant epidemics, I have unquestionable proofs. For these two epidemics began in Aberdeen at the same time, arrived at their acme together and they ceased at the same time.' Although he had a new concept of the cause of puerperal fever, his treatment of the condition continued as before. Patients were bled until they fainted; thereafter twenty or thirty leeches were attached to the patient's distended and intensely painful abdomen.

This was Gordon's only published work on puerperal fever. In 1792, when Britain began to prepare for war with France, he was recalled to the navy and in 1799 he died of tuberculosis. His observations were largely ignored, perhaps because they ran counter to what was widely regarded as the most advanced thinking of the time: that diseases were never caused by a single, supposed but unidentifiable agent, but always by a combination of three observable factors – the climate and condition of the environment; the predisposition to a disease that made one person more vulnerable than others; and some form of contact with morbid putrescent matter. There was also a great and long-persisting reluctance to believe that disease could be carried to the patient by her medical attendants. Several years later, an Edinburgh obstetrician who, in his book,[9] quoted much of Gordon's work with approval, nevertheless wrote that: 'In October 1821, I assisted at the dissection of a woman who died of the disease [puerperal fever] after an abortion in the early months. The pelvic viscera, with the external coats were removed and I carried them *in my pocket* to the classroom. The same evening, without changing my clothes, I attended the delivery of a poor woman in the Canongate and she died; next morning I went, in the same clothes, to assist some of my pupils who were engaged with a woman in Bridewell whom I delivered with forceps and she died.' As late as 1840, the highly respected Charles Meigs, Professor of Obstetrics in Philadelphia, was similarly inconsistent. He told his students that every medical practitioner should read Gordon's treatise as an excellent 'convincing and truthful' history of an epidemic of puerperal fever, but he completely rejected Gordon's conclusion that the disease was contagious. He was particularly scornful of Gordon's claim that there was a link between puerperal fever and erysipelas: 'You might as well say that a woman has iritis of her pylorus.'[10]

As we have seen (Chapter 10), Simpson disagreed with his friend

Charles Meigs on the place of general anaesthesia in childbirth; he also disagreed with him on the aetiology of puerperal fever. Simpson had been Professor James Hamilton's house physician, and from him he had absorbed the ideas on puerperal fever that Hamilton had inherited from his father. Simpson was also very familiar with the work of Alexander Gordon. And he had carried their ideas forward: he was the first to claim that puerperal fever could be transmitted to the patient on the hands of her midwife or her other medical attendants.[11] From the beginning of his career in obstetrics he had taught his students to wash their hands in chlorinated water before examining their patients.[12] He also recognised the similarity between puerperal fever and the erysipelatous infections that attacked the open wounds of surgical patients.

In January 1848, Simpson was surprised and somewhat disconcerted by a letter he received from Franz Arneth, one of the two assistants at the Vienna Lying-in Hospital. Arneth had written to draw Simpson's attention to the work of his colleague Ignaz Semmelweis, published in *Zeitschrift der Kaiserlichen und Koniglichen Gesellschaft der Arzte zu Wien* in December 1847. Semmelweis' article was entitled 'Experience of the Highest Importance Concerning the Etiology of Epidemic Puerperal Fever at the Lying-in Hospital in Vienna'.

Semmelweis was a Hungarian, born in Taba, now part of modern Budapest. He had studied medicine at Vienna University and after graduating he had taken the further degree of Mastery of Midwifery in 1844. In 1846 he had been appointed as an assistant at the Lying-in Hospital, which was part of Vienna's General Hospital. The Lying-in Hospital, the largest in the world at that time, was divided into First and Second Clinics, which received patients on alternate days. Semmelweis was the assistant in charge of the First Clinic.

Semmelweis had been able to show from hospital records that between 1784 and 1822, when post-mortems on mothers dying in childbirth were rarely performed, that the maternal mortality rate in the Lying-in Hospital was 125.[13] But when it was ordered that, for educational purposes, a post-mortem should be performed on every mother who died, the rate of maternal mortality increased sharply to 530. After the hospital was divided in 1833 into two clinics both providing instruction for medical students and midwives, maternal mortality continued virtually unchanged. But when, in 1839, it was arranged that medical students would receive instruction in the First Clinic and midwives in the Second Clinic, the mortality rate in the First Clinic increased to 984, while that in the Second Clinic fell to 388.[14] The explanation for these remarkable changes in mortality (and hence the changes in the incidence of puerperal fever, since it was by far the commonest cause of death) was suggested to Semmelweis by the sudden death of a pathologist, Professor Kolletschka. Kolletschka had cut his finger while carrying out a post-mortem, and died of an acute febrile illness; at the post-mortem on his body, the distribution and appearance of the diseased parts seemed to Semmelweis to be very similar to those found at post-mortem examination of victims of puerperal fever. He was, of course, aware that his medical students went first each morning to make, or take part in, the post-mortem examinations of those patients, usually eight or ten in number,[15] who had died the previous day; and that the students then went directly to the labour room, where they were required to make vaginal examinations of women in labour. These observations led Semmelweis to suppose that cadaveric particles adhering to the hands of his students caused the same disease among maternity patients that had killed Kolltschka, whose slip with a post-portem knife had been followed by fever and death. This hypothesis could conveniently explain the relatively very high incidence of puerperal fever in his First Clinic; the nurses being trained in the Second Clinic did not perform or attend post-mortems.

From May 1847, Semmelweis' students were required to wash their hands in a solution of chloride of lime on entering the labour room. They were not required to wash their hands between patients; that, in Semmel-weis' view, would have been 'superfluous' since the patients were alive and could not therefore contaminate the students' hands with cadaveric particles. Thereafter the maternal mortality rate in Semmelweis' First Clinic fell dramatically to a level approaching that in the Second Clinic. Nevertheless, the maternal mortality rates were still very high: 357 in the First Clinic and 306 in the Second Clinic.

Semmelweis published his findings in the *Zeitschrift der Kaiserlichen und Koniglichen Gesellschaft der Arzte zu Wien*, but his ideas attracted very little notice. When he could not be persuaded to publish his work in a more prestigious journal, his friends Carl Rokitansky, Ferdinand von Hebra, Joseph Skoda, Justus Liebeg and Franz Arneth, all distinguished members of the Vienna medical school, did what they could to disseminate the news of his work.

In January 1848 Franz Arneth, whose mother was Scottish, was delegated to write to Simpson. Simpson was far from impressed and replied by return of post. Semmelweis later wrote that his 'letter was filled with abuse. Simpson said that without the letter he knew in what lamentable condition midwifery in Germany, and especially in Vienna, still remained. He knew for certain that the cause of the high mortality lay only in the unbound carelessness with which patients were treated; as for example when they put a healthy lying-in woman into the same bed in which another patient had just died without changing the bed clothes and linen. Our letter also proved that, to us, British obstetric literature was unknown otherwise we would have been aware that in Britain it had for a long time been held that puerperal fever was a contagious disease, and they employed chlorine disinfection for its prevention. This letter did not make us feel disposed to continue the correspondence with Simpson.'[16]

Simpson's anger is, in part, explained by a letter he later wrote to his friend Francis Ramsbotham: 'A few weeks ago, I had a communication from Vienna telling me that formerly 70 in every 100 women delivered in the hospital died of puerperal disease. They delivered new patients in beds still hot and warm with the bodies of those just dead. The physician said that they had now reduced last year the deaths to 10% by using means against contagion – that is to say, they sacrificed the lives of 70% of the women delivered to their inhumane medical practices. Is it not a terrible illustration of the extent to which medical prejudices will carry men?'[17] Clearly there had been a misunderstanding. The maternal mortality in Vienna was very high, but not as unbelievably high as the figures quoted by Simpson in his letter to Ramsbotham.

The misunderstanding was only resolved three years later. Arneth had taken a year's sabbatical to visit the leading obstetric centres in Europe. In April 1851, he visited Edinburgh and there he presented a paper on the 'Evidence of Puerperal Fever Depending upon the Contagious Inoculation of Morbid Matter' to the Medico-Chirurgical Society.[18] In it he reported that the measures introduced by Semmelweis had reduced mortality at the Vienna Lying-in Hospital from 11 per cent to 2 per cent. He also reported that Semmelweis had long since been obliged to abandon his conviction that the single cause of puerperal fever was the introduction of 'cadaveric particles' into the genitalia of women in labour. In October 1847 a patient had been admitted to his ward suffering from a putrid cancer of the cervix. Unfortunately, her bed was near to the door and she was the first patient to be examined by the medical students before they went on to examine the other patients along that side of the ward; of those twelve other patients, eleven died of puerperal fever. In November 1847, this disaster was repeated after a woman with a discharging carious knee was admitted to his ward. In these two tragic incidents, neither of the women who were the sources from which the disease had spread was dead; thereafter Semmelweis conceded that puerperal fever could be carried to new patients not only by 'cadaveric particles' but also by other 'morbid matter'. And since the single washing in chloride of lime had failed to prevent the spread of the disease within the ward, he had insisted that his students should wash their hands in chloride of lime before every examination, rather than only when first entering the labour ward.

Semmelweis had not published what should have been very necessary and important amendments to his original article in *Zeitschrift der Kaiser- lichen und Königlichen Gesellschaft der Ärzte zu Wien*. Again he had relied on the efforts of his group of loyal friends in Vienna to disseminate the news of these important developments in his understanding of the spread of puerperal fever. And his friends were in a minority in Vienna. Professor Johannes Klein, the director of the Vienna Lying-in Hospital, had little time for Semmelweis, and he and his minions had always been firmly opposed to Semmelweis' new and unconventional ideas. Semmelweis' position became even more difficult in January 1848, when nationalists in Hungary rose in rebellion against the imperial government in Vienna. Semmelweis had openly identified with the nationalists and he had taken to wearing the Hungarian nationalist uniform, with its broad-brimmed hat and sweeping feather, even while attending patients at his clinic. His political sympathies and growing eccentricity told against him. In October 1850, he applied successfully for the post of Lecturer in Midwifery at the Lying-in Hospital, but the appointment was made with the humiliating condition that he should teach only the theory of obstetrics and should have no contact with patients. Abruptly and without warning, Semmel- weis abandoned his patients and his small band of friends and left Vienna to return to Budapest. He had decided that Vienna, if not the whole world, was against him; for their part, Skoda, Rokitansky and the others in Vienna who had done so much to promote his views against strong local opposition were upset by his ingratitude and appalled by his foolishness. In 1851, when Franz Arneth was in Edinburgh and presenting his paper on the aetiology of puerperal fever to the Medico-Chirurgical Society, Semmel- weis was in Budapest in an unpaid post at a small and obscure hospital, and practising as a gynaecologist rather than as an obstetrician.

It was not until 1855 that Semmelweis was appointed Director of Obstetrics at the University of Pest, and it was not until 1858 that he began work on his thesis *Etiology, Concept and Prophylaxis of Childbirth Fever*. His eccentricity was now deepening into depression, lapses of memory and paranoia, although he was still capable of periods of almost manic activity.[19] In the completed treatise he wrote: 'The birthday of my doctrine occurred in the latter half of May 1847. If we put the question to ourselves now after twelve years, did my teachings fulfil their mission, the answer has a melancholy sound.' The treatise was over 500 pages long, repetitive and somewhat disorganised. But it was clearly intended to present his own full and detailed account of his discoveries and conclusions, and to counter an increasingly popular belief that puerperal fever was a contagious disease capable of spreading as an epidemic. He wrote that: 'Puerperal fever is not contagious but it is conveyable from a sick, pregnant, parturient or puerperal woman to a healthy pregnant, parturient or puerperal woman by means of decomposed material produced by the sick pregnant, parturient or puerperal woman. Puerperal fever is not conveyable during life from every sick pregnant, parturient or puerperal woman to a healthy individual but only from those infected women who produce a decomposed material. After death puerperal fever is conveyable from every cadaver of a puerperal to a healthy individual when the cadaver has reached the necessary degree of decomposition.'

Further: 'There are no epidemic influences, atmospheric, cosmic or telluric, capable of producing puerperal fever and there never have been such epidemic causes of puerperal fever ... Before everything stands the unshakable rock on which I have raised the edifice of my doctrine concerning puerperal fever, the fact that owing to the measures which I have adopted and carried out from May 1847 until the present day in three different institutions which used to be afflicted with puerperal fever epidemics, I have brought about a condition of things as is met with only now and then. Even the most stubborn defender of the epidemic theory of puerperal fever could hardly call this state of matters an epidemic. The sickening and dying of many individuals from the same disease within the same period does not complete all that is implied in an epidemic else would every battle be an epidemic for in a battle many individuals die from the same cause in a short time.'

When Semmelweis' great thesis was published in 1860, his behaviour was deteriorating towards the insanity that led to his committal to a mental asylum in 1865. When he died later that year his passing was hardly noticed by the medical press or even by the newspapers in his native Budapest. His work had made little lasting difference to obstetric practice, even in Vienna; it had never at any time greatly influenced practice in Germany and, from the beginning, it had been almost totally rejected in France.[20] In Britain the understanding of puerperal fever continued to be based on Gordon's treatise and the example and teaching of Simpson. His long overdue *Etiology, Concept and Prophylaxis of Childbirth Fever* was seldom read; it was of little interest to a medical profession that had already been introduced to the germ theory of disease and the new science of bacteriology. Semmelweis is now best remembered for the brilliant simplicity of his original observation in 1847; for the myth that later grew up of his struggle to make his views known; and for the neglect, or even persecution, that he suffered at the hands of his colleagues in the medical profession.

Nevertheless, Semmelweis was of great importance to Simpson. His sharp and crucial observations in the Lying-in Hospital in Vienna, his understanding of the possible significance of what he had seen, and even his mistakes in interpretation, all combined to stimulate Simpson's interest in the prevalence and spread of hospital infections. This was to be the subject of Simpson's last great contributions to medical science.

FIFTEEN

Acupressure and Hospitalism

A new philosophy calls all in doubt.
John Donne

Simpson once famously commented that patients admitted to hospital for surgery were exposed to more chances of death than soldiers on the battlefield of Waterloo. The great majority of the patients who died did not die of shock, haemorrhage or some fatal error during the operation but from the febrile illness that so often followed a few days later. That illness was accurately described in a review published by the Royal College of Surgeons of Edinburgh in 1833: 'The usual symptoms are rigors, long continuing and recurring at intervals; anxiety and restlessness; occasional sickness and vomiting; pains referred to the abdomen, chest and joints; pulse weak and rapid; tongue brown and dry; abdomen painfully distended; diarrhoea and sweating; difficulty in breathing; features pinched and extremities cold.' Since these were also the symptoms and signs of puerperal fever, Simpson suggested that it would be appropriate for the illness that followed surgery to be known as surgical fever.

Semmelweis had shown that the mortality from puerperal fever could be substantially reduced by insisting that all medical attendants wash their hands in a solution of chlorine before every vaginal examination. Simpson speculated that if it could be shown that the two fevers were indeed essentially the same, as the symptoms and signs seemed to suggest, some way could probably be found to reduce the mortality from surgical fever. In 1850, he therefore made a careful study of the 'analogy between the puerperal fever and surgical fever'.[1]

In the medical literature, he found a recent report from England which claimed that as much as 87 per cent of the total mortality in childbirth was due to puerperal fever. This seemed to Simpson to be, perhaps, an unduly high estimate; in an earlier series of 2,890 deliveries at the Edinburgh Lying-in Hospital, in which 1.6 per cent of the mothers died, deaths from puerperal fever made up 77 per cent of the total mortality.[2] Again from the

medical literature, Simpson was able to cite the outcome of 4,937 operations carried out by 'the best of our civil and military surgeons' for the
amputation of one or more limbs; in all, 32 per cent of the patients died; of
these 88 per cent died of surgical fever. Although the information available
was limited, it did seem to show that surgical fever was not only a more
common disease than puerperal fever, it was at least as dangerous to life.

The 'anatomical conditions' of the two diseases were also 'in many
respects the same'. In surgical patients, the wound opened up deep tissues,
exposing the mouths of numerous arteries and veins and, if the wound was
not immediately closed, it healed slowly by the exudation of lymph and
pus over its surface and the ultimate formation of a 'skin' of new envel-
oping tissue. In the puerperal patient the whole internal surface of the
uterus was denuded by the separation of the placenta, and the mouths
of a multitude of arteries and veins were left exposed; and, as in surgical
wounds, the open site of the placenta was gradually repaired by the exudation of serum, lymph and pus. Until that repair was complete, in puerperal
patients as in surgical patients, the open mouths of the arteries and veins
remained dangerously exposed. Simpson proposed that the fever in both
puerperal and surgical cases was not caused directly by the local inflammation in the uterus or the wound but by the 'vitiated condition' of the
circulating blood, 'poisoned' by morbid and contagious matter gaining
entry through the exposed arteries and veins. He also proposed that the
morbid matter entering the bloodstream was not some common product
of the local inflammation but, on the analogy of smallpox, measles and
scarlet fever, a specific contagious agent.[3] Simpson claimed that his theory
that the phenomena of both puerperal and surgical fever were caused by
the circulation of 'poisoned' blood was supported by the post-mortem
examinations of their victims. The pathological changes that were found
were not confined to the uterus or the surgical wound but were widely
dispersed to other parts of the body, particularly the abdomen, the lungs,
the heart and the muscles and joints.

A method had been found to limit the mortality from puerperal fever. If
he could devise a method to reduce or abolish the mortality from surgical
fever, that would be a triumph to equal his achievement in advancing the
use of general anaesthesia. One possible approach would be to reduce the
time that the surgical wound remained open to invasion by potentially
fatal contagious matter. To prevent haemorrhage during the operation it
was always necessary to close off every artery (or perhaps even vein) that
had been severed by the surgical incision. This was normally done by using

silk or linen threads as ligatures to tie off the bleeding ends of the blood vessels. At the end of the operation there could be several silk ligatures left in place as irritants in the base of the wound, with their long loose ends left hanging from its edge. It was therefore impossible to close the wound immediately; gradually each ligature became swollen with accumulated, perhaps already morbid, tissue fluids; in time the constricted part of the artery became strangled, sloughed off and separated, making it possible for each of the ligatures to be pulled from the wound by its loose ends. Only then, after some weeks, was it possible for the wound to be closed. And during these weeks the patient suffered the distress of a discharging wound and the dreaded pain of repeated dressings while continuing to be exposed to the risk of surgical fever.

In December 1858, in the *Edinburgh Medical Journal*, Simpson described a new method of controlling blood loss during surgical operations that would allow the wound to be closed immediately at the end of the operation and allow it to heal, as it was said, 'by first intention'. He proposed to abandon the use of ligatures. Such a radical notion was inevitably received with considerable scepticism. A year later, on 19 December 1859, he described his new method at greater length to the Royal Society of Edinburgh. In his proposed new procedure, 'acupressure', the artery to be stopped was to be compressed by a pin just as the stem of a flower was pinned to the lapel of a coat: the flower was held against the fabric of the lapel; the pin was passed through a small fold of the fabric on one side of the stem, then across the stem and into a fold of the fabric on the other side of the stem. So, in acupressure, the artery was to be compressed against the tissues underlying the artery by a pin passed first through the underlying tissues on one side of the artery, then across the artery and into the underlying tissues on its other side. Alternatively the artery could be closed by a pin passed behind it and held compressed against overlying tissues kept firmly in place by a wire looped over the protruding sharp end of the pin, then passed across the overlying tissues and looped over the protruding blunt end of the pin. While in place the metal pins would not, like silk or linen ligatures, become impregnated with potentially morbid tissue fluids; and experience with metal sutures in closing vesico-vaginal fistula had shown that ('in despite that urine, the most irritating fluid in the body, constantly bathed one side of the wound') metal was well tolerated by deep tissues and did not provoke local inflammation. And most importantly, the pin could be removed on the second or third day, as soon as the artery was firmly closed by thrombosis, 'leaving nothing whatever in the shape of a foreign body within the wound or in the tissues composing its sides or flaps'.

Simpson had successfully tested acupressure in a number of animal experiments, but since he was not a surgeon he had been unable to try out his technique in practice. It was not until January 1860 that Dr Greig of Dundee agreed 'to give the thing a fair trial', although expressing the opinion that 'of its general adoption I have great doubts'.[4] Greig used acupressure successfully in two cases on 10 and 12 January 1860; Dr Edwards in Edinburgh followed on 30 January. In these three operations the pin was passed through the cutaneous surface of the flap of the wound, then over the line of the bleeding artery to emerge through the skin of the flap on the other side of the artery; in these cases the skin was used as the area of resistance against which the artery was compressed. On 7 July 1860, Peter Handyside, an extramural lecturer on surgery in Edinburgh and a former surgeon at Edinburgh Royal Infirmary, used the same technique in performing the amputation of a severely damaged and gangrenous leg; in all, he used four pins, all inserted through the skin. In these three cases, inserting the needles through the skin meant the wound could be closed immediately at the end of the operation; the pins were withdrawn two days later without disturbing the closed edges of the wound. The *British Medical Journal* reported that acupressure had been shown to have advantages over the ligature in preventing haemorrhage. It was easier to use, the pins did not act in the wound as an irritating foreign body, and they could be withdrawn as soon as the artery was completely closed. While 'the ligature inevitably produces ulceration, suppuration and gangrene at each arterial point at which it is applied, acupressure is not attended by any such severe and morbid consequences. The chances of the union of wounds by primary adhesion [by first intention] should therefore be greater under the arrestment of haemorrhage by acupressure than by ligature. Hence, under the use of acupressure we are entitled to expect that surgical wounds will heal more kindly and close more speedily and that surgical operations will be less frequently attended than at present by the dire effects and perils of surgical fever.'[5]

Peter Handyside continued to use and develop the technique of acupressure. In June 1861 he reported his surprise at how little pressure by the pin on the artery was required to control and stop the bleeding, and how little time was required before the pin could be withdrawn. He advised that long pins were usually unnecessary, as short pins could be used even on the largest arteries.[6] At Aberdeen, William Pirrie and William

Keith introduced no fewer than five new techniques for the application of acupressure, making it, in their experience, 'an excellent method of arresting haemorrhage and accelerating the healing of wounds'.[7] However, a number of prominent and influential surgeons published their objections. James Syme claimed that the ligature did not deserve the charges which Simpson had brought against it. He denied that the presence of a ligature in the wound delayed healing; its presence was helpful, as it acted as a drain preventing the accumulation of blood and pus in the wound. If a ligature was thought undesirable, haemorrhage could be prevented by simple torsion of the artery, and in any case acupressure could only be used to close vessels that lay close under the skin.[8] James Miller claimed it was impossible to insert the pin without the risk of damaging the accompanying vein and nerve.[9] Professor Neudorfer claimed that acupressure could only be used for amputations.[10] Sir William Fergusson thought that the benefits of early closure of the wound by first intention was overrated; it led to the patient using the limb too soon.[11] James Spence also thought early closure undesirable, since it did not allow time for all the fragments produced by the rounding-off of the bone to be extruded from the wound. Many other surgeons were equally unconvinced of the benefits of acupressure. Nevertheless, in 1862 the *British Medical Journal* reported that the practice of acupressure seemed to be gaining ground, even if only very slowly.[12] In the following years, reports of cases in which it had been used successfully continued to appear in the medical press, but almost every one of these reports ended with only the cautious recommendation that acupressure was 'worthy of a more extended trial'.[13]

At the end of December 1864, Simpson at last published his book on acupressure, *A New Method of Arresting Surgical Haemorrhage and of Accelerating Healing*. It was copiously illustrated and ran to no fewer than 580 pages. It included a section entitled 'Answers to the Various Objections Against Acupressure of the Temporary Metallic Compression of Arteries Adduced by Professors Miller, Erichsen, Neudorfer, Spence and Syme', which was also published separately as a pamphlet. In it Simpson gave a full and convincing answer to every objection. To counter Syme's statement that the presence of ligatures in the wound did not delay healing, Simpson quoted from Syme's own article in the *Lancet* of 5 May 1860. Syme's other objections he dismissed completely, as they 'merely proved that Mr Syme simply and entirely misunderstood the subject'.

Soon after the publication of Simpson's pamphlet setting out his 'Answers', an Edinburgh newspaper, the *Edinburgh Daily Review*, commented: 'It is often stated that when Paracelsus wished to show his aversion to any particular author, he immolated the writing he dissented from in the presence of his pupils. We are not aware that this mediaeval practice has ever been adopted in any of our Scottish Universities till last week when it was followed in one of the class-rooms of the University of Edinburgh . . . Mr Syme took [Simpson's] pamphlet into his class-room and without attempting to answer the rather unanswerable arguments it contains in favour of acupressure, he scolded at the author and declared the pamphlet to be a piece of "vulgar insolence". Then came the denouement; with firm hand, teeth compressed, pale lines around his orbits and altogether a most determined and savage expression, he tore up the pamphlet with his fingers, and gave the fragments to his assistant to be consigned to the sawdust box with the other surgical remains.'

The squabble continued. Some months later the *British Medical Journal* reported that 'if a report in an Edinburgh newspaper were to be believed it would seem to be correct that acupressure was just superseding the ligature with the majority of surgeons in Scotland'.[14] James Syme immediately wrote to the editor of the *Journal* to object to its publication of a 'puff to show that acupressure is fully established in Scotland. The truth is that in a few operations it is sometimes possible to arrest bleeding by means of needles although without any advantage and not without the risk of very serious bad consequences. When some obscure surgeon cuts off a leg or an arm in the normal way he has no pretext for sounding his little trumpet. But when he uses acupressure he may send the result to a learned journal or even have the happiness of seeing his name printed in the newspapers.'[15]

Simpson responded, again in a letter to the editor of the *British Medical Journal*. 'In the last number of your Journal you have inserted from my colleague, Professor Syme, a letter animadverting upon acupressure. As his remarks on this subject are only calculated to mislead both you and your readers you must kindly grant me adequate space to reply to them. Let me begin by observing that Mr Syme has no knowledge whatsoever of the subject of acupressure practically, for he has never once yet tried it himself nor ever once seen it employed by others. All the objections which he has ever yet adduced against it are hypothetical and not real. His observations, brief though they are, like all his previous observations on the same subject, grievously inexact in several ways.'[16] Simpson's demolition of Syme's case against acupressure then continued in a further seven and a half columns (over three pages) of the *Journal*. At its end, the editor added an extraordinary note: 'Professor Simpson's letter would have appeared in the Journal of last week had it not, as originally forwarded to us, contained some very personal allusions which we declined to publish.'

Simpson's and Syme's unseemly squabble continued thereafter, but it had no obvious influence on the popularity of acupressure, which was in use in Britain and in most parts of the British Empire, Europe and America. But the extent to which it had taken the place of the ligature was quite uncertain. On 20 June 1868, the *British Medical Journal* announced the appointment of a committee to 'investigate by the collection of clinical facts the value of acupressure as a means of arresting surgical haemorrhage'. If the committee ever met it did not succeed in publishing a report. Whether or not acupressure was ever in more general use than the ligature, it continued to be used in surgical practice for at least a further twenty-five years; a new and improved design of the acupressure pin was introduced as late as 1891.[17] By then, however, new and safer ligatures had already come into use. These new ligatures were the product of many years of experimentation by James Syme's son-in-law, Joseph Lister.

Joseph Lister had been Syme's house surgeon in 1853 and had later married his daughter. He had been an assistant surgeon at Edinburgh Royal Infirmary for four years before being elected Professor of Surgery at Glasgow in 1860. For some years he had been actively interested in the causes of suppuration, but it was one of his new colleagues at Glasgow, the Professor of Chemistry, Thomas Anderson, who drew his attention to the works and writing of Louis Pasteur. From Pasteur he learned that putrefaction was a form of fermentation caused by the growth of minute microscopic beings or 'germs' carried freely in the air. Lister related what he had discovered from Pasteur to the putrefaction that developed in the tissues surrounding ligatures implanted in surgical wounds. The silk or linen thread used as ligatures was soft and porous, clearly capable of absorbing tissue fluids in their interstices but presumably capable also of carrying 'germs' into the wound, giving rise to putrefaction in the tissues with which they came into contact. Lister concluded that ligatures would no longer be a source of putrefaction if they could be rendered free of 'germs' before being inserted into the wound.

He put his theory to the test in December 1867. He tied off the carotid artery of a horse with a piece of purse-silk that had been steeped for some time in a watery solution of carbolic acid. The wound healed cleanly without any evidence of suppuration; when the horse died of old age six weeks later, Lister dissected out the part and found the ligature intact but encased in dense fibrous tissue. Encouraged by this observation, he tried his technique on his first human patient, a lady of fifty-one suffering from an aneurism of the iliac artery. To tie off the artery he used a silk thread that had been steeped for two hours in a strong solution of carbolic acid. He cut both ends of the ligature short and closed the wound completely. The operation went well, but six weeks later the patient died of an aneurism in a different part of her body. At post-mortem, Lister found that the fibrous mass that contained the ligature also contained a small quantity of yellow fluid that, on microscopic examination, contained pus cells. Disappointed, Lister decided to use animal material as his ligature. In an experiment on a calf he found, when the animal was sacrificed, that the ligature appeared at first to be intact; on closer examination it was seen that the ligature had been completely replaced by fibrous tissue without the least evidence of putrefaction. However, ordinary catgut soaked in carbolic was unsuitable for use in practice. It was soft and slippery, difficult to handle, and did not tie into a tight and secure knot. In a long course of experiments over the next several years he tried other antiseptic substances – tannin, chromic acid, chromic alum with sublimate, bichromate of potash and many others – to prepare his catgut ligatures and tried to find the optimum time that they should be immersed in the antiseptic. None of his experimental ligatures proved to be entirely satisfactory. Then in 1870, a year after he had returned to Edinburgh as Professor of Clinical Surgery, he received some chance but crucial assistance from an old itinerant fiddler who came to the Royal Infirmary to play to the patients. One day the old fiddler explained that his fiddle would not work properly because the weather was wet and his fiddle strings were not sufficiently seasoned. Lister discovered that when his catgut was properly seasoned it became 'drier and denser' when steeped in antiseptic fluid, while unseasoned catgut became moist and swollen. Thereafter, in a very lengthy and complicated series of experiments, Lister prepared trial ligatures of seasoned catgut, each batch steeped in one of his various antiseptic substances for various periods of up to a maximum of one year. His final preferred ligature was of properly seasoned catgut that had been steeped in chromic acid and corrosive sublimate for at least two months. He did not decide on this as the best possible ligature until 1908. By then acupressure had already faded from conventional surgical practice.

There can be no doubt that Simpson succeeded in establishing a vogue for acupressure that lasted for almost thirty years. But during that time there was no lessening of the appalling mortality rates in Britain's hospitals; indeed the very limited evidence then available indicated that the death rates were continuing to climb. Simpson attributed this ever-increasing problem to the introduction of general anaesthesia. Surgeons were now able to perform new and adventurous operations that could never have been contemplated without the benefits of anaesthesia, and more and more patients were now ready to submit themselves to even complex surgical treatment, confident in the knowledge that their treatment would not entail almost unendurable agony. These advances in surgery had created a continuing increase in the number of patients seeking admission to hospitals that were already crowded.

Simpson had drawn attention to the risks created by overcrowding in his *Report of the Edinburgh Royal Maternity Hospital* for the years 1844 to 1846.[18] The hospital at No. 3 St John Street was on three storeys, with two rooms on the first and second flats and three on the third flat. The hospital was too small to provide adequate accommodation for the patients as well as for the resident house surgeons and the matron. All of its rooms had low ceilings and were poorly ventilated. During the two-year period under review, 374 patients had been delivered in the hospital, while 1,101 had been delivered in their own homes in various parts of the city. The overall maternal mortality rate was not unduly high for that time (6.3 per 1,000). However the maternal mortality rate among patients delivered in hospital was 18.7 per 1,000; that is, five times the rate for patients delivered at home (3.6 per 1,000).

In his report Simpson wrote: 'Everyone acquainted with hospital practice is well aware of the great liability among patients to febrile inflammatory attacks whenever the wards are overcrowded. I have often stated and taught that, if our hospitals were changed from being crowded palaces with a layer of sick in each flat into villages or cottages with one or at most two patients in each room, a great saving of human life would be effected. And if the village were constructed of iron instead of brick or stone it could be taken down and rebuilt every few years, a matter apparently of much moment in hospital hygiene. It could be erected in any vacant space of ground within or around a city that chanced to be unoccupied and in cases of epidemics the accommodation could always be at once and readily increased.'[19]

Simpson's concept of a prefabricated iron-frame building was not original. It had been described in detail in the second edition of J.C. Loudon's *The Encyclopedia of Cottage, Farm, Villa Architecture* published in 1846. Loudon, who was born in Cambuslang near Glasgow in 1783, had studied botany and chemistry (as it applied to agriculture) at Edinburgh and gone on to make a very successful career as a landscape and city planner. In 1851, Joseph Paxton added low timber walls, roof guttering and an efficient ventilation system in a complex version of Loudon's plan for his glass and iron-framed Crystal Palace for the Great Exhibition. During the Crimean War, Isambard Kingdom Brunel used a simpler variant of Loudon's design to build a prefabricated iron-frame hospital that was erected at Renkioi, near the Scutari Hospital in Turkish Anatolia, in February 1855.

In 1852, Simpson almost succeeded in persuading the Marchioness of Bute to build iron-frame cottages and cottage hospitals on her vast estates in various parts of Britain. Thereafter he continued to advocate the construction of prefabricated iron-frame hospitals in his lectures to students but did not publish his ideas again until 1869, when planning began for a new Royal Infirmary. The existing Edinburgh Royal Infirmary had been built by William Adam in 1741. It had been planned to provide accommodation for only 228 patients; a new 'surgical hospital' had been added in 1832, but a new and larger infirmary was now clearly necessary. Where and how the new infirmary was to be built had become a matter of public debate. On 12 January 1869 Simpson wrote a long letter to the *Scotsman*, Edinburgh's leading newspaper, in which he advised against the construction of a single, grandiose hospital building. Large hospitals, he argued, were dangerous. The source and agency of that danger were still unclear. As we have seen, Pasteur had shown that micro-organisms ('germs'), seemingly present everywhere in the atmosphere, could, in certain circumstances, cause putrefaction – but that germs were the cause of the putrefaction that so commonly developed in surgical wounds had still not been proved. Simpson talked not of germs but of 'morbid emanations', or 'morbific materials'. He believed that patients in hospitals were in danger of acquiring surgical fever, puerperal fever or putrid wounds from morbid emanations from the bodies of other patients who had already become victims of these potentially fatal disorders. He believed that the danger was greatest in the largest hospitals and increased further as the number of sick patients crowding into the hospital went up. And, over the years, as the hospital aged, the morbid emanations from the bodies of sick patients penetrated and accumulated in the fabric of the walls of the hospital, which then became an increasingly potent and ever-present source of risk.

In an investigation to test the validity of his theory, Simpson had already collected the reports of over 1,000 amputations performed in country and provincial practice: he found that 1 in 9 of the patients had died following their operations. This he compared with the results of 1,000 similar amputations performed in the teaching hospitals of Edinburgh, Glasgow and London; in these large and elderly hospitals, 1 in 3 patients

had died. He also noted that in the first years after the new University
College Hospital, London was opened in 1834, only 1 in 7 patients had
died following amputation of a limb, but twenty years later that death
rate had risen to 1 in 3. He concluded that not only were large hospitals
dangerous, they became even more dangerous after they had been in use for
some years. He urged that the new infirmary should be constructed in the
form of a number of temporary single-storey blocks that could be conveniently replaced every few years.

Simpson sent a copy of his *Scotsman* letter to Thomas Holmes, surgeon
at St George's Hospital who, with John Bristowe of St Thomas's Hospital,
in 1864 had written a report for the Privy Council on the hospitals in the
United Kingdom.[20] Holmes replied at length in a letter to the *British
Medical Journal*.[21] He challenged the validity of Simpson's somewhat
sketchy statistics and protested: 'I cannot therefore, at present, admit that
Professor Simpson has proved the startling proposition on which he founds
so sweeping a proposal for the reformation of our hospital system; and I
cannot but regret that such damaging imputations should be cast upon our
great charities in the public press by an author of Professor Simpson's reputation before they have undergone proper discussion in professional circles.'
Holmes' views were widely shared. Simpson's long-standing practice of
communicating his ideas directly to the general lay public before submit-
ting them to the scrutiny of the profession had always caused annoyance.
And surgeons everywhere, together with their physician colleagues, were
reluctant to accept from him judgements that threatened to denigrate the
reputations of the hospitals at which they had all been trained. Even if the
problem Simpson described did exist, his proposed solution was seen as
unduly radical. In the medical press his whole proposition was described
as 'fierce', 'intemperate' and 'nonsense'.

When Holmes questioned his statistics on 23 January 1869, Simpson
had not yet completed the enquiry to which he had referred in his letter to
the *Scotsman*, but he immediately published in the *British Medical Journal*
a short article entitled 'Effects of Hospitalism upon the Mortality of Limb
Amputations'.[22] In it he drew attention to evidence that was already available which supported his case. During the Austro-Prussian War in 1866,
many of the sick and wounded had been cared for in temporary huts and
tents with better results than had been achieved in Germany's 'mansioned
and palatial' hospitals. Since then, 'cottages' had been used with similar
success in association with major hospitals in Berlin, Leipzig, Heidelberg,
Darmstadt, Frankfurt and Kiel. During the civil war in America, more

than a million patients had been treated in small temporary hospitals, and the surgeon-general, William Hammond, reported that they proved to be 'far healthier than permanent buildings'. Simpson was also able to quote from the *Sixth Report of the Medical Officer to the Privy Council* written by Holmes and Bristowe in 1864; from the data in that report Simpson was able to calculate that in large metropolitan hospitals in the United Kingdom at that time, in 1 in every 3 cases of amputation the patient died; in smaller provincial hospitals the ratio was 1 in every 4; and in rural hospitals it was less than 1 in 5.

Simpson presented the statistics on which he rested his case in a series of articles entitled 'On Our Existing System of Hospitalism and its Effects' published in the *Edinburgh Medical Journal* in March, June and December 1869.[23] The statistics derived from a large survey that he had carried out across the United Kingdom on the mortality that resulted from amputations of the thigh, leg and arm. These were the most commonly performed major operations, and deaths following amputations were among the most tragic. Many amputations were performed because of some crippling or life threatening disease of the limb. But the majority were performed on healthy men, women and children who had suffered an accident that had caused the fracture of one or possibly more bones. If the fracture left the overlying skin intact, the bone could be expected to heal. But if the fractured bone had penetrated the skin and left an open wound it was almost inevitable that the wound would suppurate and become a threat to life; it was therefore the normal practice to amputate limbs that had suffered such a 'compound' fracture. Unfortunately, the amputation itself could then cause the death of a previously healthy and active person.[24]

Simpson's survey was intended to discover both the number and the distribution (in private country practice; in provincial hospitals; or in large metropolitan hospitals) of deaths that followed the amputation of a limb. He first sent a printed schedule to 'numerous medical men' in country practice in England and Scotland, in which they were asked to record the number of amputations that they had carried out and the number of deaths that resulted. In England the schedule was sent chiefly to practitioners employed by the Poor Law service; in Scotland schedules were sent to practitioners of his own acquaintance. A number of practitioners failed to return the schedule. Others could not recall the exact number of amputations they had performed, but reported that few if any of their patients had died. In all, 374 country practitioners returned complete records of a total of 2,098 cases in which they had performed amputations of legs (at thigh level), lower legs, arms or forearms. Simpson published their results in full and careful detail. In summary, he reported that the overall mortality from amputations carried out by country practitioners in the patients' homes was 10.8 per cent, or approximately 1 in 9.

Simpson next investigated the mortality following amputations performed in Britain's largest and most prestigious teaching hospitals (Guy's, St Bartholomew's, St George's, the London, Middlesex, King's College, St Mary's, Westminster and Royal Free in London, and, in Scotland, the Royal Infirmaries of Glasgow and Edinburgh). He found the relevant information in the published reports of these institutions. The reports showed that in these large hospitals the mortality following the amputation of legs damaged in accidents was 2 in 3 (64.4 per cent). Even the lesser operation of a forearm amputation carried a mortality of 1 in 6.7 (14.7 per cent). In all, of the total of 2,089 amputations performed in these eleven large hospitals, 855 resulted in the death of the patient.

Simpson wrote: 'Out of 2,089 amputations in hospital practice 855 died; out of 2,098 amputations in country practice 226 died; giving an excess in hospital practice of 629 deaths. This excess in the same class of operations and in the same limited number of patients – in hospital practice as compared with rural practice, in our palatial hospitals as compared with our rural cottages, in large wards as compared with isolated rooms – is certainly much greater than I myself expected. But must the calling of this dismal death role still go on unchallenged and unchecked? Shall this pitiless and deliberate sacrifice of human life to conditions that are more or less preventable be continued or arrested? Do these terrible figures plead eloquently and clamantly for a revision and reform of our hospital system?'

Thomas Holmes immediately protested against the accusation that Britain's great hospitals were deliberately sacrificing the lives they were founded to preserve.[25] It was, he wrote, unfortunate that Simpson's name carried far more weight with the public than did his arguments. His heavy charge against the hospitals was now causing the public to direct their charity elsewhere, in the assumption that the statistics produced by so eminent an author were satisfactory. As Holmes proceeded to show, this was not the case. The statistics Simpson had offered on amputations carried out in rural private practice were totally unreliable. He had not published the number of country surgeons who had been sent his printed schedule, or the number who had failed to return it. Only 374 country surgeons had completed and returned the schedule, and it was natural that those who had done so were those whose operations had been unusually successful and who were glad to have the opportunity to make their successes known.

On the interpretation of the statistics, Holmes wrote: 'Professor Simpson argues about the amputations by a method of reasoning exactly like that [which] would be applied by a statistician to cattle or inanimate objects just as if amputation was an entity. The fact is that an amputation is a process and its success and failure depends on the nature of the case to which it is applied.' From his own hospital, St George's, Holmes was able to produce records that showed that, of all the patients who had been treated for erysipelas, cellulitis or purulent sloughing of their wounds, 38 per cent had been affected before they were admitted to hospital. Clearly, in his view, the life threatening septic condition of their wounds had not been caused by 'hospitalism'.

Simpson was aware that, in suggesting that the splendid hospitals built for the care of the sick poor were less beneficial in practice than they were benevolent in their intentions, he was committing 'medical heresy'. Certainly his articles in the *Edinburgh Medical Journal* criticising 'Our Existing System of Hospitalism' immediately came under attack in the medical press, and not only by Thomas Holmes. In the *British Medical Journal*,[26] Richard Holmes Coote objected to Simpson's quoting one combined mortality for all eleven of Britain's large hospitals; he claimed that, when taken alone, the results at his own hospital, St Bartholomew's, were no worse than those quoted by Simpson for private country practice. In the *Lancet*, George Callender, also of St Bartholomew's Hospital, claimed that the figures given by Simpson for mortality following amputation in provincial hospitals 'did not represent the actual state of the case and no reliance could be put on them';[27] he had figures from an enquiry of his own that flatly contradicted them. Even James Matthews Duncan, Simpson's former assistant, expressed disagreement with his arguments.

As the correspondence continued in the medical press, Simpson stoutly and cogently defended himself against every attack, but it became clear that he was gaining little or no support. Lawson Tait,[28] Simpson's former pupil and assistant and his most loyal supporter, thought the case had been badly presented. The use of the word 'hospitalism' in the title of his articles had been unfortunate; 'hospital' should not have been used as the root of a term that had since become one of reproach. To seem to accuse hospitals of 'sacrificing' large numbers of patients was unnecessarily offensive. But the principal weakness in Simpson's case had been in presenting returns from private practitioners anonymously; had the names been published, the returns would not have been so open to suspicions of exaggeration and bias.

The hostility of the medical profession became apparent at the Annual Meeting of the British Medical Association at Leeds in July 1869. Two days of the meeting were devoted to a debate on 'The Construction of Hospitals'. Apart from Simpson himself, eighteen members made important contributions to the debate, but not one gave more than the most limited support for Simpson's case. John Hughes Bennett rejected Simpson's case completely. He was unwilling to proceed 'on the basis of vague opinion and fallacious assumptions. The Royal Infirmary of Edinburgh was one of the best ever planned and as far as he knew no epidemic had ever originated there.' The other speakers all agreed that Simpson had drawn attention to a real and pressing problem, but no one believed that such a radical solution as he proposed was necessary or even possible: big hospitals would always be required to serve towns and cities with large populations. Some claimed that the only thing necessary to make hospitals safe was to build them with effective systems of ventilation. Others proposed that cases of surgical fever, puerperal fever, and even inflamed or septic wounds should all be treated as cases of contagious disease and isolated in a specially designed area within the hospital; yet others proposed that they should be isolated in separate and specially designed 'cottages' within the grounds of the hospital. Professor Evory Kennedy of Dublin agreed with Simpson that the 'habitat of disease' gradually accumulated in hospitals as they aged until their walls were saturated and dangerous. But he believed this could be prevented by building hospitals of concrete; nevertheless he recommended that patients at risk of puerperal or surgical fever should be admitted not to the general hospitals but to specially constructed isolation pavilions. But much more significantly, Dr Macleod from Glasgow claimed that a solution to Simpson's problem had already been found. Since Professor Joseph Lister had introduced the use of carbolic acid as an antiseptic at Glasgow Royal Infirmary,[29] 'cases of compound fracture had been saved which would have had no chance of being saved by any other method'. Macleod had himself performed no fewer than fifty amputations, with only one death. Simpson's work on 'hospitalism' was already on the point of being sidelined by the introduction of antiseptic surgery.

Nevertheless, from July until November 1869 Simpson continued to defend his position against the onslaught of his many critics in the pages of the *Lancet* and the *British Medical Journal*. Then, in December, he published the last of his articles on Hospitalism in the *Edinburgh Medical Journal*.[30] From 74 hospitals across the United Kingdom, he had collected reports of the outcome of 3,077 cases of limb amputation. He

Table 15.1 Mortality from Limb Amputations and Hospital Size

Size of Hospital (No. of Beds)	Deaths Rate
300 to 500	1 in 2.4
201 to 300	1 in 3.5
101 to 200	1 in 4.4
26 to 100	1 in 5.6
25 or less	1 in 7.1
Patient's home	1 in 9.2

then compared the mortality from operations in hospitals of different sizes (Table 15.1).

In large hospitals of between 300 and 500 beds, 1 patient in 2.4 had died; in hospitals with 25 or fewer beds it was 1 in 7.1. And once again, in spite of all the objections that had earlier been made to his method of obtaining his statistics, he included the mortality in operations carried out in the patients' homes; this he again quoted as 1 in 9.2.

In a final paragraph, now in language less deliberately provocative than the language he had used when first launching his campaign against the lethal dangers of 'hospitalism', Simpson set out the principle that had always been at the heart of his campaign:

> The data establish the general fact or general law in hospital hygiene, that the death rate accompanying amputation of the limbs – and as we may infer, the death rate accompanying other surgical operations and many medical diseases – is regulated in a great and marked manner by the size of the hospitals and the degree of aggregation or segregation in which the patients are treated. But like all other general laws in medicine, this law is subject to many exceptions. Thus a small hospital, if overcrowded with beds and patients, becomes as insalubrious as a large hospital under one roof. On the other hand, a large hospital would be generally made almost as salubrious as a small institution provided that few beds were left scattered over its wards and these wards were well ventilated and often changed. But such exceptions only establish the great and important hygienic law. That, in the treatment of the sick, there is ever a danger in their aggregation and safety only in their segregation; and that our hospitals should be constructed so as to avoid as far as possible the former and secure as far as possible the latter condition.

SIXTEEN

Triumph and Decline

I have touched the highest point of all my greatness
and from that full meridian of my glory I haste now to my setting.
Shakespeare

More than twenty years after his discovery of chloroform, Simpson had still received no honour from the nation to mark his achievement. In Norway, however, he had been made a Knight of the Order of St Olaf. He applied for permission to use the title 'Sir' in Britain but the College of Arms informed him that there was no Royal Licence that would him to allow him to do so.[1] Nevertheless, Simpson proceeded to buy an estate in Linlithgowshire and to matriculate arms simply as James Young Simpson of Strathavon. This setback was very soon corrected. On 6 January 1866, Simpson received a letter from his friend Earl Russell who, only three months earlier, had become Prime Minister in a Whig administration:

Osborne, 3rd January 1866

Dear Dr Simpson,

Your professional merits, especially your introduction of chloro-form, by which difficult operations in surgery have been rendered painless, and which has in many cases made that possible which would otherwise have been too hazardous to attempt, deserve some special recognition from the Crown.

The Queen has been pleased to command me to offer you on these grounds the rank of Baronet. I trust it will be agreeable to you to accept the honour.

I remain,
Yours very truly,
Russell.

For Simpson, a baronetcy was even more acceptable than a knighthood. It conferred a hereditary rank, and that difference was crucially important.

Even while he was still a child, his mother had looked to him to restore the family to the place in society that generations of her ancestors had once enjoyed but that she, in her generation, had lost. A baronetcy would not only honour him, it would also confer a prestigious rank that would pass to future generations of the family. And like his first armorial bearings as James Young Simpson, his new arms, Sir James Y. Simpson, Bart. of Strathavon and the City of Edinburgh, were 'differenced' to include the goshawk Argent that had been part of the arms of his mother's family.

Scottish medical men and Scottish university professors had been knighted before, but none had ever achieved the rank of baronet. When Simpson's honour was announced in the *London Gazette*, messages of congratulation poured in from every part of Britain, the British Empire, Europe and North America. In a letter to his son Walter, Simpson wrote that 'all Edinburgh has apparently been set mad with joy. I have shaken hands for two or three days till my arm is weary and sore.' Together the President of the Royal College of Physicians, the President of the Royal College of Surgeons and the Principal of the university planned a great public dinner to celebrate his award. But the celebration had to be cancelled.

When Simpson received his letter from the Prime Minister, his son David was already very ill. He was suffering from appendicitis for which, at that time, the only treatment was rest, opium and a regime of enemas. At least two thirds of patients could be expected to die of the disease, but after a week David seemed to be recovering. Then suddenly, on 14 January, David died. This was a dreadful blow. Simpson had been immensely proud of his oldest son. David had been a distinguished student at Edinburgh and had taken his MD degree in 1863. In the same year, he was also awarded the licences of both the Royal College of Physicians and the Royal College of Surgeons of Edinburgh. After a short appointment as a house physician at Edinburgh Royal Infirmary, his father had sent him to spend some time at the leading hospitals in Berlin, Vienna and Prague. When he returned in March 1865, he joined his father as one of his assistants. He became Senior President of the Royal Medical Society, and had already published his first article in the medical literature. When he became ill in January 1866, he was already managing his father's practice and it had seemed probable that, in time, he would inherit not only his father's title but also his practice and his chair as Professor of Midwifery.

At David's death, Simpson's seventeen-year-old daughter Jessie was distraught. From infancy she had been chronically unwell.[2] She had always been particularly close to David, and in the months after his return from the Continent she had come to rely on him for comfort as her health gradually worsened. Only David had been trusted to change the dressings on the weeping sores that covered so much of her body. When he died, her condition deteriorated rapidly and four weeks later, on 13 February, she too died. Simpson had loved Jessie even more tenderly than his other children, and her loss, added to the loss of his son and heir, was hard to bear.

Even before the award of his baronetcy and the loss of two of his children, his personal life had already begun a slow decline into sickness, grief and disappointment. From the age of fourteen, when he left home to become a student at Edinburgh, he had suffered periods of depression as well as periods of elation and hyperactivity; and when depressed or frustrated, he often retired to bed for three or four days because of brief attacks of 'rheumatism' or 'low fever'. His first session as Professor of Midwifery had been marred by recurring rancorous confrontations with the more senior members of the Medical Faculty; when the session ended, he suffered a particularly prolonged attack of 'low fever' and kept to his room for almost two weeks. Then, in 1855, his physical symptoms changed. He began to suffer attacks of acute chest pain, and although they were still attributed to 'rheumatism', he was not slow to think that his symptoms might have a more sinister significance. When his daughter Eve was born in December of that year, he arranged for her godmother, Lady Blantyre, to become her legal guardian in the event of his death.

In the years that followed he had further frequent attacks of crushing chest pain, but he was able to continue his otherwise full and active life until August 1865. He then suffered a more protracted and crippling attack of pain. His recovery, on this occasion, was slow, and when his symptoms at last subsided, he spent almost two months resting at Captain Petrie's house on the Isle of Man before returning to Edinburgh in the autumn for the new academic session. When David, then Jessie, died in January 1866, Simpson was still not completely well.

It was not possible for Simpson to share his problems and his anxieties with his wife. Even before Eve was born, Jessie had begun to withdraw to the solace of her religious tracts and comforting whiffs of chloroform; a pane of glass was later fitted in the door of her room so that her behaviour could be supervised.[3] Simpson continued to speak to and of her in terms of loyalty and affection, but she now lived an emotional and very personal life at a distance from his. Simpson felt alone with his grief. Of his nine children, only four were now still alive. His second son, Walter, who had been sent abroad for a year to improve his French and German, had extended his tour and was now exploring archaeological sites in Egypt. William, Magnus, and Eve (aged fourteen, twelve and ten) were either away at school or at Viewbank under the care of his wife's sister. Simpson turned to his religion and his church.

Many years before, in 1843, Simpson had been one of those who walked out of the meeting of the General Assembly of the Church of Scotland at St Andrew's Church in George Street and, led by Thomas Chalmers, had then marched down to Tanfield Hall in the Canonmills to form a new Free Church of Scotland.[4] The split in the Church had followed ten years of differences between the 'Moderates', for whom religion was a matter of social decency, private virtue and a quiet accommodation with the state, and the 'High Flyers', who were eager to promote Evangelism, and who organised active public charity and the extension of the Church to serve the new poor of Scotland's soulless industrial towns. But, in 1843, the immediate difference was over Church government. For many years the Moderates had been the dominant party but, in 1833, the High Flyers at last became the majority party in the General Assembly. The General Assembly now challenged the right of the patrons of a parish church (the Crown or the local landlords) to appoint a minister against the preferences and wishes of the congregation. The matter was referred to the Court of Session in Edinburgh, which ruled in favour of the rights of the patrons; on appeal, the ruling of the Court of Session was upheld by Parliament. However, the evangelical High Flyers within the Church took as their preferred authority the Confession of Faith of 1646 and insisted that 'in all matters touching the doctrine, government and discipline of the Church, her judicatories possess an exclusive jurisdiction founded on the Word of God'. When they walked out of the General Assembly of the Church of Scotland in 1843 to form a Free Church, free of the interference of the state, Simpson walked with them. Although he had private reservations on important matters included in the Confession of Faith, he believed that the church should be free of state interference, and he agreed with the High Flyers' policy on public charity. He therefore left St Stephen's Church in the New Town[5] and joined the Rev. Thomas Guthrie's congregation at the Free St John's Church at Castlehill.

Simpson was invited to become an elder of the new Free Church, but this would have required declaring himself bound by belief in all the doctrines of the Westminster Confession of Faith. Simpson explained that while he most heartily and sincerely believed in the general theology laid down in the Westminster Confession, there were certain doctrines in the

Confession from which he felt obliged to differ. Chapter IV of the Confession stated that: 'It pleased God the Father, Son, and Holy Ghost, in the beginning, to create or make of nothing the world, and all things therein, whether visible or invisible, in the space of six days.' Simpson could not subscribe to the belief that 'nothing of this world existed some six or seven thousand years ago'. Chapter XXI stated that 'prayer, being one special part of religious worship, is by God required of all men'. Simpson could not accept that the practice of prayer could alter the settled purpose of an unchanging God. He therefore felt unable to be an elder of his Church.

He continued as a loyal member of the congregation, but his friend (and chosen mentor on matters of religion), the Rev. John Duns, Professor of Natural Philosophy at New College, Edinburgh,[6] saw Simpson's religion as simply 'baptized heathenism'[7] and his regular church attendance no more than part of a 'system of becomingness' proper to a Christian physician. Certainly, at this time, religion did not have a central role in Simpson's life and thought. When, in the late 1840s, he became interested in mesmerism and also curious about the relationship between the human spirit and the human body, he chose to consult not a theologian but the philosophers Professor Sir William Hamilton and Professor Samuel Brown, as well as the works of Thomas De Quincey.

However, as his periods of illness increased in the 1850s, his thoughts began to turn more and more to mortality and 'the relationship of the soul to God'.[8] He had already witnessed the deaths of two of his children – but Maggie died at the age of four and Mary at the age of two, both of them too young to express an awareness of God or the hereafter. But his friend John Reid had died in 1849, at the age of forty, after a year of misery and suffering caused by cancer of the tongue. Simpson had been profoundly moved by Reid's saying many times during his illness that he found comfort in the certainty that, in the end, the world would 'be behind' and that he would be saved by 'the atoning sacrifice of his Saviour'. But Simpson was unable to share John Reid's faith and certainty. As he explained to John Duns: 'I wish to come to Christ but I do not see him.' He found what he saw as the 'wildly extravagant' claims and views of the Free Church's Evangelical ministers very unhelpful. 'Why do they not preach the gospel and not give out views that spring from the influence of a diseased body on the mind?' he asked. But the chief intellectual barrier was not the extravagant style of Evangelical preaching, but Simpson's inability to accept the Biblical version of the Creation. To overcome this difficulty, John Duns re-introduced Simpson to the concept of Natural Theology. Paley's *Natural Theology* was one of the books that Simpson bought when he was a first-year student in 1825, and he had discussed the *Bridgewater Treatises*[9] in his correspondence with his future wife in 1838, but for Simpson, in those years, theology was no more than a casual and passing interest.

William Paley first published his *Natural Theology; or, Evidences of the Existence and Attributes of the Deity* in 1802. Later, in the 1830s, his ideas were taken up by the editors of a number of radical and scientific journals, notably Thomas Wakley of the *Lancet*, and by the Society for the Promotion of Christian Knowledge. Interest in Natural Theology had increased even further in response to the publication of *Vestiges of the Natural History of Creation* in 1844. Natural Theology held that true belief in God need not come by divine inspiration and by close and persistent attention to the study of the Bible. The existence of God could be induced by reasoning upwards from the observation of nature and from a true 'scientific' perception of the mechanics and intelligent design of the universe; the design and benevolence of God were to be seen everywhere in the natural world.[10]

After many intense discussions with John Duns, Simpson came to accept that a 'day' in the text of the Bible should be equated with an 'epoch' in the natural world. And the evolution of the earth, and everything on the earth, was part of God's design and the proof of His existence, His power and His wisdom.

At Christmas 1861, after a long struggle with his beliefs, Simpson felt he had at last found God and was 'saved'. It was, he said, 'My first happy Christmas. My only happy one.' Duns advised him that, before attesting to his new-found faith in public, he should take time to study the Bible and review his understanding of its texts and its often obscure truths. However, this would have been against Simpson's nature. He at once made his new faith abundantly clear in his correspondence and in everyday conversation. That same faith gave him comfort when, little more than a month after his conversion, his third son, James, died after a lifetime of ill health. Simpson was able to write: 'I gave him over into the arms of Christ in the full faith that he was utterly safe in His keeping, and that after all, though here we all loved him dearly, God loves him more, infinitely more.'[11] Two weeks later, he was invited to preach at one of a series of Special Religious Services at the Queen Street Hall. To an audience of almost 2,000 he 'spoke for Jesus'. He talked at length of the careless souls living regardless of their future. 'Is it not one of the astounding things to be seen around us that men, actively engaged in the pursuit of this life and neglecting nothing which can secure success in these pursuits, should yet be found so entirely to forget to make their peace with God.' Only a few days later he addressed a medical students' meeting arranged by the Edinburgh Medical Missionary Society. He talked to them of sin: 'An unnecessary angry thought is sin. An unchaste thought is sin. Every idle word is sin. How many then are our sins? God not only knows every action, but he reads every thought of our hearts. Let us remember that in the sight of God, our sins deserve death.' In 1862, he published a pamphlet entitled *Dead in Trespasses and Sins*. He was now expressing the views that he had so recently thought of as extravagant in the preaching of Evangelical ministers. Many of his medical colleagues, who had known him as he made his way in his profession, regarded this very public and very sudden profession of his faith as a piece of eccentric cant.[12] But those who knew him best never doubted his sincerity. Until his death the events of Simpson's life were acted out against a background of his religion and his declining health.

In June 1866, he was invited to go to Oxford to receive the degree of Doctor of Civil Law. He was well enough to go, and being conferred with the degree gave him great pleasure and pride. But on the way home by way of Liverpool he had a sudden and lasting pain in his left leg which made it almost impossible for him to walk. He did not recover during the summer, and when the new academic session began he was obliged to apply to the Senatus for leave of absence and permission to employ a locum to take charge of his classes. When the university classes re-assembled in the new year of 1867 he was still weak and experienced difficulty in walking, but he felt able to take his own classes. However, he was unable to climb even one flight of stairs, and a lecture theatre had to be found for him on the ground floor.

In April, he enjoyed a week in Switzerland, and before returning home he reported to his family that he felt much better and stronger than when he had left home, and that 'I walked more than I ever expected to do in life again'. By the summer he was once again attending to his private patients, lecturing at the university and teaching medical students at the bedside at the Royal Infirmary. He was also preaching at Evangelical meetings in Edinburgh, in the neighbouring counties and, on occasion, even further afield. But his old physical vigour had gone, and in December he suffered a further blow. In a letter to Walter he wrote: 'I am in great distress. You cannot imagine the pain I have felt in weeks past as the idea came burning back on me by night and by day that I have used you so ill by squandering the money which I should have collected for you as my heir. Often I wish I could unbaronet myself.' His estates in Tobago had proved unprofitable, and suddenly a shale-oil company that he owned in Linlithgowshire failed completely. Walter's reply was comforting: 'If I were offered a baronetcy and £5,000 or no baronetcy and £50,000 I should prefer the former.'

Simpson was now frequently confined to his room for several days at a time. However, he did not allow the time to go to waste, writing two more important works on archaeology: *Is the Great Pyramid of Gizeh a Meteorological Monument?* and *Archaic Sculpturing of Cups, Circles etc upon Stones and Rocks, in Scotland, England and other Countries.*[13] For the *Medical Gazette* he wrote a thoughtful but uncontroversial article on measures to control the spread of smallpox. But thereafter, when writing on professional and academic matters, his style changed. Until now, in all his many publications, he had been sharply belligerent only when defending himself from unfair or ill-informed criticism; in 1867 he became the attacker.

Between March and April of that year Joseph Lister published a series of articles in the *Lancet* on the use of carbolic acid as an antiseptic in the practice of surgery, and in September he presented an overall account of the subject to a meeting of the British Medical Association in Dublin. His paper was reported in full in the *Lancet*.[14] Simpson responded in a piece also published in the journal.[15] He stated that Lister's 'use and application of [carbolic] and his theories of its mode of action were not in any way original'. It had been used in France by Lemaire since 1863, and in Edinburgh by Professor Spence since 1864. Lister had written that of all those who had visited Glasgow Royal Infirmary to view his treatment of wounds, abscesses, compound fractures, etc. with carbolic, 'not one had ever expressed the slightest doubt that the system in question was not original'. Simpson commented that he regretted 'the strange and almost incomprehensible want of knowledge with which Mr Lister charges his professional visitors and if Mr Lister had taken the slightest trouble to search the English literature alone, he would have convinced himself of his grave error'. This was unfair. Lister had not claimed to be the first to use carbolic; as he had made clear, it was his 'system', the way in which he used it, that was original.

Lister also reported that since he had introduced his system of antisepsis, 'wounds and abscesses no longer poison the atmosphere with putrid exhalations, my wards have changed completely their character so that, during the last nine months, not a single incidence of pyaemia, hospital gangrene or erysipelas has occurred in them'. Simpson pointed out that in Aberdeen, of twelve cases of excision of breast tumours treated by Professor Pirrie with acupressure, eight of the resulting wounds had closed without the formation of a single drop of pus. He asked if Mr Lister 'had ever met in the Glasgow Hospital with one single case of such healing when the ligature and carbolic acid were used'. And Professor Pirrie had also reported that since he had introduced the routine use of acupressure, pyaemia had disappeared from his wards. As criticism of Lister this was not only unkind, it was irrelevant. Lister had reported his experience of his own system, but he had not attempted any comparison with alternative forms of treatment.

The content and style of Simpson's attack in the *Lancet* caused great annoyance, particularly in Edinburgh, where Lister had made many friends during his six years there; it infuriated his father-in-law, Professor Syme. Simpson also angered almost all the professors of Edinburgh with a powerful paper presented to the Edinburgh Philosophical Institution at the end of 1867. Simpson was President of the institution but, because of his poor health, he had been absent from many of its recent meetings. He was absent in November when Robert Lowe MP lectured on the relationship between education and the state, but he prepared a long and powerful paper on the same subject for presentation at the institute's next meeting in December. He later explained to John Duns that his intention was simply to suggest that study of the classics should not be 'imperative on all' university students but should be taught to the highest level to all those whose tastes or careers made it necessary; and that modern languages should be 'imperative to all not only as classics now are but conversationally; that natural science should have pre-eminence assigned to it by demanding a knowledge of one branch at least from every student before he is sent into work where such information is valuable.' However, the manner in which he presented his case to the meeting was calculated to cause maximum offence.

He claimed that the best speakers in the House of Commons were John Bright and Richard Cobden (both Radicals), and they could speak English very well without a knowledge of Latin or Greek; that half of the magazine literature of the day was written by women who had, of course, no Latin or Greek; and that many of the most financially successful novelists of the day were women, who did not acknowledge any need of Latin or Greek. It was so often said that Latin and Greek were necessary to impart the highest kind of taste and imagination, yet Bunyan and Shakespeare were not classical scholars. He suggested that, if students were to study Latin and Greek because those languages were the origin of some English words, it would better for them to study Anglo-Saxon, which was the origin of many more.

He argued that the classics provided dreadful descriptions of the seething sea of demoralisation which had prevailed in ancient Greece and Rome, and that the books put into the hands of the young – those by Horace, Ovid, Martial, Juvenal, etc. – were obscene and should be withdrawn from sale. If mothers knew the improprieties in some of the works given to their children as textbooks and prizes, they would rise in rebellion. It was so often claimed that Latin and Greek were the best means of training the mind; Simpson insisted that they tended to make the mind stunted and deformed instead of developing it: they cultivated memory and left uncultivated the higher powers of observation so necessary for science and for life. Students of Latin and Greek expended their powers on words and names invented by man, instead of on the works and wonders of God as revealed in nature.

This diatribe could not have upset the feelings, convictions and prejudices of the great majority of the professors of the university at a more unfortunate time. In February 1868, Sir David Brewster, the Principal of Edinburgh University, died. When he was appointed in 1859, Simpson had been his most prominent supporter; when he died, the Royal Society of Edinburgh called on Simpson to give the oration in his honour. It was generally assumed in Edinburgh that Simpson would be his successor. Robert Christison, who had been a professor at Edinburgh for almost forty years and was a member of every one of the university's influential committees, could have commanded considerable support, but he chose not to allow his name to go forward for election. The two candidates were therefore Simpson and Sir Alexander Grant, Bart., a former Professor of History and Political Economy, and now Principal of Bombay University.

The power to appoint the Principal was vested in the Court of Curators, a committee of seven members, four of whom were nominated by the university and three by the Town Council. The university was represented by John Inglis, the Lord Justice General; Sir William Gibson Craig, MP for Midlothian; Adam Black, formerly MP for Edinburgh; and the advocate David Milne Home. The Town Council was represented by the Lord Provost, Baillie Russell and Baillie Fyfe. During the canvass the members of the Court of Curators made no secret of their voting intentions, and it became clear that on 18 July, the day originally fixed for the election, Simpson could expect to win by a majority of one. But, as the *Lancet* reported, 'the appointment of the Principal of the University of Edinburgh was one of the most unseemly things that had occurred for years'.[16]

At the eleventh hour, the Court of Curators received a petition signed by twelve senior professors, including seven medical professors, stating that 'having heard with regret that it is the intention of the Curators to appoint Sir James Simpson to the office of Principal of the University and having reason to believe that the Curators were proceeding under the impression that this appointment would be acceptable to the Senatus generally we deem it our duty to express the conviction that it would not be to the advantage of the University'. According to a report in the *Lancet*, their 'principal objections to Simpson were that he was a physician, especially an obstetric physician, who had disparaged the importance of classics in education'. But it was perhaps also relevant that the seven medical professors who signed the petition all had personal differences with Simpson that had never been completely resolved.[17] The Curators understood the petition from as many as twelve professors was a threat that a substantial number, even a majority, of the university's leading professors would withdraw from the Senatus should Simpson be appointed. They postponed the election until 6 July.

Within three days of their decision they received a petition from over 800 graduates of the university, who stated that Simpson's appointment would not only add lustre to the university but would be highly advantageous to its interests and prosperity. However, there were further irregular and unpleasant objections to his election. Professor Robert Christison delivered to a member of the Court of Curators a communication that he had received from one of his colleagues. It was found to contain defamatory comments on Simpson's character; the elector passed the document to the clerk of the Court of Curators, who destroyed it.[18] Later, a member of the public, who had no connection with the university, wrote a letter to the Curators attacking Simpson's moral character and the sincerity of his religious professions. The letter and its contents were investigated on Simpson's behalf by an advocate, Thomas McKie; a former President of the College of Physicians, Alexander Wood; and Simpson's friend, John Pender of Crumpsall House, Manchester. They found the letter to be clearly libellous, but Simpson refused to take legal action. When the letter's writer was discovered and confronted, he retracted all of his accusations and apologised. However, the damage was done. Adam Black decided to withdraw his support from Simpson and to vote instead for Sir Alexander Grant. At the election on 6 July, only the Lord Provost and the two Baillies voted for Simpson, who therefore lost the office of Principal of Edinburgh University by a single vote. The *Lancet* commented that: 'If such men are not to be honoured by our universities, so much the worse for the universities.'[19] The Provost, Magistrates and Council of the City of Edinburgh promptly demonstrated their profound disagreement with the decision of the university's Court of Curators: they awarded Simpson their highest honour, the Freedom of the City.

Simpson was not only disappointed at his failure to be elected Principal of Edinburgh University, he was also deeply humiliated by the underhand and demeaning campaign that had been mounted against him. But it became clear to his family and friends that he no longer had the strength and confidence to counter or shrug off the injustice and slanders of his enemies.[20] It also soon became evident that he was unable to demonstate his former vigour in promoting his ideas for the advance of medicine and surgery. He was convinced that his new plan to eliminate 'hospitalism' was even more important than his discovery of chloroform, but he failed to push it forward with any of his old spirit and determination.

Nevertheless, Simpson was still ready to take up yet another cause. In 1869, the only woman medical graduate who was registered to practise in Britain was Elizabeth Blackwell. After graduating from Geneva College, New York in 1849, she travelled to Europe for two years of further study. Her reception in Paris was hostile. In London, she was treated as an interesting, even amusing, anomaly. Simpson, however, was sympathetic; he made public his support for the admission of women to the medical profession and invited her to Edinburgh. In 1851, Elizabeth Blackwell returned to America. When, three years later, her sister Emily graduated from Case Western Reserve University, she contacted Simpson, who agreed to take Emily as his assistant for a year. The experiment proved very successful, and it attracted notice and comment. Simpson became recognised as one of the few senior members of the profession in Britain who believed that women should have their place in the practice of medicine.

Some years later, in 1869, Sophia Jex-Blake, unable to find a medical school in England willing to accept women as students, applied for admission to Edinburgh and wrote to Simpson asking for his support. Simpson invited to her to breakfast. Later that day she wrote to a friend: 'He was, of course, quite favourable to my application and I am to breakfast with him again tomorrow and hear what he will do about it. He is so unreliable though I don't know how to make sure of his doing it.' Miss Jex-Blake, aware that Simpson was about to leave for a short holiday in Rome, feared that he would not find time to help. However, before leaving he persuaded the Medical Faculty to agree that 'as an experiment', Miss Jex-Blake should be allowed to attend the class of any professor who was willing to teach her.[21]

The new Principal of the University, Sir Alexander Grant, later wrote that this was 'an imprudent step that led to disaster.'[22] When the matter was referred to the University Court, it decided that: 'for one lady alone no change could be made in the University custom; that ladies could not be admitted to study medicine in the same classes as the students; but that, if sufficient number of ladies could be brought together and if any medical professors would give them lectures at separate hours, there could be no objection.' Miss Jex-Blake found no difficulty in recruiting five other young women who wished to join her, but it soon emerged that a number of the medical professors who had large and lucrative practices were unwilling to give up time to teach their subjects to only half a dozen fee-paying students. However, the regulations of the university allowed the women to complete the curriculum for the MD degree by studying, at Edinburgh's extramural schools, the subjects they had not been able to study at the university. But when the women had duly completed the full four-year curriculum, the Senatus of the university ruled that that they could not graduate. The women challenged this decision in the courts, at first with success, but on appeal a majority of the judges ruled that the university had no power of admitting women to its degrees.

This unfortunate and frustrating outcome of his efforts in support of the education of women could not have been foreseen when, in April 1869, Simpson returned to Edinburgh after a pleasant few weeks visiting the antiquities of Rome. He was well enough to resume his private practice, but recurring attacks of crushing pain in the chest and upper arms were now, at last, recognized as *angina pectoris*. And he was soon drawn into the stress of his part in one of the great scandals of Victorian times: the birth of an illegitimate child to Lady Mordaunt of Walton d'Eiville in Warwickshire.

Harriet Mordaunt was the daughter of Sir Thomas Moncreiffe of Moncreiffe House near Perth. In 1866, at the age of eighteen, she married the much older Sir Charles Mordaunt. Sir Charles preferred country life, shooting and fishing on his estates in England; the beautiful and vivacious Harriet was already a member of the fashionable set centred on the Prince of Wales and, before the marriage, it was agreed that she would be allowed to continue in the way of life she had come to enjoy, and that her friends would always be welcome at Walton.[23] Later that year she became pregnant, and when the child was born, one month before term on 27 February 1867, she seemed confused and greatly distressed. She showed little affection for her baby daughter and was convinced that the discharge from the baby's eyes was due to gonorrhea. Dr Orford, who had been in charge of Harriet's delivery, decided that both the child's small size and the discharge from her eyes were probably attributable to gonorrhea, and that Harriet's strange behavior was due to hysteria. Harriet continued to behave oddly and on 8 March, she suddenly informed her husband that the child was not his and that she had 'done very wrong with Lord Cole, Sir Frederic Johnstone and the Prince of Wales and with others often in open day'. Sir Charles was deeply shocked but did not believe her, accepting Dr Orford's conclusion that she was simply hysterical. Her father was not convinced, however, and asked Simpson to see her.

On 15 April 1868 Simpson travelled to Warwickshire, and there he showed some of his old fire. After talking at some length to Harriet, and examining the baby's eyes and measuring her weight and length, he announced the baby had been born six weeks prematurely and showed no evidence of gonorrhea; he also announced that Harriet was suffering from puerperal insanity. He reprimanded Dr Orford for having failed to measure the baby, and when Orford continued to insist that Harriet was only hysterical and not insane, Simpson warned him that her father might bring an action for conspiracy.

Simpson was aware of the rift developing between Harriet's husband and her father. Sir Charles had calculated that at the probable time of the baby's conception he had been in Norway, and his servants confirmed that all three of the men named by Harriet had spent time alone with Harriet during his absence. He decided to divorce his wife. Sir Thomas hoped to avoid divorce proceedings and the resulting scandal by establishing that Harriet was insane and unable to respond to a petition for divorce.

While preparations for a divorce trial dragged on, Harriet was kept isolated under the care of a nurse. By April 1869, the lawyers acting in her husband's interest believed that they had accumulated evidence enough to convince a jury that Harriet was sane, and they lodged his petition for divorce. However, in May, her father asked Simpson to visit Harriet again in London; he found her even more profoundly insane than she had been the previous summer.

The trial was set for 12 February 1870. On the evening of 11 February, Simpson had already left home to travel overnight to London when a telegram arrived at midnight to inform him that the trial had been postponed until 16 February. In London, Simpson visited Lady Mordaunt, at the house at Bickley where she was confined, and returned to Edinburgh. There he saw a few patients before travelling south again overnight on 15 February.

When he was called to give evidence, the barrister acting for the Moncreiffe family reminded the court that Sir James Simpson had a reputation that reached far beyond the United Kingdom. Simpson presented his evidence that Harriet was insane, and was later supported by Dr Alderson, President of the College of Physicians of London; Dr Gull, personal physician to the Royal Family; and the eminent psychiatrist John Tuke. Their evidence was accepted. The Prince of Wales was now able, without fear of competent contradiction, to tell the court (to loud applause) that he had had 'no improper familiarity with Harriet'. Since Harriet was insane she could not answer to her husband's petition for divorce. Sir Charles remained married, and Harriet remained confined in the care of a mental nurse.

Simpson returned overnight to Edinburgh on 17 February. During the journey he suffered a severe attack of chest pain, which passed off slowly when he lay down on the carriage floor. Next day, as arranged, he visited a patient in Forfar and had to wait for his train at a very cold and windy station at Perth. When he reached home he had to be helped to his room and into bed. He was now in heart failure. He was breathless, his ankles were swollen, his heartbeat was irregular and his chest pain came and went. For three weeks he welcomed visitors and was pleased to listen to what they had to say but was hardly able to reply. In April, he asked to be moved to the drawing room, which he thought would be more suitable for receiving those who wished to see him. He knew he was dying, and his most frequent and most comforting companion was his nephew Robert, who shared his deep religious faith.[24] On 5 May, he was barely conscious and could no longer recognise members of his family. Jessie, his brother Alexander and other members of his family were with him when he died peacefully on 6 May 1870.

Letters of condolence addressed to Jessie flooded in, it seemed from everywhere and from every rank in society, from the Queen to the poorest of his former patients. Processions of friends and complete strangers called at 52 Queen Street to pay their respects. It was too much for Jessie. For several years she had not played a central role in Simpson's life. What evidence survives suggests that they had long been on affectionate but somewhat distant terms. In the accounts of his life written by the members of his family and the friends who knew them best, she seems only a shadowy figure.[25] While her sister Williamina and her son, now Sir Walter, remained in charge in Edinburgh, Jessie was taken north into the care of the Rev. Alexander Stewart and his wife at Killin in Perthshire. Only a few weeks later, on 17 June, she died. Tragically, the cause of her sudden and unexpected death, as recorded on the death certificate, was 'cardiac syncope', the fatal disorder that John Snow had identified as a hazard of the inhalation of chloroform.

In May, every medical journal carried an obituary of Simpson. The *Lancet* found that much of what was written about him was in error, either in the direction of worshipping him as a man divinely inspired, or in the direction of disparaging even his greatest merits.[26] The journal conceded that he had failings, but held that his failings were far outweighed by his virtues and achievements. It commended his humanity and his concern for those in pain or at risk of a miserable and perhaps unnecessary death. It praised his remarkable ability to conceive of possibilities to bring them relief. It also admired Simpson for having maintained 'an activity, a power of work, which almost constituted greatness of itself, a power of work which was all the more wonderful because he was not strong and was frequently laid aside for a day or two together by headaches and prostration; and an activity that bore him through thirty years of such anxious, original, responsible and successful practice as has perhaps no precedent.'

Public opinion in Britain demanded that Simpson should be buried in honour in Westminster Abbey. The Dean conveyed the offer to his family, but Sir Walter decided that his father should be buried in Edinburgh alongside his children. During the funeral on Friday 13 May, all business stopped in Edinburgh, flags on every public building flew at half-mast and bells tolled from every church. On its way from Queen Street to the cemetery at Warriston, the coffin was followed by the Lord Provost, Magistrates and Council of Edinburgh, the Town Council of Bathgate, the Fellows of the Royal College of Physicians and the Royal College of Surgeons, the Senate and officers of the University, the Faculty of Advocates, the Writers to the Signet, and representatives of over thirty other learned societies and corporate bodies in Edinburgh. It was the largest funeral there had ever been in the city. The hundreds who walked in the long procession were outnumbered by the many thousands – some said 80,000, some said 100,000 – who lined the streets. People came from every part of Britain to pay their respects to a physician who had touched and eased the lives of every one of them, and the lives of many thousands more in almost every part of the world.

Epilogue

Lord, now lettest thy servant depart in peace, according to thy word.
St Luke

Very early in his life, Simpson had been chosen by his mother as the son who could recover for the family the distinguished position in society that her forebears had once held. At the end of his life, he had good reason to be satisfied that he had done all that his mother had required of him. But if he had ever nurtured an ambition to found a medical dynasty at Edinburgh University on the model of Alexander Monro *primus*, Alexander Monro *secundus* and Alexander Monro *tertius*, that ambition came to nothing. Five of his nine children had predeceased him and he was not, as he had once hoped, succeeded in his university chair by his son David. He was succeeded by his nephew, Alexander Simpson, and although Alexander occupied the chair for twice as many years as his uncle, he never did so with anything approaching the same distinction.

However, already in his own career Simpson had achieved greatness. Two hundred years after his birth, his contributions to the science and practice of medicine are still admired and celebrated. Much less is now remembered of the person behind the achievements. At his death, he was mourned by many members of his profession as a Prometheus among physicians. But he did not have the divine gift of vision and forethought that the name implies. Since childhood, he had shown qualities that promised success: intelligence, prodigious memory, industry and a strong sense of purpose, but the source of his greatness was a combination of ambition and desperation.

His mother had fired his ambition. Almost randomly, at the age of fifteen, he had chosen a career in the medical profession as his route to the eminence that was expected of him. But he soon became aware of the difficulties that faced him as a young man without family or political influence. He witnessed the persecution and destruction of his friend Robert

Knox. Knox was the leading comparative anatomist of his time, but he had no family influence and he held political views that were not acceptable to the established authorities in Edinburgh. Simpson was also aware of the remarkable skill and patience that had been required of his mentor, John Thomson, in overcoming these same disadvantages.

Throughout his career, Simpson never doubted his ability, his judgement or his purpose, but he continued to fear that he might be denied success by the political prejudice, personal antipathy or simple inadequacy of others. That constant fear led to feelings of desperation and behaviour that was resented as arrogance. As written in St Matthew, Simpson firmly believed that he who was not for him was against him. And many were against him. He was a reformer. He was able to see opportunities for much-needed advances in medical and surgical practice at a time when the conservative majority of the medical profession was not ready for change. He repeatedly infuriated that conservative majority by publishing pamphlets with the deliberate aim of enlisting the power of public opinion to force change upon them. And he was especially infuriating when he strayed from his own professed discipline of obstetrics to promote change in branches of medicine and surgery in which he had no personal experience or acknowledged authority. He provoked quarrels and made enemies; and as he was never willing to yield to opposition or to accept defeat, he earned a reputation as a man who never forgave his enemies. His frustrations and his quarrels had their cost, 'laying him aside for days together by headaches and *prostration*.'[1]

Yet this belligerent pattern of behaviour did not extend beyond his life as a desperately ambitious medical scientist. It was an aspect of his character that his legions of charmed and devoted patients could hardly have imagined. His house in Queen Street was the centre of a large community of friends and acquaintances. And it was well known that anyone of distinction, women as well as men, visiting or passing through Edinburgh, was welcome at 52 Queen Street. Florence Nightingale,[2] John Ruskin, Earl Russell, Elizabeth Gaskell, David Livingstone, William Makepeace Thackeray, Caroline Norton, Hans Andersen, Sarah Siddons and many others were happy to discuss their work, their experiences, their plans and their opinions at his table.

He greatly enjoyed the many times he spent as the guest of the greatest and most cultivated of Scotland's aristocratic families, the Argylls, Sutherlands and Hamiltons. He was confident enough of his own greatness never to feel insecure in their company. They shared many of his interests and, equally, he could talk easily in their language. But he took no liberties, just as he never expected liberties from his many friends among the fisher folk of Newhaven or among the poor of Edinburgh.

He greatly valued all the many honours that he received, but he took particular pride in those that had been awarded not by medical institutions, but by civic bodies; first among these were his Order of St Olaf, his Freedom of the City of Edinburgh and his baronetcy. He was also flattered by the large sums that he could earn from his private practice; a single fee of £300 (the equivalent of £22,500 now) was not unknown. He found great satisfaction in being able to afford everything that he thought worth having. But it was never his purpose to gather in full the material rewards of his success. In his everyday life, he was careless with money. He invested heavily in his brother-in-law's shipping ventures, in the development of the new shale oil industry in his native Linlithgowshire and, after slavery had been abolished, in plantations in the West Indies; but he did so because he was attracted by the idea rather than in the need or expectation of profit. He was never clear about what he owned. When, towards the end of his life, he suddenly informed his son Walter that he had lost everything, he was quite mistaken.

Simpson had devoted his adult life to making his name as a reformer striving to make hospital care everywhere in the world more humane, more effective and, above all, less dangerous. Not every project ended in personal triumph. His work on acupressure and on hospitalism, his twin campaigns to overcome the dreadful toll of death from hospital infection, were overtaken and sidelined by the introduction of antiseptic surgery. This was a cause of regret to Simpson, who had believed that his work to overcome hospitalism would prove to be even more important to the advance of medical and surgical practice than his work on the promotion of general anaesthesia. And, in the last years of his life, he championed a new cause. But his efforts to have women admitted to the medical profession were made too soon. Tradition and public opinion were against him; women were not accepted as medical students at Scotland's universities until twenty-two years after his death.

Throughout his life Simpson had never been without a cause, and he had often faced vigorous opposition. But in the end he knew that he had won the admiration of his medical peers and the gratitude of patients everywhere. He was at the last able to be at peace in the comfort of his religion and in the love and pride of his children. He could look back on his life with satisfaction. But it had all been more turbulent that it need have been.

The Last Illness of Sir James Y. Simpson

During Simpson's last illness, his nephew, Robert Simpson, spent many hours at his bedside. In 2008, bound holograph notes made by Robert Simpson during those weeks were discovered and are now in the archives of the Royal College of Physicians of Edinburgh. They are published here for the first time.

Notes on the last illness of Sir James Y. Simpson

On Friday the 11th day of February 1870 Simpson went to London to give evidence in the Mordaunt Divorce Case. At midnight a telegram arrived stating that the trial was put off till Wednesday the 16th but Sir James had left Edinburgh two hours before the telegram arrived. When in the south he went to see Lady Mordaunt at Bickley so as to be able to give evidence about her condition, and returned to Edinburgh on the 14th.

Sir James was very busy after his return and had to go once or twice to the country to see patients between his first and second visits to London. On 15th February he again went to London and on 16th he was examined as a witness for Lady Mordaunt. Reports of his evidence were in all the papers. Descriptions of him as he appeared at the trial were in the 'Daily News' of 17th February.

He returned to Edinburgh fatigued with travel but wonderfully fresh and vigorous. He gave us a most animated account of the trial and his visit to London. On 18th he was called to Perth to see a patient – the last of his countless professional journeys. On Friday 25th February he took to bed and never left the house again. He was alarmingly ill several times, especially at night and on more than one such occasion during the early part of his illness it was feared he would be taken away.

One Sunday morning, Eve told me in Church that her Papa had been very ill during the night, and on going to the house at mid-day I found him in a somewhat critical condition however he soon rallied.

Saw him very often and spent much of my spare time with him. It was always delightful to be with him in health or sickness. But during this last illness, even amid intense pain, his wonderful kindness and intense interest in the welfare of all whom he loved were most marked.

One Saturday evening, I spent three or four hours with him alone. When leaving he said in his loving way, 'Thank you for spending so much time with me' as if he and not I had been the gainer. That same evening he spoke of his letter about the cause of his death appended to Dr. Hanna's work and said he would like to make some corrections on it if republished, and asked me to look out the book for him.

At his request I wrote to Sir Thomas Moncrieffe's solicitor for £400 in payment of his fees for attending as a witness in Lady Mordaunt's case. Also to the MP for Blackburn with copy of his essays on 'Hospitalism' which were at the time attracting attention.

He took a great interest in my future. Constantly asking about my arrangements for commencing business. Eve was writing an essay on 'Animals in History'. He spoke to her about it as was his wont, and reminded her of Bruce and the Spider. He had often given his children suggestions for their essays when this was allowable but never composed for them.

I told him of Carrubers Close Mission where the subject of how to deal with the anxious was under consideration. He spoke of difficulties.

He showed me a letter from the Rev. Robert Young about Rome. I told him that Dr. Guthrie had gone. He said, 'If I had known he was going I would have given him introductions to my friends there.'

I told him of Mr Young's having gone to Spain. He said if he recovered he would like to visit Spain to see its antiquities. He got books and read a great deal about Spain.

When he felt himself worse than he at first supposed he gave up thought of Spain and spoke of going to Buxton but that too had to be abandoned.

He was removed in end of March or beginning of April from his bedroom to the Drawing Room. He used the front Drawing Room for a sitting room, and the back Drawing Room for his bedroom. He died in the latter.

On 3rd April (Sunday) I spent the day while not at Church with him. I told him that after my Sunday Evening School, I was going to the House of the Industrial Brigade in Grove Street to speak to the lads. In my Sunday School and the Brigade boys he took a deep interest. He often asked me what my subject of address was to be. He always gave me a story or a suggestion which I found helpful. On this particular night in reply to his usual question I told him that my text was to be 'Out of the Heart are the issues of Life'. He told me about the ossification of the heart and showed how I might illustrate my subject by it.

Aunt Jessie read part of the story of Orfie Sibbald (Christian or Family Life) to him. He was so charmed with the story that he asked me to get a copy of the Treasury and send it to Miss Williams of York, an intimate personal friend. This story (cleaning away infidel doubts) was greatly appreciated by him and he had it read out to him chapter by chapter during his last illness.

On Tuesday (5th April) he had a severe attack of breathlessness. Father saw him and was struck by his increasing illness.

Friday 8th April. He spoke to me as if he would not live long with great calmness, and asked me to write a Codicil to his Will adding Mr Pender as one of his Trustees.

Saturday 9th April. After leaving the office at 2.45 I went to Queen Street with his Trust Deed. Found him suffering, and ill at ease. I wrote out a Codicil to his Will making Mr Pender one of his Trustees. When the Codicil was signed he was greatly relieved, and having got his worldly affairs arranged as far as possible he unburdened himself about his spiritual concerns. He became calm and collected. Among other things he said to me, 'I have not lived so near to Christ as I should have liked. I have led a busy active life and have not had so much time to think about eternal things as I should have wished and should have sought. Yet I know it is not my merit that I am to trust to for eternal life. Christ is all. I have not got far in the divine life,' he added with a sigh of regret.

'But dear Uncle,' I said, 'you have learned the one great truth of salvation through the blood of the Lamb. He is made unto us wisdom and righteousness, sanctification and redemption. We are complete in Him.' 'Yes, that's it,' he replied with a smile. 'There is a hymn often on my mind at present which just expresses my thoughts – just as I am with one plea but that Thy blood was shed for me. I so much like that hymn.' He spoke of not having a mind for theology. 'I like the plain simple gospel truth, and do not care for giving into quest beyond that.'

He spoke most tenderly of all his family, of Aunt, Walter, Willie, Magnus and Eve. He seemed much concerned about Eve. She was not to be sent to a boarding school as her health might break down. Nor was she to be pressed with work unduly, as her mental energy is greater than her physical strength. He said he intended to write to Mr Pender to get Mrs Pender to ask Eve to visit them occasionally. Asked me to see Mrs Hayed (Ainslie Place) and to write to Mrs Close, Killiny Castle Dublin, and Mrs Ainsworth about Eve.

He wished Mr McKie (advocate) to get some memento from him for his great kindness in connection with the Principalship. I suggested that he should get the drawing copy of Daniel Webster's works: 'Just the thing,' he said. Also Mr Imlach was to get books. He desired that his tracts on Hospitalism should be published together. He expressed his regret at his inability to complete this work.

As to his Library he said that his Medical Tracts were very valuable. Alex was welcome to use all his medical books and was to get them if Magnus does not study medicine.

In regard to the letters about Principalship he asked me to keep the printed copies. If occasion arise, they are to be published but not unless it was absolutely necessary. Pender, McKie and I are to consider about this.

I asked, 'Who is to be your Biographer?' 'You. Aren't you collecting materials?' 'Yes, I should be glad to help but some else must write the Memoir.' 'I should like Dr. Black to write a letter for insertion in it with his estimate of me.' Nothing further was said on this subject, and I did not care to revert to it.

I spoke of Mr Spurgeon's approaching visit. (Uncle went to London, twice I think, to see Mrs Spurgeon and he has a great admiration of Spurgeon's writings.) 'It would give me much pleasure to see him, but I fear I will not be able.' I mentioned the subject of his sermon on a previous subject having seen it in the dining room. 'When they had looked round about they saw no man any more save Jesus only with themselves.' 'Will you get it and read it to me?'

I read part of the sermon. As he was suffering a good deal he could not listen attentively to all I read, but his face at times lit up with emotion and he said, 'That's very nice. Read it again.'

Father came in from Bathgate at 7. Uncle was glad, as usual, to see him. Of Alex he spoke with much affection. 'He should come forward as a candidate for the chair although at first it might be a sacrifice to him. Duncan will of course be a candidate. He would seek to reverse my teaching. Alex would help to perpetuate it.'

Uncle dictated to me this evening the letter to Dr. Storer of Boston. His patience under his severe suffering was very remarkable and his kindness and consideration for all was most notable.

In the course of the evening he said to Walter (who had come home from Cambridge to be with his father and who with Dr Munro and the faithful Jarvis nursed him most tenderly and affectionately during this last illness). 'Dr Munro and you did very well last night.' I left him to go home about 10 o'clock. He was then somewhat easier.

Sunday 10th April. Went over to see Uncle in the morning before going to Church. Rather worse. He had not slept well during the night. Dr. Munro was giving him a little chloroform to allay pain.

Before leaving for the Sabbath School in the evening, I went to say good night. 'Come back,' said he 'and stay all night. I do not think I will be long here, and I should like you to remain till the end.' He added, 'From extreme pain I have not been able to read or even to think much to-day but when I think it is of the words you read yesterday. "Jesus only", and really that is all that's needed is it not? Jesus only.'

On returning from the School, I found him somewhat better. He asked about the School, and the lessons.

When Eve and I were alone with him he spoke of the probability of his being taken away. 'I've been telling Eve and all of them about Jesus only. Read a hymn,' said he after some of the others had come in. I read 'Rock of Ages'. 'A beautiful hymn that but I like "Just as I am" best. Read it please.'

He went to bed about 11, and I was with him till between 1 and 2. He could not rest in bed, and got feverish and breathless. After being, as he thought, impatient he said, 'Excuse me because I am suffering a good deal.' 'Dear Uncle,' I said. 'I am so sorry to see you suffering so much.' He replied with great submissiveness, 'It's all for the best.' I said, 'Your sufferings work out for you a far more exceeding, even an eternal weight, of glory.' 'Yes,' he said, 'an eternal weight of glory.'

'Read me some nice texts,' he said. Knowing that the 14th Chapter of John was a favourite with him I repeated several verses of it. Though he knew these words of the Lord Jesus so well, some parts seemed as if new to him, new light being shed on the words by the suffering he was undergoing and the prospect of death near at hand. The thought of the many mansioned house of Jesus and the loved ones from his own fireside who had gone before cheered him amidst the paroxysms of pain. When I came to the verse 'I am the way,' he wanted me to stop that he might think of it. After a short pause he said, 'What a wonderful redemption this is. Christ's blood can float a cork or a man of war. It can bear every one to heaven.' Continuing as he wished to repeat some portions of scripture, I quoted from Timothy. This is a faithful saying and worthy of all acceptance. 'If Paul had to speak of himself as chief of sinners well may I make use of the words too. But yet it is not a question of degree, for all have sinned.' He then spoke with much enthusiasm of the power of Christ's blood. I shall never forget our conversation. How he was cheered and comforted amid pain and weariness by his Saviour's grace I cannot rightly describe.

It was heaven begin on earth. He who had seen suffering in so many forms and had done so much to alleviate the pain of others was now in the furnace of affliction. But there he was sustained by the presence of the Son of Man. He who had so often stood by the bed of death and softened so many dying pillows was now face to face with the last enemy. Yet there was no murmuring under suffering, no terror in prospect of death. He had learnt to count these afflictions as but for a moment. He had been taught the secret of victory over death. More than once he said to me that he wished it was all over, as he knew from the nature of his disease that he would have to undergo much suffering but he bowed with meek submission to the will of God and looked forward to death without a tinge of fear or alarm. In former illnesses he was sometimes fractious. There was nothing of this in his last illness. Jarvis, remarking upon this one day to Dr. Wood, said he thought this was a bad sign. I repeated some verses of the hymn 'Forever with the Lord'. He spoke with joy of being with the Lord. He again spoke with great tenderness of Eve and asked me to take an interest in her. 'You know her so. She is the cleverest of them all and I should like to see her rightly trained.' He hoped that Alex would marry Margo Barbour, of whom uncle spoke very highly. Of Mrs Barbour, then at Cannes, 'She is a dear lady. Write her to say since my illness I've often been thinking of her and that I've read her last and New Years addresses with much pleasure.'

Monday 11th April. Read and prayed with him before going to the office. Very ill. Didn't rest well during the night. Got easier during the day.

It was suggested that Magnus (who was in Geneva) should be telegraphed for. Averse to this, he did not wish to give him any unnecessary pain.

Dr. Duns called. He told me that he enjoyed the Dr's visit but had felt a remark he had made about taking opium. 'As regards that,' he said, 'I am entirely in my doctor's hands.'

Went to Queen Street at 4.30 and found him calm and peaceful. 'I am so well,' he said with a smile. Walter, who watched unweariedly during these anxious days, was with him. He employed us in examining the proof sheets of the (2nd) letter to Dr Bigelow in which he was much interested.

Occasional fits of breathlessness. Spoke of Walter's future. Strongly in favour of his joining the bar, unless something specially good in the mercantile line turns up.

Walter left for a walk. He wrote a letter to Mr Pender which he handed to me and asked me to send off when I thought that all hope of recovery was gone. Spoke of his unshaken confidence in Jesus. 'I have mixed a great deal with men of all shades of opinion. I have heard men of science and philosophy raise doubts and objections to the gospel of Christ but I have never for one moment had a doubt myself.'

I gave him a message from Mr Jenkinson for whom he had a great regard – to rest entirely in the finished work of Christ. 'That's it,' he said, 'that is what I desire to do.' I repeated a verse of Mrs Cousin's beautiful hymn which Mr Jenkinson gave me for him.

> I stand upon him best
> I know no other stand
> Not even where glory dwellest
> In Immanuel's land.

'Repeat it again,' said he. After repeating it he said, 'Thank him for me, I should so much like to shake hands with him again.'

He asked me to get the whole poem which I afterwards did with an account of Rutherford's last illness and dying words. He enjoyed the reading of it.

At his request, finished the reading of Spurgeons' sermon on 'Jesus Only'. 'Read that again,' he frequently said when I came to some passage full of Christ. At the close, he said that the sermon – especially the last part of it – had given him great comfort and these words 'Jesus Only' were often on his lips.

Walter, Eve and Dr Munro joined us, and at his request I read a Chapter from Orfie Sibbald.

On returning from the office at 9.30 I found him fully well. Dr. Wood, Dr. Moir, Mr Coghill, Mr Philip and Mr Drummond all saw him. Mr Philip prayed with him.

Walter read part of Oliver Underwood. About 11.30, he asked me to read 'Just as I am'. I also read Dr Bonar's hymn 'I heard the voice of Jesus say'. He enjoyed it, especially the first verse about rest. 'Mr Morgan,' said he, 'told me to rest my head in Jesus' bosom as John did at the Supper table. I cannot just do that. I think it enough if I have hold of the hem of his garment.' I read Oliver Underwood until he slept and I left him with Walter at 1. He slept well during the night.

Tuesday 12th April. Read Revelation VIII and prayed. Alex came from Glasgow to see him. He enjoyed his visit very much. Dr. Morgan also saw him. I went to Queen St at 4.30 and found him very well. Read 'Little Will' to him – a simple story of a boy's faith in rhyme. Greatly pleased with it.

Dr Parker of Andover had told him the story. Willie arrived from the Isle of Man. Asked him all about the friends there and spoke about his future. Read about Rutherford's last days.

Evening

Dr Wood and Dr Moir came at 10.30. Told them of Walter's intention to study law. He was glad they approved of it. Long talk with them about olden times. Told me that he had been reading parts of 'Jesus Only' himself. I read Ephesians I and prayed. Read Teddie's 'First and Last Sacraments'. Liked it greatly. Then Oliver Underwood until he slept. Slept from 12 to 8 with slight interruptions.

Wednesday 13th April. Read John III. When I came to the words 'Wind Bloweth Where It Listeth' that had been the means of Benjamin Bell's conversion. When I read the 16th verse, 'Read that again,' said he, 'read it again'. Prayed. Great peace and calmness.

Evening.

Read Hebrews XII and John Ashworth's *Strange Tales* till he slept.

Thursday 14th April. Passed a good night. Waked between 3 & 4 somewhat heated but soon fell asleep again. Read last Chapter of Matthew and prayed. After prayer he said, 'Do you know I felt during the worst of my illness that special united prayer was being offered up to God for me and that I heard it.' I then told him about the prayer meetings which had been held for his recovery. Dr Black came from London in the morning and left in the evening. Greatly pleased to see him.

Saturday 16th April. In much the same condition.

Sunday 17th April 1870. Before going to school he asked me what was to be the subject of my address. I told 'Jesus Christ the Same as Yesterday'. Gave me a story of a native preacher in India telling story of redeeming love to his countrymen in the street of one of the large towns when a British officer rode up and called to the preacher, 'How is your friend Jesus Christ today?' 'Jesus,' he replied, 'is the same yesterday, to day and for ever.' The words touched the officer's heart and led him to seek pardon and peace from this unchanging saviour.

Read XXII chapter of Revelation at worship. Afterwards I repeated to him the hymn 'There is a name I love to hear'. New to him and delighted with it.

Wednesday 20th April 1870. Got offer of partnership with Mr Gifford. Told uncle of it. Greatly delighted and advised me at once to accept it. Talked very cheerily.

Thursday 21st April 1870 (Fast Day). Went to Bathgate to see father. Took good account of uncle.

Friday 22nd April. Arranged finally with Mr Gifford. Uncle could talk of nothing else almost. Told all the Drs and others seeing him about it.

Saturday 23rd April. Uncle very well and happy to-day.

Sunday 24th April (Communion Sabbath). Told Uncle about the service. Read John X at worship.

Monday 25th April. Willie and Eve left for Killin. Uncle, who was wonderfully well, embraced Eve with great affection. 'God bless you my darling,' he said and, as she left the room, his eyes followed her with melting tenderness. It was the last time they spoke together on earth.

Tuesday 26th April. Father came in at night.

Wednesday 27th April. Uncle very well. Slept better than he has done for a week. Slept in Front Drawing Room in a sitting attitude.

Thursday 28th April. Went to Conference in Glasgow. Uncle sent his love to all there.

Friday 29th April. Remarkably well. Read Luke XV in the evening. Told Uncle I proposed to go to Killin next morning if he felt well. Said 'go by all means' and gave my messages to Eve. Read him asleep.

Saturday 30th April. Left early for Killin without seeing Uncle. Alex came from Glasgow to-day to see him. Got suddenly much worse in the evening. Mind wandered sometimes.

Sunday 1st May. Worse.

Monday 2nd May. No signs of improvement.

Tuesday 3rd May. I returned from Killin in the evening. Having had no news of Uncle in my absence I was horrified to find him so much worse. He knew me however, and asked kindly about Eve. Then relapsed into torpor.

Wednesday 4th May. Father came in and Alex also. Uncle's mind wandered very much. Father sat up most of the night with him. Sat on the pillow with Uncle's head on his knee. It was most touching to see the elder brother – 14 years older than the younger and who watched his progress with such affection – watching by the death bed. 'Oh Sandy, Sandy,' Uncle repeatedly said showing he knew who was beside him. Said little more.

Thursday 5th May. Went to Killin and brought Eve home, but he did not know us. Dr. Hanna and Mr Morgan saw him during the day and prayed at his bedside.

Friday 6th May 1870. Gradually sinking. After dinner I went up to his room (Back Drawing Room) where Aunt Jessie and Miss Grindlay were watching. While Aunt and I were whispering together, we heard a longer drawn sigh than usual. Saw he was dying. Aunt rang the bell for the others to come up. I moistened his lips and while the others came in his spirit passed away. No struggle – no pain.

The Last Illness of Sir James Y. Simpson

On Medical Subjects

Presented here is a brief selection from the vast number of papers on medical subjects published by Simpson in medical journals and, as was his practice, reprinted and published privately as pamphlets for sale to the public.

On the evidence of the occasional contagious propagation of malignant cholera, which is derived from cases of its direct importation into new localities by infected individuals. *Edinburgh Medical and Surgical Journal*, 1838, 49:355–408. Reprinted Edinburgh: John Stark [1838].

Contributions to intra–uterine pathology. Part I. Notices of cases of peritonitis in the foetus in utero. *Edinburgh Medical and Surgical Journal*, 1838, 50:390–416. Reprinted Edinburgh: John Stark [1838].

Contributions to intra-uterine pathology. Part II. On the inflammatory origin of some varieties of hernia and malformation in the foetus. *Edinburgh Medical and Surgical Journal*, 1839, 52:17–36. Reprinted Edinburgh: John Stark [1839].

Case of amputation of the neck of the womb followed by pregnancy; with remarks on the pathology and radical treatment of the cauliflower excrescence for the os uteri. *Edinburgh Medical and Surgical Journal*, 1841, 55:104–12. Reprinted Edinburgh: John Stark [1841].

Contributions to the pathology and treatment of diseases of the uterus. Part I. Propositions regarding uterine diagnosis. *Monthly Journal of Medical Science*, 1843, 3:547–56. Reprinted Edinburgh: Balfour and Jack [1843–4].

The same. Part II. Proposals for the improvement and elucidation of uterine diagnosis by means of a sound or bougie passed into the uterine cavity. *Monthly Journal of Medical Science*, 1843, 3:701–15. Reprinted Edinburgh: Balfour and Jack [1843].

The same. Part III. On the measurement of the cavity of the uterus as a means of diagnosis in some of the morbid states of that organ. *Monthly Journal of Medical Science*, 1843, 3:1009–27. Reprinted Edinburgh: Balfour and Jack [1843].

The same. Part IV. On the measurement of the cavity of the uterus as a means of diagnosis in some of the morbid states of that organ. *Monthly Journal of Medical Science*, 1844, 4:208–17. Reprinted Edinburgh: Balfour and Jack [1844].

On the alleged infecundity of females born co-twins with males; with some notes on the average proportion of marriages without issue in general society. *Edinburgh Medical and Surgical Journal*, 1844, 61:107–19. Reprinted Edinburgh: John Stark [1844].

Memoir on the sex of the child as a cause of difficulty and danger in human parturition. *Edinburgh Medical and Surgical Journal*, 1844, 62:387–439. Reprinted Edinburgh: Stark [1844].

On the expulsion and extraction of the placenta before the child in placental presentations. *Provincial Medical and Surgical Journal*, 1845, 9:82–6. Reprinted Worcester: Deighton [1845].

Some remarks on the treatment of unavoidable haemorrhage by extraction of the placenta before the child. With a few observations on Dr Lee's objections to the practice. *London Medical Gazette*, 1845, 1:1009–16. Reprinted London: Wilson and Ogilvy [1845].

Additional observations on unavoidable haemorrhage in cases of placental presentation. *London Medical Gazette*, 1845, 1:1193–5. Reprinted London: Wilson and Ogilvy [1845].

Clinical lectures on midwifery and the diseases of women and children. Taken in short-hand by Charles D. Arnott, Esq., student of medicine, London. *Monthly Journal of Medical Science*, 1845, 5:109–22. Reprinted Edinburgh: Balfour and Jack [1845].

Memoir on the spontaneous expulsion and artificial extraction of the placenta before the child in placental presentations. Section I. Dangers of placental presentations – Opinions of authors – Statistical evidence of the fatality of these presentations. *Monthly Journal of Medical Science*, 1845, 5:169–204. Reprinted Edinburgh: Andrew Jack [1845].

Some suggestions regarding the anatomical source and pathological nature of post-partum haemorrhage. *Northern Journal of Medicine*, 1846, 4:1–6. Also published as: Anatomical source and pathological nature of post-partum haemorrhage. *Monthly Journal of Medical Science*, 1846, 6:137–41. Reprinted Edinburgh: Hugh Paton [1846].

Clinical lectures on midwifery and the diseases of women and infants during the session 1845–6. Collated from the notes of students. *Northern Journal of Medicine*, 1846, 4:216–39. Reprinted Edinburgh: Hugh Paton [1846].

Observations regarding the influence of galvanism upon the action of the uterus during labour. *Monthly Journal of Medical Science*, 1846, 6:33–48. Reprinted Edinburgh: Sutherland and Knox [1846].

On the nature of the membrane occasionally expelled in dysmenorrhoea. *Monthly Journal of Medical Science*, 1846, 6:161–5. Reprinted Edinburgh: Sutherland and Knox [1846].

Discovery of a new anaesthetic agent more efficient than sulphuric ether. *Provincial Medical and Surgical Journal*, 1847, s1–11:656–8 (1 December 1847). Also published as: On a new anaesthetic agent, more efficient than sulphuric ether. *Lancet*, 1847, 2:549–50; and in *London Medical Gazette*, 1847, 5:934–7.

Anaestetic and other therapeutic properties of chloroform. *Monthly Journal of Medical Science*, 1847, 7:415–7. Reprinted Edinburgh: Sutherland and Knox [1847].

Case of delivery, without operative aid, through a pelvis extremely deformed by malacosteon; child, at the ninth month of uterogestation, passing through an oblong aperture under 1 inch in its narrow, and 2 ½ in its long diameter. *Monthly Journal of Medical Science*, 1847, 7: 22–38. Reprinted Edinburgh: Sutherland and Knox [1847].

Etherization in surgery. Part I. Its effects; objections to it, &c. *Monthly Journal of Medical Science*, 1847, 7:145–66. Reprinted Edinburgh: Sutherland and Knox [1847].

The same. Part II. Proper mode of investigating its effects; statistical propositions and results; &c. Value and necessity of the numerical method of investigation as applied to sugery. *Monthly Journal of Medical Science*, 1847, 7: 313–33. Reprinted as: *Some Remarks on the Value and Necessity of the Numerical or Statistical Method of Inquiry as Applied to Various Questions in Operative Surgery*. Edinburgh: Sutherland and Knox [1848].

The same. Part III. Does etherization increase or decrease the mortality attendant upon surgical operations? *Monthly Journal of Medical Science*, 1848, 8:697–710. Reprinted Edinburgh: Sutherland and Knox [1848]

Notes on the anaesthetic effects of chloride of hydrocarbon, nitrate of ethyle, benzin, aldehyde, and bisulphuret of carbon. *Monthly Journal of Medical Science*, 1848, 8:740–4. Reprinted Edinburgh: Sutherland and Knox [1848].

Local anaesthesia; notes on its artificial production by chloroform, &c., in the lower animals and in man. *London Medical Gazette*, 1848, 7:62–8. Reprinted Worcester: Deighton [1848].

Report on the early history and progress of anaesthetic midwifery, *Monthly Journal of Medical Science*, 1848, 8:209–51. Reprinted Edinburgh: Sutherland and Knox [1848].

Letter in reply to Dr Collins, on the duration of labour as a cause of danger and mortality to the mother and infant. *Provincial Medical and Surgical Journal*, 1848, s1–12:601–6. Reprinted Worcester: Deighton [1848].

Local anaesthesia; notes on its artificial production by chloroform, &c., in the lower animals and in man. *Provincial Medical and Surgical Journal*, 1848, s1–12:365–71. Reprinted Worcester: Deighton [1848].

Remarks on the alleged case of death from the action of chloroform. *Lancet*, 1848, 1:175–6. Reprinted as: *Remarks on the Alleged Fatal Case of Chloroform-Inhalation*. Edinburgh: Murray and Gibb [1848].

Report of the Edinburgh Royal Maternity Hospital from 1844 to 1846. *Monthly Journal of Medical Science*, 1848–9, 9:329–38. Reprinted Edinburgh: Sutherland and Knox [1848].

The attitude and positions, natural and preternatural, of the foetus in utero, acts of the reflex or excito-motory system. *Monthly Journal of Medical Science*, 1849, 9:423–41, 639–55, 863–86. Reprinted Edinburgh: Sutherland and Knox [1849].

On a suction-tractor; or new mechanical power, as a substitute for the forceps in tedious labours. *Monthly Journal of Medical Science*, 1848–9, 9:556–9, 618–20. Reprinted Edinburgh: Sutherland and Knox [1849].

On the detection and treatment of intra-uterine polypi. *Monthly Journal of Medical Science*, 1850, 10:3–21. Reprinted Edinburgh: Sutherland and Knox [1850].

Some notes on the analogy between puerperal fever and surgical fever. *Monthly Journal of Medical Science*, 1850, 11:414–29. Reprinted Edinburgh: Sutherland and Knox [1850].

Inquiry relative to the external use of oil in the prevention and treatment of scrofula, phthisis, etc. *Monthly Journal of Medical Science*, 1853, 17:316–30. Reprinted Edinburgh: Sutherland and Knox [1853].

Inaugural address to the Medico-Chirurgical Society on the modern advancements in practical medicine and surgery. *Monthly Journal of Medical Science*, 1853, 16:354–66. Reprinted Edinburgh: Sutherland and Knox [1853].

The propriety and morality of using anaesthetics in instrumental and natural parturition; in a letter to Prof Meigs, of Philadelphia. *Association Medical Journal*, 1853, 528–9. Reprinted London: T. Richards [1853].

Valedictory address to the newly made medical graduates of the University of Edinburgh, 1 August, 1855. *Association Medical Journal*, 1855–6, 1:224–33. Also published in *Lancet*, 1855, 2:289–91.

Acupressure, a new method of arresting surgical haemorrhage. *Edinburgh Medical Journal*, 1859–60, 5: 645–51. Reprinted Edinburgh: Sutherland and Knox [1860].

On acupressure in amputations. *Medical Times and Gazette*, 1860, 1:137–9. Reprinted Edinburgh: Sutherland and Knox [1860].

Our existing system of hospitalism and its effects, *Edinburgh Medical Journal*, 1869, 817–1115. Reprinted Edinburgh: Sutherland and Knox [1869].

Hospitalism; Its influence upon limb amputations in the London hospitals. *British Medical Journal*, 1869, 1:533–5. Reprinted Edinburgh: Sutherland and Knox [1869].

Publications on Archaeological Subjects

Antiquarian notices of leprosy and leper hospitals in Scotland and England. Part I. *Edinburgh Medical and Surgical Journal*, 1841, 56:301–30.

Antiquarian notices of leprosy and leper hospitals in Scotland and England. Part II. The nosological nature of the disease. *Edinburgh Medical and Surgical Journal*, 1842, 57:121–56.

Antiquarian notices of leprosy and leper hospitals in Scotland and England. Part III. The etiological history of the disease. *Edinburgh Medical and Surgical Journal*, 1842, 57:394–429.

Notices of ancient Roman medicine-stamps. *Monthly Journal of Medical Science*, 1851, 12:39–50, 235–55, 338–54.

Notes on some ancient Greek medical vases for containing lykion; and on the modern use of the same drug in India. *Monthly Journal of Medical Science*, 1853, 16:24–30.

Was the Roman Army Provided with Medical Officers? Edinburgh: Sutherland and Knox; 1851.

On an old stone-roofed cell or oratory in the Island of Inchcolm. *Proceedings of the Society of Antiquaries of Scotland*, 1857, 2:489–528.

On the Cat-Stane, Kirkliston: Is it not the tombstone of the grandfather of Hengist and Horsa? *Proceedings of the Society of Antiquaries of Scotland*, 1861, 4:119–65.

Notes on Scottish curing-stones and amulets. *Proceedings of the Society of Antiquaries of Scotland*, 1861, 4:211–24.

Pyramidal structures in Egypt and elsewhere; and the objects of their erection, *Proceedings of the Royal Society of Edinburgh*, 1868, 6:243–68.

Address on archaeology. *Proceedings of the Society of Antiquaries of Scotland*, 1861, 4:5–51. Reprinted as: *Archaeology: Its Past and its Future Work; being the Annual Address to the Society of Antiquaries of Scotland, Given January 28, 1861*. Edinburgh: Neill and Company [1861].

Notes

Chapter 1 The Ambition to Rise

1 Sir James Y. Simpson, Bart. was Physician to the Queen in Scotland, Past President of the Royal College of Physicians of Edinburgh, the Royal Medical Society, the Royal Physical Society, the Obstetric Society of Edinburgh and the Medico-Chirurgical Society of Edinburgh.

His many other honours included DCL Oxon; Honorary MD, Dublin; Honorary Fellow of the King's and Queen's Colleges of Physicians in Ireland; Laureate of the Imperial Institute of Prague; Laureate of the Imperial Institute of France; Knight of the Order of Norway; Foreign Member of the Academies of Medicine of France, Belgium and New York, and of the Academy of Science of Sweden, of the American Philosophical Society, of the Medical Institute of Egypt, and of the Medical Societies of Constantinople, Athens, Bohemia, Norway, Stockholm, Copenhagen, Ghent, Massachusetts, Lima and Bombay; Foreign Member of the Societies of Surgery and Biology of Paris; Honorary Fellow of the Obstetric Societies of London, Leipzig and Berlin.

2 *The Lancet*, 1 April 1871.

3 *The Lancet*, 13 May 1870.

4 Now West Lothian.

5 A hardy variety of barley grown for baking into bannocks rather than for malting.

6 The landlord received farm produce as payment of rent 'in kind'.

7 This system had survived from a previous age, when the land had been worked by men whose most valued skill was as soldiers rather than as farmers and when, for the landlord, his land and his farms were a source, not of revenue, but of military power.

8 In 1699, Sir Robert Sibbald described his observations of the famine in his *Provision for the Poor in Time of Dearth and Scarcity*.

9 The first college offering a three-year course on animal medicine was opened in 1791. The Army Board recognised the category of veterinary surgeon in 1804.

10 D. Buchan (ed.), *Folk Tradition and Folk Medicine in Scotland* (Edinburgh, 1994), p. 28.

11 M. Simpson, *Simpson the Obstetrician* (London, 1972), p. 20.

12 M. McCrae, *The National Health Service in Scotland* (Edinburgh, 2003), p. 5. *Domestic Medicine* was almost as frequently to be found in Scottish homes as

the Bible.

13 I. H. Adams, *The Mapping of a Scottish Estate* (Edinburgh, 1971), p. 5.

14 P. Rogers (ed.), *Boswell and Johnson in Scotland* (Yale, 1993) p. 121.

15 Now the 2nd Earl, the 1st Earl having died in 1767.

16 T. M. Devine, *Clearance and Improvement: Land, Power and People in Scotland 1700–1900* (Edinburgh, 2006), pp. 113–25.

17 Alexander Simpson, born 1750, died 1820.

18 John Simpson, born 1752, died 1812.

19 In 1755 the population was 1,265,380; in 1801 it was 1,608,000. B. P. Lenman, *Integrations and Enlightenment: Scotland 1746–1832* (Edinburgh, 1986), p. 2.

20 Homespun grey or black cloth.

21 'The more elegant and luxury among farmers, I observe, in equal proportion the rudeness and stupidity of the peasantry.' R. L. Brown, *Robert Burns' Tour of the Highlands and Stirlingshire 1787* (Ipswich, 1973), p. 16.

22 Thomas, born 1757, died 1844.

23 Margaret was born in 1800. Her twin sister died within a few days of birth.

24 When distilling became unprofitable for a time after 1805 they emigrated to Australia.

25 David, born 1760, died 1830.

26 George, born 1764, died 1832.

27 W. Haig, *William Pitt the Younger* (London, 2004), p. 278.

28 J. Duns, *Memoir of Sir James Y. Simpson, Bart.* (Edinburgh, 1873), p. 8.

29 For a time it seemed possible that the Revolution in France might spread to Britain. Later the war with France created some hardship at home.

30 D. J. Brown, *The Politicians, The Revenue Men and the Scottish Distillers, Review of Scottish Culture*, No 12, 1999–2000, p. 55.

31 A. Clow and N. L. Clow, *The Chemical Revolution* (London, 1952), p. 573.

32 On his birth certificate he was named simply James Simpson. He became James Young Simpson while a student at Edinburgh. The reason is unclear.

33 Sir A. R. Simpson, Memories of Sir James Simpson, *Edinburgh Medical Journal*, 1911, Vol. 6, No 6, p. 491.

34 Duns, *Memoir*, p. 17.

35 N. Ferguson, *Empire* (London, 2004) p. 33.

36 Bathgate Academy was opened in 1833.

37 Sir John Sinclair, *Statistical Account of Scotland 1791–1799* (Wakefield, 1975), p. 694.

38 Main Street, Brown Square, Engine Street, Livery Street, Gideon Street, Drumcross and Armadale.

39 Duns, *Memoir*, p. 17.

40 A. M. Bisset, *History of Bathgate* (Bathgate, 1906), p. 194.

41 A. R. Simpson, *Memories*, p. 498.

42 Duns, *Memoir*, p. 17.

43 H. L. Gordon, *Sir James Simpson* (London, 1897), p. 19.

Chapter 2 A Sense of Exclusion

1 *The Topographical, Statistical and Historical Gazetteer of Scotland* (Glasgow, 1842), Vol. 2, p. 438.
2 Sir A. Grant, *The Story of the University of Edinburgh* (London, 1884), p. 492.
3 The licensing body was the Church of Scotland.
4 B. Hilton, *A Mad, Bad and Dangerous People: England 1783–1846* (Oxford, 2006), p. 410.
5 H. Cockburn, *Memorials of His Time, 1779–1830* (Edinburgh, 1910), p. 74.
6 The police force was established in 1805. In 1812, Edinburgh had Scotland's first detectives.
7 The Argethelians, supporters of the Hanoverian and led by the Duke of Argyll, and the Squadrone Volante, who were not Jacobites but were not fully committed to the House of Hanover.
8 M. Fry, *The Dundas Depotism* (Edinburgh, 2004), p. 15.
9 The title of Prime Minister was not yet in use.
10 Fry, *Dundas Depotism*, p. 242.
11 Others in England included: The Society for Promoting Constitutional Information, Sheffield Constitutional Society, The Corresponding Society, the Norwich Revolutionary Society, The Manchester Constitutional Society. In Scotland the radical movement was much less well organised.
12 Hilton, *Mad, Bad and Dangerous*, p. 65.
13 The 'Massacre of Peterloo' in 1819.
14 The 'Radical War' in 1829.
15 In the previous century the word Tory had indicated a Jacobite.
16 R. P. Gillies, *Memoirs of a Literary Veteran* (London, 1851), Vol. 3.
17 Later the judge Lord Jeffrey.
18 Later co-founder of the *Edinburgh Review*.
19 Later the Lord Chancellor.
20 Cockburn, *Memorials*, p. 249.
21 Hilton, *Mad, Bad and Dangerous*, p. 208.
22 M. Simpson, *Simpson the Obstetrician* (London, 1972), p. 29.
23 M. H. Kaufman, *Medical Teaching in Edinburgh in the 18th and 19th Centuries* (Edinburgh, 2003), p. 10.
24 Sir Robert Christison, quoted by Grant, *Story*, p. 438.
25 Lisa Rosner, Monro, Alexander, *tertius* (1773–1859) *Oxford Dictionary of National Biography*, (Oxford, 2004).
26 His students gave him the nickname 'Old Cyclops'.
27 I. Rae, *Knox the Anatomist* (Edinburgh, 1964), p. 2.
28 He did not retire completely from the army until 1832.
29 F. J. Knox, *The Anatomist's Instructor and Museum Companion* (Edinburgh, 1836), p. 7.
30 R. Knox, Letter to the Right Honourable the Lord Provost of Edinburgh, 6 July 1837. RCPE Library.
31 Ibid.

32 Quoted by Rae, *Knox the Anatomist*, p. 50.

33 G. Wilson, *Life of Dr John Reid* (Edinburgh, 1852), p. 30.

34 Ibid., p. 56.

35 M. Simpson, *Simpson the Obstetrician*, p. 32.

36 Bodies received for dissection were normally without a name and without a history.

37 Rae, *Knox the Anatomist*, p. 66.

38 Comparative anatomy was then called philosophical anatomy. See Janet Browne, *Charles Darwin* (London, 1995), p. 53.

39 H. L. Gordon, *Sir James Simpson* (London, 1897), p. 25.

40 In 1835 he had been elected a Corresponding Member of the French Academy of Medicine, an honour that was rarely conferred on foreigners.

Chapter 3 Revival

1 The parish schoolmaster received £30 per annum; the surgeon's salary would have been less than £50.

2 Robert Carswell (later Sir Robert) was a medical student at Glasgow when first employed by Thomson. In 1828 he was appointed to the chair of Pathological Anatomy and curatorship of the medical museum at the new London University. In 1837 he published *Pathological Anatomy: Illustrations of the Elementary Forms of Disease,* which included illustrations made during his European tour commissioned by Thomson.

3 Obituary, *The Monthly Journal of Medical Science*, 1847, Vol. 7, p. 395.

4 For this translation I thank Professor Iain Donaldson. Previous biographers of Simpson (Dunns, M. Simpson, Laing) all translate the title of his thesis as 'death from inflammation'. This is unsatisfactory since it implies something much more general than Simpson's title, missing the significance of both 'proxima' and 'quibusdam'.

5 It was not until 1833 that candidates could opt to be examined in English.

6 It is believed that the nickname was the invention of Robert Knox.

7 W. Thomson, Memoir of Dr John Thomson, *Edinburgh Medical and Surgical Journal*, 1847, Vol. 67, p. 131.

8 Dr White to William Thomson, quoted in the *Edinburgh Medical and Surgical Journal*, 1847, Vol. 67, p. 132.

9 Ibid., p. 134.

10 John Allen was a Whig intellectual and member of the Holland House set. He was also a physiologist whose ideas on the part played by the unconscious mind were disputed by Dugald Stewart, since they denied man the freedom to choose between good and evil.

11 Lord Cockburn, *Memorials of His Time* (Edinburgh, 1856), p. 45.

12 Allen later abandoned a promising career in Edinburgh as a physician and lecturer on physiology to move to London and devote himself to politics as a member of the Holland House set. L. S. Jacyna, *Philosophical Whigs* (London 1994), p. 74.

13 Ibid, p. 85.

14 W. Thomson, *Edinburgh Medical and Surgical Journal*, 1847, Vol. 67, p. 151.

15 Dundas was accused of financial irregularities while Treasurer of the Navy in the 1780s and was censured by the House of Commons on the casting vote of the Speaker.

16 As a regius chair it had been created by the government, and the appointment of the professor was made by the government.

17 Anon, *Monthly Journal of Medical Science*, 1847, Vol. 7, p. 395.

18 The extramural classes were continued by his son.

19 Traditionally at Edinburgh, surgery had been taught by the Professor of Anatomy.

20 B. Hilton, *A Mad, Bad and Dangerous People: England 1783–1846* (Oxford, 2006), p. 208.

21 Founded in 1771 'for the promotion of zoology and other branches of natural history'.

22 J. Duns, *Memoir of Sir James Simpson*, Bart. (Edinburgh, 1873), p. 46.

23 Later Sir Andrew Douglas Maclagan, Professor of Forensic Medicine at Edinburgh and president of the Royal College of Physicians of Edinburgh in 1884–87.

24 Clift was an expert on the structure of the placenta.

25 In 1841 John Reid was appointed Chandos Professor of Anatomy at St Andrews.

26 Letter, Simpson to Alexander Simpson, 1 April 1835.

27 Elizabeth Fry, quoted by D. H. Tuke, *The History of the Insane in the British Isles* (London, 1882), p. 329.

Chapter 4 Professor of Midwifery

1 The Royal Medical Society was founded in 1734 by Edinburgh's medical students to provide a forum for their own independent efforts to advance their education and training.

2 *Scotsman*, 10 May 1870.

3 *Edinburgh Medical and Surgical Journal*, 1836, Vol. 127, pp. 266–310.

4 Anon [William Thomson], Of John Thomson, in J. Thomson, *Life of Cullen* (Edinburgh, 1859), Vol. l, p. 71.

5 When John Thomson resigned from the chair of General Pathology in 1842, he was not succeeded by his son but by William Henderson.

6 His collection of teaching material.

7 *Edinburgh Medical and Surgical Journal*, 1838, Vol. 50, No. 127, pp. 390–416.

8 *Edinburgh Medical and Surgical Journal*, 1839, Vol. 52, No. 140, pp. 17–35.

9 R. B. Todd (ed.), *Cyclopaedia of Anatomy and Physiology* (London, 1839), Vol. 2, p. 691.

10 J. Duns, *Memoir of Sir James Y. Simpson, Bart* (Edinburgh, 1873), p. 76.

11 All of Simpson's correspondence quoted in this and subsequent chapters is either found in the Duns *Memoir* (the originals of which are no longer to be found) or in the archive of the Royal College of Surgeons of Edinburgh.

12 Letter, Simpson to Jessie Grindlay, 27 June 1838.

13 The Test Act and the Corporation Act had been introduced in the seventeenth century to exclude Roman Catholics and Non-Conformists from civil or military office under the Crown.

14 These were the 'Regius Chairs' of which the chair of Midwifery was not one.

15 The originals of the testimonials are in the archive of the Royal College of Surgeons of Edinburgh.

16 J. A. Shepherd, *Simpson and Syme of Edinburgh* (Edinburgh, 1969), p. 53.

17 The calculation is based on Research Paper 06-009 issued by the House of Commons Library in 2006.

18 The designation was changed when Hamilton, after a long and bitter legal battle, prevailed over the Senatus of the university to have midwifery made a compulsory subject for medical students intending to graduate at Edinburgh.

19 Sir A. Grant, *The Story of the University of Edinburgh* (Edinburgh, 1884), pp. 416–7.

20 Letter, J. Hope to W. Grindlay, RCSE Archive.

21 Letter, Simpson to the Misses Grindlay. RCSE Archive.

22 In his biography Duns claims (p. 94) that during this very brief visit JYS and Jessie Grindlay became engaged. If so, neither family was informed.

23 Letter, Simpson to Walter Grindlay, RCSE Archive.

24 Duns, *Memoir*, p. 134.

25 James Syme had been appointed Professor of Clinical Surgery in 1833.

Chapter 5 Physician to the Queen

1 The correspondence referred to in this chapter is in the archive of the Royal College of Surgeons of Edinburgh, or amongst family letters.

2 A. D. C. Simpson, James Hamilton's Lying-In Hospital at Park House and the Status of Midwifery Instruction in the Edinburgh Medical School, *Book of the Old Edinburgh Club*, 1994, New Series Vol. 1, p. 136.

3 It was widely assumed that the principal, if not the only, beneficiaries would be the town's prostitutes.

4 Park House was built in 1738 by William Adam on a site at the south-east corner of the city wall where Bristo Street is now; the park included the area now covered by George Square.

5 A. M. Nuttal, The Edinburgh Royal Maternity Hospital and the Medicalisation of Childbirth in Edinburgh, 1844–1914, PhD Thesis, Edinburgh University (2003), p. 42.

6 J. Moir, Royal Maternity Hospital, Minutes of Directors Meetings, 26 September 1895, Lothian Health Board Archive.

7 Nuttall, The Edinburgh Royal Maternity Hospital, p. 44.

8 Edinburgh Royal Maternity Hospital, Minutes of Directors Meeting, 17 March 1856.

9 Chapel House, which had been Andrew Melrose's grocery shop, was in Chapel Street, near the present site of the university's Appleton Tower.

10 Edinburgh Royal Maternity Hospital, Minutes of Directors Meeting, 11 May 1870.

11 Edinburgh Royal Maternity Hospital, Indoor Case Book, 1844–71, RCPE Archive.

12 His younger brother, David, lent him a small sum to help pay for the furniture.

13 Simpson refers to it as his 'drosky', but it was a two-wheeled carriage drawn by only one horse and was described by others as a curricle. J. Duns, *Memoir of Sir James Young Simpson, Bart.* (Edinburgh, 1873), p. 120.

14 His brother John had always been his lawyer, but he was now very ill and died a few months later.

15 E. B. Simpson, *Sir James Y. Simpson* (Edinburgh, 1896), p. 37.

16 Ibid., p. 74.

17 The technique of percussion had been invented by Auenbrugger in 1761 but had subsequently been forgotten.

18 J. Y. Simpson, Proposals for the Improvement and Elucidation of Uterine Diagnosis, *London and Edinburgh Monthly Journal of Medical Science* 1843, Vol. 3, p. 701.

19 The dukes of Hamilton were, and are still, the Hereditary Keepers of the Palace of Holyroodhouse.

20 The marquises of Breadalbane also had apartments in the palace.

21 The Duke of Hamilton's estate on Arran.

22 Letter, Simpson to Alexander Simpson.

23 Agent (Manager) of the Royal Bank of Scotland in Bathgate.

24 David (b. 1842), Walter (b. 1843), James (b. 1847). His daughters Margaret (b. 1840) and Mary (b. 1845) died at the ages of four and two.

Chapter 6 Experimental Medicine: Galvanism and Gynaecology

1 W. Bynum, S. Lock and R. Porter (eds), *Medical Journals and Medical Knowledge* (London, 1992), p. 30.

2 *The Edinburgh Medical and Surgical Journal* was published by the Royal College of Physicians of Edinburgh.

3 The number of copies printed and distributed by his publisher was on occasions no more than 250, but in the case of the first 'Notice' of his introduction of chloroform, his publisher, Sunderland & Knox of Edinburgh, sold over 4,000 copies. Large numbers were also printed and published in London and America.

4 J. Y. Simpson, Observations Regarding the Influence of Galvanism upon the Action of the Uterus during Labour, *Monthly Journal of Medical Science*, 1846, Vol. 1, pp. 33–48.

5 G. Herder, *Diagnostische Praktisce Beitrage zur Ertwieterung der Gebirtshole* (Leipzig, 1903).

6 T. Radford, On Galvanism Applied to the Treatment of Uterine Haemorrhage, *Provincial Medical and Surgical Journal*, 24 November 1844, p. 424.

7 Simpson, Observations, p. 42.

8 V. B. Green-Armytage in J. Munro Kerr, R. Johnstone and M. Philips (eds), *Historical Review of British Obstetrics and Gynaecology, 1800–1950* (Edinburgh, 1954), p. 358.

9 It was said that two fortunes could be made in gynaecology, one by those who inserted pessaries and one by those who took them out.

10 This was not reported in the medical press until 1816.

11 The meeting, held on 14 December, was reported in full in the *Monthly Journal of Medical Science* for January 1843.

12 In Glasgow hospitals, in a series of 276 amputations (thigh, leg or arm) carried out between 1795 and 1840, the mortality was 37 per cent.

13 In Paris, in a series of 484 amputations between 1836 and 1842, the mortality was 56 per cent.

14 J. Y. Simpson, Case of Amputation of the Neck of the Womb followed by Pregnancy, *Edinburgh Medical and Surgical Journal*, 1841, Vol. 50, pp. 104–12.

15 R. Gooch, *An Account of Some of the Most Important Diseases Peculiar to Women (London, 1829)*.

16 D. Davis, *Principles of Obstetric Medicine (London, 1836)*.

17 Gooch, *An Account*.

18 M. Boivin and A. Duges, *The Diseases of Women* (Paris, 1833).

19 Davis, *Principles*.

20 Colombat de L' Isere, *Traite de Maladies des Femmes* (Paris, 1834).

21 Boivin and Duges, *Diseases of Women*.

22 F. Dupaecque, *Traite theorique et pratictique* (Paris, 1832).

Chapter 7 Library Medicine: Evolution of Disease

1 The full text was published in the *Transactions of the Royal Society of Edinburgh* in 1788.

2 B. Hilton, *A Mad, Bad and Dangerous People: England 1783–1846* (Oxford, 2006), p. 447.

3 James Hutton was Adam Smith's literary executor.

4 Both were published in the *Transactions* of the society.

5 Father of Charles Darwin.

6 The comment was made in a hostile review of Walter Scott's *Marmion*.

7 *The Edinburgh Medical and Surgical Journal*, 1841, Vol. 56, pp. 301–30; 1842, Vol. 57, pp. 121–56; 1842, Vol. 57, pp. 394–29.

8 Ibid., 1841, Vol. 56, p. 324.

9 Ibid., 1842, Vol. 57, p. 406.

10 Ibid., 1842, Vol. 57, p. 407.

11 J. Browne, *Charles Darwin: Voyaging* (London, 1995), p. 457.

12 Hilton, *Mad, Bad and Dangerous*, pp. 438–54.

13 T. Carlyle, Signs of the Times (Article VII), *Edinburgh Review*, June 1829, p. 442.

14 The immediate and ostensible dispute was over church patronage. On that issue a substantial number of Evangelical minsters remained within the established

church. But the underlying difference was over Evangelism, and all of those who left were Evangelicals.

15 R. Chambers, *Vestiges of the Natural History of Creation* (Edinburgh, 1884), p. 152.

16 Ibid., p. 12.

17 This procedure was carefully followed in all nine editions of the book published between 1844 and 1853.

18 The reactions of the press are described in Browne, *Charles Darwin*, pp. 462–64.

19 Hilton, *Mad, Bad and Dangerous*, p. 442.

20 Browne, *Charles Darwin*, p. 461.

21 J. Duns, *Memoir of Sir James Y. Simpson, Bart.* (Edinburgh, 1873), p. 126.

Chapter 8 Library Medicine: On Cholera

1 Thomas Watson, *Lectures on the Principles and Practice of Physic* (London, 1843), Vol. 1, p. 15.

2 The seven members appointed were the elite of the Royal College of Physicians of London, all successful physicians and all able to count members of the royal family and numbers of the highest ranks of London society among their patients. The *Lancet* later dismissed them as drones, sycophants and courtiers who had never had any experience of treating cholera.

3 *Lancet*, 1831–2, Vol. 1, p. 304.

4 The teams were drawn from an 'Association' of 150 doctors.

5 In 1831 he was commissioned by the Royal College of Surgeons in London to investigate the outbreak of cholera in Sunderland.

6 W. B. O'Shaughnessy, *Lancet*, 1831–2, Vol. 1, p. 401; W. B. O'Shaughnessy, *Report on the Chemical Pathology of Malignant Cholera* (London, 1832).

7 *Lancet*, 1831–2, Vol. 2, p. 274.

8 N. MacGillivray, Dr Latta of Leith: Pioneer in the Treatment of Cholera by Intravenous Saline Infusion, *Journal of the Royal College of Physicians of Edinburgh*, 2006, Vol. 36, p. 82.

9 *Edinburgh Medical and Surgical Journal*, 1838, Vol. 49, p. 408.

10 J. Y. Simpson, On the Evidence of the Occasional Propagation of Malignant Cholera, Which is Derived from its Direct Importation into New Localities by Infected Individuals, *Edinburgh Medical and Surgical Journal*, 1838, Vol. 49, pp. 355–408.

11 When the ships of the Royal Navy lying in the Medway in 1831 suffered an outbreak of cholera the debate was whether the disease had been caused by a miasma arising 'from a peculiar condition of the soil and atmosphere there or from some miasma communicated to the air or by exhalations from vessels newly arrived from Riga'. *Edinburgh Medical and Surgical Journal*, 1832, Vol. 37, pp. 295–308.

12 It was often claimed that those most affected were the *inebriated* poor.

13 He had treated the miners infected with cholera at Killingworth Colliery near Newcastle in 1832.

14 J. Snow, *On the Mode of Communication of Cholera* (London, 1849).

Chapter 9 Ether

1 Father of the more famous Oliver Wendell Holmes, the Supreme Court Justice.
2 Stinking nightshade or Hyoscyamus.
3 Mandrake or Mandragora officinarum.
4 Letter, Charles Meigs to Simpson. Simpson Papers, Royal College of Surgeons of Edinburgh Archive.
5 Simpson Papers, RCSE Archive.
6 He eventually recorded his experience in the *Southern Medical and Surgical Journal* in 1849.
7 L. Stratman, *Chloroform* (Stroud, 2003), p. 15.
8 F. D. Moore, John Collins Warren and his Act of Conscience, *Annals of Surgery*, 1999, Vol. 229, pp. 187–96
9 H. J. Bigelow, Insensibility During Operations Produced by Inhalation, *Boston Medical and Surgical Journal*, 1846, Vol. 35, pp. 309–17.
10 He also published his results in the April edition of the *Monthly Journal of Medical Science* in 1848.
11 For some years general anaesthesia was generally known as etherisation, no matter whether the agent used was ether, chloroform or even nitrous oxide.
12 William Huskisson, who had recently been President of the Board of Trade, was crushed by a train at the opening of the Liverpool to Manchester Railway on 15 September 1830.
13 Ole Selcher, Hans Andersen and James Young Simpson, *British Journal of Anaesthesia* 1972, Vol. 44, No. 11, p. 1212.
14 Here Simpson took encouragement from the thought that 'the motor nervous powers of the uterus belong to the spinal system and are not in any necessary dependence on the brain', and from reports in the medical literature that in women paralysed by paraplegia, parturition proceeded regularly in its course and without conscious pain.
15 The number was not reported. Later, in April 1847, a correspondent in London, Dr Protheroe Smith, asked Simpson for the exact number of cases included in his series, but there is no record of any reply.
16 Simpson, April 1848 edition of *Monthly Journal of Medical Science*, p. 726n.
17 J. Duns, *Memoir of Sir James Simpson*, Bart. (Edinburgh, 1873), pp. 207, 208.
18 J. Y. Simpson, *Account of a New Anaesthetic Agent as a Substitute for Ether* (Edinburgh, 1847), p. 6.

Chapter 10 Chloroform

1 B. Silliman, *American Journal of Science*, 1830, Vol. 21, p. 405.
2 B. Silliman, *Elements of Chemistry in the order of lectures given in Yale College* (New Haven, 1830), pp. 19–20.
3 L. Stratman, *Chloroform: The Quest for Oblivion* (Stroud, 2003), pp. 19–30.
4 J. W. Dundee, David Waldie: Facts and Fiction, *Anaesthesia*, 1953, Vol. 8, p. 219.
5 D. Waldie, *Pharmaceutical Times*, 1848, Vol. 3, p. 202.
6 In February 1832 Guthrie succeeded in finding a method of separating his

'chloric ether' from the alcohol in which it had been carried through the process of production.

7 Simpson acknowledged the part played by Waldie in the introduction of chloroform only in a footnote of two lines on page 6 of his *Account of a New Anaesthetic Agent as a Substitute for Ether*. Simpson did not credit Samuel Guthrie with the discovery of chloroform; he cites only the work of Soubeiran in 1831 and Liebeg in 1832.

8 Professor James Miller, quoted by Simpson's daughter in E. B. Simpson, *Sir James Y. Simpson* (Edinburgh, 1896), p. 58.

9 M. Simpson, *Simpson the Obstetrician* (London, 1972), p. 130.

10 This list of advantages and surrounding discussion reported in *Monthly Journal of Medical Science*, December 1847 issue.

11 Simpson, *Simpson the Obstetrician*, p. 131.

12 *Account of a New Anaesthetic Agent as a Substitute for Sulphuric Ether in Surgery and Midwifery*.

13 It appeared in the 21 November edition.

14 *Times*, 12 October 1854.

15 Richard Mackenzie was at the beginning of what promised to be a very successful career as a surgeon in Edinburgh. He died of cholera a few days after the battle at Alma. His place in Edinburgh was taken by another promising surgeon, Joseph Lister.

16 The poison gas used in France during World War I.

17 Letter, A.W. Cockburn to Simpson, Royal College of Surgeons of Edinburgh Archive.

18 Letter, Dr Gream to Simpson, RCSE Archive.

19 John Bird Sumner was appointed in 1848.

20 Thomas Chalmers was appointed in 1832.

21 In January 1848, Thomas Chalmers had already assured Simpson's colleague, Professor Miller, that those with religious objections to the use of chloroform were 'small theologians and should be ignored'.

22 Letter, A. C. Cockburn to Simpson, RCSE Archive.

23 Letter, Dr A. Tytler to Simpson, RCSE Archive.

24 The same John Snow who had played such an important part in explaining the spread of cholera in London in 1854.

25 J. Snow, On the Fatal Cases of Inhalation of Chloroform, *Edinburgh Medical and Surgical Journal* 1849, Vol. 72, pp. 75–84.

Chapter 11 Fortune, Family and Fame

1 Letter to Simpson from Robert Grindlay, Simpson Papers, Royal College of Surgeons of Edinburgh Archive.

2 Simpson Papers, RCSE Archive.

3 M. Simpson, *Simpson the Obstetrician* (London, 1972), pp. 160–1.

4 J. Duns, *Memoir of Sir James Young Simpson, Bart.* (Edinburgh, 1873), p. 117.

5 Ibid., pp. 116 and 119.

6 The house was originally called Starview; later it became Viewbank. Later still, when Simpson was made a baronet, the name was changed to Strathavon Lodge.

7 *The Monthly Journal of Medical Science*, 1853, Vol. 16, pp. 354 and 366.

Chapter 12 Homoeopathy, Mesmerism and Blackmail

1 The statement was made by the city's Provost during the ceremony at which Simpson was made an honorary burgess of Edinburgh.

2 F. Black, *A Treatise on the Principles and Practice of Homoeopathy* (London, 1842).

3 J. Y. Simpson, *Homoeopathy: Its Tenets and Tendencies*, 3rd edition (Edinburgh, 1853).

4 *Lancet*, 20 September 1851, p. 284.

5 B. Hilton, *A Mad Bad and Dangerous People: England 1783–1846* (Oxford, 2006), p. 452.

6 *Lancet*, 20 September 1851, p. 283.

7 Simpson also wrote that he totally disbelieved in any of the so-called related phenomena such as transference of senses or clairvoyance. To the editor he wrote: 'to show the sincerity of my belief I will if you allow me, place five boxes or packets, each of them containing a line of Shakespeare, in your hands and in the hands of a small committee of medical men who you and I shall conjointly agree upon and who with you shall be the judges and make all the necessary arrangements; and I now offer through you £500 for the reading of these included five lines by any clairvoyant.'

8 *London and Edinburgh Monthly Journal of Medical Science*, 1845, Vol. 51, No. 3, pp. 169–204.

9 *Medical Gazette*, 9 September 1846.

10 *Lancet*, 8 May, 1847, pp. 479–80.

11 *Lancet*, 14 August, 1847, p. 185.

12 *Lancet*, 13 November 1847, pp. 517–21.

13 J. Y. Simpson, *Homoeopathy: Its Tenets and Tendencies, Theoretical, Theological and Therapeutical* (Edinburgh, 1852).

14 Rumours and false accusations were used against him during the election of a new Principal of Edinburgh University in 1868 (see Chapter 16).

Chapter 13 Influence and Power

1 Letter from the Queen to her uncle, King Leopold, quoted by C. Hibbert, *Queen Victoria: A Personal History* (London, 2000), p. 216.

2 Ibid., p. 217.

3 He had not yet succeeded and was then the Marquis of Lorne.

4 Louis Agassiz, Professor of Zoology and Geology at Harvard, 1847–73.

5 J. Duns, *Memoir of Sir James Y. Simpson, Bart.* (Edinburgh, 1873), p. 360.

6 L. J. Jacyna, Sharpey's Fibres: The Life of William Sharpey, The Father of Modern Physiology in England, *Medical History*, 2003, Vol. 42, p. 265.

7 T. Laycock, quoted in M. Barfoot (ed.), *To Ask the Suffrages of the Patrons: Thomas Laycock and the Edinburgh Chair of Medicine, 1851* (London, 1955), p. 70.

8 Barfoot, *To Ask the Suffrages of the Patrons*, p. 33.

9 Ibid., p. 110.

10 William Russell, quoted in R. Hudson, *William Russell, Special Correspondent of The Times* (London, 1995), p. 10.

11 T. Royle, *Crimea: The Great Crimean War 1854–1856* (London, 1999), p. 247.

12 M. Bostridge, *Florence Nightingale: The Woman and Her Legend* (London, 2008), p. 205.

13 Mackenzie died of cholera soon after the Battle of the Alma. Joseph Lister succeeded to his place on the staff of Edinburgh Royal Infirmary.

14 M. McCrae, The Great Highland Famine: The Lack of Medical Aid, *Review of Scottish Culture*, 2001–2002, No. 14, p. 62.

15 G. Clark, *A History of the Royal College of Physicians of London; Volume Two* (London, 1966), p. 628.

16 P. Bartrip, *Themselves Writ Large: The British Medical Association 1832–1966* (London, 1996), p.72.

17 Ibid, p. 339, quoting Professor George Watt of Glasgow.

18 An authority vested in the Archbishop of Canterbury in 1533 and never repealed.

19 Bartrip, *Themselves Writ Large*, p. 80.

20 Lord Elcho, son and heir of the Earl of Wemyss and MP for Haddington.

21 Thomas Headlam, barrister and Liberal MP for Newcastle upon Tyne.

22 This was a view shared by medical corporations in Scotland; see M. McCrae, *Physicians and Society* (Edinburgh, 2007), p. 212.

23 Bartrip, *Themselves Writ Large*, p. 90.

24 Storrer's many reports are among the Simpson Papers in the archive of the Royal College of Surgeons of Edinburgh.

25 Letter, Storrer to Simpson, RCSE Archive.

26 To prevent Scotland from being over-represented on the council, Edinburgh and Aberdeen universities together elected one member, and Glasgow and St Andrews together elected one member.

27 Duns, *Memoir*, p. 385.

Chapter 14 Private Practice, Archaeology and Semmelweis

1 On one occasion a firm of pharmaceutical chemists found it had on its hands a large stock of a rare and expensive drug that Simpson had been prescribing for his patients but had suddenly abandoned as useless. A partner in the firm explained the situation to Simpson, who replied: 'I will put that right.' He began to prescribe again until the stock was used up. B. Ashworth, *The Bramwells of Edinburgh: A Medical Dynasty* (Edinburgh, 1986), p. 73.

2 At night he used a cab.

3 M. Simpson, *Simpson the Obstetrician* (London, 1972), p. 169.

4 See Appendix 1.

5 Royal College of Physicians of Edinburgh Archive.

6 I. Loudon, *The Tragedy of Childbed Fever* (Oxford, 2000), p. 6.

7 Ibid., pp. 60–3.

8 A. Gordon, *Treatise on the Epidemic Puerperal Fever of Aberdeen* (Aberdeen, 1795).

9 W. Campbell, *A Treatise of the Epidemic of Puerperal Fever as it Prevailed in Edinburgh in 1821–22* (Edinburgh, 1822) quoted by Loudon, *Tragedy of Childbed Fever*, p. 45.

10 C. D. Meigs, *Females and their Diseases: A Series of Letters to his Class* (Philadelphia, 1847), p. 591.

11 Loudon, *Tragedy of Childbed Fever*, p. 85.

12 Sir William Sinclair, *Semmelweis: His Life and His Doctrines* (Manchester, 1909)

13 The Maternal Mortality Rate was the number of maternal deaths per 1,000 births.

14 Loudon, *Tragedy of Childbed Fever*, p. 93.

15 F. H. Arneth, Evidence of Puerperal Fever Depending upon the Contagious Inoculation of Morbid Matter, *Monthly Journal of Medical Science*, 1851, Vol. 12, p. 506.

16 Sinclair, *Semmelweis*, p. 73.

17 Loudon, *Tragedy of Childbed Fever*, p. 95.

18 Arneth, Evidence of Puerperal Fever Depending upon the Contagious Inoculation of Morbid Matter, *Monthly Journal of Medical Science*, 1851, Vol. 12, pp. 505–11.

19 Loudon, *Tragedy of Childbed Fever*, p. 103.

20 Ibid., p. 108.

Chapter 15 Acupressure and Hospitalism

1 J. Y. Simpson, Some Notes on the Analogy between Puerperal Fever and Surgical Fever, *Monthly Journal of Medical Science*, 1850, Vol. 11, p. 414.

2 The total mortality in the Edinburgh series was unusually low, only 1.6 per cent. It may be that the estimate of the percentage of deaths due to puerperal fever that Simpson thought too high was in fact more representative of general experience in Britain.

3 Simpson, Some Notes, p. 421.

4 *Medical Times & Gazette*, 11 February 1860.

5 *British Medical Journal*, 14 January 1860.

6 *Edinburgh Medical Journal*, 1861–2, Vol. 7, p. 717.

7 W. Pirrie and W. Keith, *Acupressure: An Excellent Method for the Arresting of Haemorrhage and of the Accelerating the Healing of Wounds* (Edinburgh, 1867).

8 *Lancet*, 5 May 1860, p. 446.

9 *Edinburgh Medical Journal* 1860, Vol. 6, p. 568.

10 J. Neudorfer, *Handbuch der Kriegschirurgie*, 1867, p. 213.

11 *Lancet*, 24 January 1863, p. 94.

12 *British Medical Journal*, 12 April 1862, Vol. 1, p. 391.

13 This recommendation followed even the most enthusiastic account of the advantages of acupressure. *British Medical Journal*, 2 September 1865.

14 *British Medical Journal*, 18 November 1865, p. 544.

15 Ibid., 19 December 1865, p. 595.

16 Ibid., 23 December 1865, p. 672.

17 Ibid., 22 August 1891.

18 *Monthly Journal of Medical Science*, November 1848, No. 24, pp. 329–38.

19 J. Y. Simpson, Report of the Edinburgh Royal Maternity Hospital, *Monthly Journal of Medical Science*, 1848, No. 24, pp. 329–38.

20 *Sixth Report of the Medical Officer to the Privy Council* (1864). The Medical Officer to the Privy Council was John Simon. He commissioned Holmes and Bristowe to prepare his report.

21 *British Medical Journal*, 23 January 1869, pp. 87–8.

22 J. Y. Simpson, Effects of Hospitalism upon the Mortality of Limb-Amputations, *British Medical Journal*, 30 January 1869, p. 93. This was the first time that the word 'hospitalism' had been used.

23 *Edinburgh Medical Journal*, 1869, Vol. 14, pp. 816–30; Vol. 14, pp. 1084; Vol. 15, 523–32.

24 J. Y. Simpson, On Our Existing System of Hospitalism and its Effects, *Edinburgh Medical Journal*, 1869, Vol. 14, p. 1114.

25 T. Holmes, On 'Hospitalism', being a Criticism on Some Papers by Sir J. Y. Simpson in the Edinburgh Medical Journal for March and June 1869, *Lancet*, 1869, Vol. 2, p. 194.

26 R. Holmes Coote, On Hospitalism, *British Medical Journal*, 27 March 1869.

27 G. W. Callender, Note on Amputations in Hospitals, *Lancet*, 18 September 1869.

28 L. Tait, A Consideration of the Criticisms Advanced on Sir J. Y. Simpson's Papers on Hospitalism, *Lancet*, 1 April 1871, p. 443.

29 Joseph Lister first described his antiseptic system of surgery in articles in the *Lancet* between March and July 1867. The first of these articles described the use of carbolic acid in the management of compound fractures.

30 J. Y. Simpson, On Our System of Hospitalism and its Effects, *Edinburgh Medical Journal*, 1869, Vol. 15, pp. 523–32.

Chapter 16 Triumph and Decline

1 For this information I am indebted to Bruce Gorie, Secretary to Lyon Office.

2 No diagnosis has been recorded for illnesses suffered by Simpson's children James and Jessie, but from the little information available about their illnesses and the entries in the death certificates it seems probable that both had atopic dermatitis and severe chronic asthma.

3 M. Simpson, *Simpson the Obstetrician* (London, 1972), p. 218.

4 His portrait appears in David Octavius Hill's huge painting, 'The Disruption

General Assembly', which now hangs in the offices of the Free Church of Scotland on the Mound in Edinburgh.

5 Although the minister, Dr Muir, was an Evangelical he was unwilling to leave the Church of Scotland and give up his parish.

6 After the Disruption, the Free Church founded New College as an institution for educating a learned ministry, to guide the nation through a new Reformation, reasserting the spiritual independence of the Church.

7 J. Duns, *Memoir of Sir James Y. Simpson, Bart.* (Edinburgh, 1873), p. 125.

8 Ibid., p. 404.

9 *The Bridgewater Treatises*, published in 1836, had been commissioned in the will of Francis Egerton, the eccentric Earl of Bridgewater who wished to promote a modified version of Paley's *Natural Theology*.

Treatise I: Thomas Chalmers, *The Adaptation of External Nature to the Moral and Intellectual Constitution of Man.*

Treatise II: John Kidd, *On the Adaptation of External Nature to the Physical Condition of Man.*

Treatise III: William Whewell, *On Astronomy and General Physics.*

Treatise IV: Charles Bell, *The Hand: Its Mechanism and Vital Endowments as Evincing Design.*

Treatise V: Peter Mark Roget, *Animal and Vegetable Physiology Considered with Reference to Natural Theology.*

Treatise VI: William Buckland, *Geology and Mineralogy Considered with Reference to Natural Theology.*

Treatise VII: William Kirby, *On the History, Habits, and Instincts of Animals.*

Treatise VIII: William Prout, *Chemistry, Meteorology, and the Function of Digestion.*

10 Charles Bell, *The Hand.*

11 Letter, Simpson to his brother Sandy.

12 E. B. Simpson, *Sir James Y. Simpson* (Edinburgh, 1896), p. 127.

13 J. Y. Simpson, *Is the Great Pyramid of Gizeh a Meteorological Monument?* (Edinburgh, A & C Black, 1867). Presented at the Royal Society of Edinburgh in January 1868; and J. Y. Simpson, *Archaic Sculpturing of Cups, Circles etc upon Stones and Rocks, in Scotland, England and other Countries* (Edinburgh, A. & C. Black, 1868).

14 J. Lister, On the Antiseptic Principle in the Practice of Surgery, *Lancet*, 21 September 1867, p. 353.

15 Sir J. Y. Simpson, Bart., Carbolic Acid and Its Compounds in Surgery, *Lancet*, 2 November 1867, p. 546.

16 *Lancet*, 11 July 1868, p. 58.

17 These were James Syme, Robert Christison, John Hughes-Bennet, Thomas Laycock, James Spence, Douglas Maclagan, Sir Lyon Playfair.

18 This was a revival of the accusations that Simpson fathered the child adopted by the Quintons in 1854. There was also a second rumour that he had an illegitimate son. Lawson Tait, one of Simpson's students, who later became Professor

of Midwifery at Birmingham, frequently took pleasure in drawing attention to the remarkable similarity of his facial features and body shape to those of the great J. Y. Simpson. It was only after Simpson died that he began to claim Simpson was his father as well as his mentor, a claim that was usually treated as a joke. It was also something that Lawson Tait's parents and Simpson's family never took seriously.

19 *Lancet*, 11 July 1868, p. 58.

20 E. Simpson, *Sir James Y. Simpson* (Edinburgh, 1896), p. 143.

21 Myrtle Simpson, *Simpson the Obstetrician* (London, 1972), p. 279.

22 Sir A. Grant, *The Story of the University of Edinburgh* (London, 1884), p. 159.

23 E. Hamilton, *The Warwickshire Scandal* (London, 1999), p. 22.

24 Robert kept a diary of Simpson's last few weeks, which is reproduced in Appendix 1.

25 Simpson, in his will, had set aside a fourth part of his estate to provide a very comfortable annuity for Jessie but he did not leave her outright any funds or property that she would be required to manage herself.

26 *Lancet*, 14 May 1970, p. 704.

Epilogue

1 *Lancet*, 14 May 1870, p. 704.

2 E. Simpson, *Sir James Simpson* (Edinburgh, 1896) p. 140.

Bibliography

COLLECTIONS, LETTERS AND PAMPHLETS

Book of the Old Edinburgh Club
Jamaican Archives and Records Department
Royal College of Physicians of Edinburgh
Royal College of Surgeons of Edinburgh
University of Edinburgh
West Lothian Local History Library

JOURNALS

British Medical Journal
Edinburgh Medical Journal
Edinburgh Review
Journal of Obstetrics and Gynaecology of the British Empire
Journal of the Royal College of Physicians of Edinburgh
Journal of the Royal College of Surgeons of Edinburgh
Journal of the Royal Society of Medicine
Lancet, the
Medical Gazette
Monthly Journal of Medical Science
New England Journal of Medicine
Obstetrics and Gynaecology
Provincial Medical and Surgical Journal
Review of Scottish Culture
Scottish Medical Journal

PAMPHLETS

Anon. *John Newland*, Jamaican Archives and Records Department. BB/B/Newland.
Anon. *Sir James Young Simpson*. London (Monthly Tract Society) 1870.
Anon. *Memoir of Sir James Y. Simpson, Bart. With an account of the Funeral and Funeral Sermons*. Edinburgh (J. Mclaren) 1870.
Anon. *Sir James Young Simpson: The Man of Science, the Man of God*. (Reprinted in Bullock, The Crown of the Road, 1884.).
Anon. *Sir James Young Simpson*. London (Religious Tract Society) 1912.

BOOKS

Adams, I. H. *The Mapping of a Scottish Estate*. Edinburgh (Edinburgh University Press) 1971.

Aitchison, P. and Cassell, A. *The Lowland Clearances*. East Lothian (Tuckwell Press) 2003.

Aldini, G. *An Account of the Late Improvements in Galvanism Containing the Author's Experiments On the Body of a Malefactor Executed at Newgate*, London. London (Cuthill & Martin; John Murray) 1803.

Asherson, N. *Stone Voices: The Search for Scotland*. London (Granta Publications) 2002.

Atkinson, R. S. *James Simpson and Chloroform*. London (Priory Press) 1973.

Banwell, P. E. *Sir James 'Young' Simpson and the History of an Idea: Acupressure in Context*. London (Wellcome Institute for the History of Medicine) 1991.

Barfoot, M. *To Ask the Suffrages and Patrons: Thomas Laycock and the Edinburgh Chair of Medicine, 1855*. London (Wellcome Institute for the History of Medicine) 1995.

Bartrip, P. *Themselves Writ Large: The British Medical Association 1832–1966*. London (BMJ Publishing) 1996.

Baxter, S. *Revolutions in the Earth: James Hutton and the True Age of the World*. New York (Tom Docherty) 2003.

Bissett, A. M. *History of Bathgate*. Bathgate (West Lothian County Council) 1906.

Black, F. A. *Treatise on the Principles and Practice of Homoeopathy*. London (Drysdale and Russel) 1842.

Black, J. W. (ed.). *Selected Obstetrical & Gynaecological Works of Sir James Y. Simpson*. Edinburgh (Adam & Charles Black) 1871.

Boivin, M. and Duges, A. *The Diseases of Women*. Paris, 1833.

Bostridge, M. *Florence Nightingale: The Woman and Her Legend*. London (Viking) 2008.

Brown, R. L. *Robert Burns' Tours of the Highlands and Stirlingshire 1787*. Ipswich (The Boydell Press) 1973.

Brown, T. *Observations on Zoonomia by Erasmus Darwin, M.D*. Edinburgh (Mundell & Son) 1798.

Browne, J. *Charles Darwin: Voyaging*. London (Jonathan Cape) 1995.

Buchan, D. (ed.). *Folk Tradition and Folk Medicine in Scotland*. Edinburgh (Canongate) 1994.

Bynum, W. F., Lock S. and Porter, R. *Medical Journals and Medical Knowledge*. London (Taylor and Francis) 1992.

Campbell, W. *A Treatise of the Epidemic of Puerperal Fever as it Prevailed in Edinburgh in 1821–22*. Edinburgh (Bell & Broadfute) 1822.

Cecil, D. *Melbourne*. London (Constable) 1965.

Chambers, R. *Vestiges of the Natural History of Creation*. London (John Churchill) 1884.

Clark, G. *A History of the Royal College of Physicians of London*. London (Oxford University Press) 1966.

Clow, A. and Clow, N.L. *The Chemical Revolution*. Philadelphia (Gordon and Breach) 1952.

Cockburn, Lord. *Memorials of His Time*. Edinburgh (Adam and Charles Black) 1856.

Cosh, M. *Edinburgh: The Golden Age*. Edinburgh (John Donald) 2003.

Darwin, E. *Zoonomia or the Laws of Organic Life*. Dublin (Dugdale) 1800.

Davidson, T. *Bathgate Academy 1833–1933*. West Lothian (West Lothian County Council) 1933.

Davis, D. *Principles of Obstetric Medicine*. London (Taylor and Watson) 1836.

Desmond, A. and Moore, J. *Darwin*. London (Michael Joseph) 1991.

Devine, T. M. and Mitchison, R. (eds). *People and Society in Scotland 1760–1830*. Edinburgh (John Donald) 1988.

Devine, T. M. *The Scottish Nation*. London (Allen Lane) 1999.

Devine, T. M. *Clearance and Improvement*. Edinburgh (John Donald) 2006.

Dodgson, R. A. *Land and Society in Early Scotland*. Oxford (Oxford University Press) 1981.

Donnachie, I. *A History of the Brewing Industry in Scotland*. Edinburgh (John Donald) 1979.

Duns, J. *Memoir of Sir James Young Simpson, Bart*. Edinburgh (Edmonston and Douglas) 1873.

Fenton, A. *Country Life in Scotland: Our Rural Past*. Edinburgh (Birlinn) 1999.

Ferguson, N. *Empire*. London (Penguin) 2004.

Franklin, T. B. *A History of Scottish Farming*. Edinburgh (Nelson) 1952.

Fry, M. *The Dundas Despotism*. Edinburgh (Edinburgh University Press) 1992.

Galvani, L. *De Viribus Electricitatis in Motu Musculare Commentarius*. Bologna, 1791.

Gauldie, E. *The Scottish Country Miller, 1700–1900*. Edinburgh (John Donald) 1981.

Gibbon, J. *History of Western Science*. London (Folio Society) 2006.

Gillies, R. P. *Memoirs of a Literary Veteran*. London (Richard Bentley) 1851.

Godlee, Sir R. J. *Lord Lister*. Oxford (Clarendon Press) 1924.

Grant, Sir A. *The Story of Edinburgh University*. London (Longman, Green & Co.) 1884.

Hutton, J. *Theory of the Earth with Proofs and Illustrations*. Edinburgh (Dickson) 1788.

Gooch, R. *An Account of Some of the Most Important Diseases Peculiar to Women*. London (The New Sydenham Society) 1829.

Gordon, A. *Treatise on the Epidemic Puerperal Fever of Aberdeen*. London (G.G. and J. Johnson) 1795.

Gordon, H. L. *Sir James Young Simpson and Chloroform (1811–1870)*. London (Fraser Unwin) 1897.

Graham, D. *John Newland*. Arbroath (Brodie and Salmond) 1901.

Graham, H. G. *The Social Life of Scotland in the Eighteenth Century*. London (A & C Black) 1928.

Grant, Sir A. *The Story of the University of Edinburgh*. London (Longman, Green & Co.) 1884.

Haig, W. *William Pitt the Younger*. London (Harper Collins) 2004.

Hamilton, D. *The Healers: A History of Medicine in Scotland*. Edinburgh (Canongate) 1981.

Handley, J. E. *Scottish Farming in the Eighteenth Century*. London (Faber and Faber) 1953.

Hendrie, W. F. and Mackie, A. *The Bathgate Book*. Bathgate (West Lothian County Council), 2001.

Houston, R. A. and Knox, W. W. J. *History of Scotland from the Earliest Days to the Present Time*. London (Allen Lane) 2001.

Hurd, D. *Robert Peel: A Biography*. London (Weidenfeld & Nicolson) 2007.

Jacyna, L. S. *Philosophical Whigs*. London (Routledge) 1994.

Kaufman, M. H. *Medical Teaching in Edinburgh in the Eighteenth and Nineteenth Centuries*. Edinburgh (Royal College of Surgeons of Edinburgh) 2003.

Kerr, J. M., Johnstone, R. and Philips, M. (eds.). *Historical Review of Obstetrics and Gynaecology*. Edinburgh (E. & S. Livingstone) 1954.

Knox, F. J. *The Anatomist's Instructor and Museum Companion*. Edinburgh (Adam and Charles Black) 1836.

Dodgshon, R. A. *Land and Society in Early Scotland*. Oxford (Clarendon Press) 1981.

Hilton, B. *A Mad, Bad and Dangerous People: England 1783–1846*. Oxford (Clarendon Press) 2006.

Hurd, D. *Robert Peel: A Biography*. London (Weidenfeld & Nicolson) 2007.

Lonsdale, H. *A Sketch of the Life and Writings of Robert Knox*. London (Macmillan) 1870.

Loudon, I. *The Tragedy of Childbed Fever*. Oxford (Oxford University Press) 2000.

Meigs, C. D. *Females and their Diseases: A Series of Letters to his Class*. Philadelphia (Lea and Blanchard) 1848.

Miller, J. *Sir James Young Simpson and the Discovery of Chloroform*. Canada Lancet and Practitioner, 1926.

Muir, C. *Mercat Cross and Tollbooth*. Edinburgh (John Donald) 1988.

Paterson, R. *Memorials of the Life of James Syme*. Edinburgh (Edminston and Douglas) 1871.

Pirrie, W. *A Practical Treatise on Acupressure*. London (John Churchill & Sons) 1867.

Pirrie, W. and Keith, W. *Acupressure: An Excellent Method for the Arresting of Haemorrhage and Accelerating the Healing of Wounds*. Edinburgh (John Churchill & Sons) 1867.

Priestley, W. O. and Storer, H. R. *The Obstetric Memoirs and Contributions of J.Y. Simpson*. Edinburgh (Adam & Charles Black) 1856.

Rae, I. *Knox the Anatomist*. Edinburgh (Oliver and Boyd) 1964.

Roberts, S. *Sophia Jex-Blake: A Woman Pioneer in Nineteenth Century Medical Reform*. London (Routledge) 1993.

Rogers, P. (ed.). *Boswell and Johnson in Scotland*. New Haven (Yale University Press) 1993.

Royle, T. *Crimea: The Great Crimean War*. London (Little, Brown and Company) 1999.

Shaw, J. *Water Power in Scotland 1550–1870*. Edinburgh (John Donald) 1984.

Shepherd, J. A. *Simpson and Syme of Edinburgh*. Edinburgh (Livingstone) 1969.

Sibbald, Sir R. *Provision for the Poor in Time of Dearth and Scarcity*. Edinburgh, 1699.

Silliman, B. *Elements of Chemistry in the Order of Lectures given in Yale College*. New Haven (Yale University Press) 1830.

Simpson, E. B. *Sir James Y. Simpson*. Edinburgh (Oliphant, Anderson and Ferrier) 1896.

Simpson, M. *Simpson the Obstetrician: A Biography*. London (Gollancz) 1972.

Simpson, J. Y. *Homoeopathy: Its Tenets and Tendencies, Theoretical, Theological and Therapeutic*. Edinburgh (Sutherland and Knox) 1852.

Sinclair, Sir W. *Semmelweis: His Life and his Doctrines*. Manchester (Manchester University Press) 1909.

Small, H. *Florence Nightingale*. London (Constable) 1998.

Snow, J. *On the Mode of Communication of Cholera*. London (John Constable) 1849.

Stratman, L. *Chloroform: The Quest for Oblivion*. Stroud (Sutton Publishing) 2003.

Symon, J. A. *Scottish Farming, Past and Present*. Edinburgh (Oliver and Boyd) 1959.

Thomson, J. *An Account of Life, Lectures and Writings of William Cullen*. Edinburgh (William Blackwood) 1859.

Todd, R. B. (ed.). *Cyclopaedia of Anatomy and Physiology*. London (Longman, Brown, Green, Longman and Roberts) 1839.

Topographical, Statistical and Historical Gazetteer of Scotland. Glasgow (Fullarton & Co.), 1842.

Tuke, D. H. *The History of the Insane in the British Isles*. London (Kegan Paul) 1882.

Turner, A. L. *The Story of a Great Hospital: The Royal Infirmary of Edinburgh, 1729–1929*. Edinburgh (Oliver and Boyd) 1937.

Young, D. *Improvements Upon Agriculture*. Edinburgh (John Bell) 1785.

Young, G. M. *Victorian England: Portrait of an Age*. London (Oxford University Press) 1936.

Index

Aberdeen Obstetric Dispensary 194
Abernethy, John 23
acupressure 204–9, 226, 236
Adam, Alexander 19
Adam, Robert 6, 13, 79
Adam, William 211
Agassiz, Louis 170
Air Tractor forceps 159
Aitkin, John 22, 24
Alderson, Dr 232
Alexander, Robert 34
Alison, Dr W. P. 28, 62, 154, 155,
    171, 172
Allen, John 35, 36
Allman, Professor George 170
*American Journal of Medical
    Science* 99
American Medical Monthly 125
amputations, mortality from 212–17
anaesthesia 105–16, 117–37, 188,
    193, 196
    see also chloroform and ether
Andersen, Hans Christian 111, 235
Anderson, Thomas 208
Anstruther, Lady 65
antiseptics 225
Apothecaries Act, 1815 181
Apothecaries Hall, Liverpool 118,
    119
Apothecaries Society 181
Archaeological Institute of
    London 187
Aretaeus 94, 106
Argyll, Dukes of 6, 66, 67, 168, 170,
    178, 235

Aris's Gazette 114
Army Medical Department 23, 36
Arneth, Franz 196–9
Arnott, Neil 88
Ashwell, Dr Samuel 153
Association Medical Journal 179
Auchenskioch Estate 140
Austro-Prussian War, 1866 212

Babbage, Charles 20
'baby sucker' forceps 159
Baillie, William of Polkemmet 11
Balbardie 8
Ballingall, Sir George 109, 178, 191
Bank of England 139
Barbour, Margo 242
Barclay, John 23
Barker, Dr 125
Bathgate 9–15, 27, 30–2, 88, 95, 244
    cholera in 95
    Parish School 11, 12
Batista Porta 106
Battle of Alma 177
Battle of Waterloo 23, 41
Bauchope, Miss Maria 49
Becker, Dr 98
Beddoe, John 178
Beddoes, Thomas 106, 107
Bede, the Venerable 191
Bell, John 74
Bennett, Professor John
        Hughes 171–6, 216
Bethlehem Hospital, London
        (Bedlam) 42
Bett, Dr 118, 119

Bigelow, Dr Henry 108, 153, 242
objection to JYS as inventor of
chloroform 153
bills to regulate medicine in the
UK 180–6
Black, Adam 227, 228
Black, Professor Joseph 18, 79
Blackwell, Elizabeth 229
Blackwell, Emily 229
Blackwood's Magazine 20, 26
Blair, Professor Hugh 18, 79
Blantyre, Lady 220
Blantyre, Lord 67
bloodletting 41
bodysnatchers 24
Boece, Hector 85, 191
Boivin, M. 77
Bonnymuir slaughter 17
*Boston Medical and Surgical
Journal* 153
Boswell, James 5
Boyer, Professor 23
Breadalbane, Marchioness of 66
Brewster, Sir David 227
Bright, John 226
Bristowe, John 212, 213
British Linen Bank 34
British Lying-In Hospital 160
British Medical Association 184,
186, 216, 225
British Medical Journal 205–8, 212,
215, 216
British Museum 150, 191
Brodick Castle 66
Brodie, John 68
Brougham, Henry 19, 36
Brown, Professor Samuel 222
Broxburn 95
Brunel, Isambard Kingdom 211
Burke, William 22, 25–7
Burke and Hare trial 22, 25–7
Burns, John 77
Burns, Robert 7, 49
Bute, Marchioness of 211

Callender, George 215
Cambridge, Duke of *see* Prince
George
Campbell, William 54
carbolic acid, use of as
antiseptic 225, 226
Carlyle, Thomas 86
Carmichael, William 173, 175
Carstairs, Jane 121
Carswell. Robert 32, 37, 40
Case Western Reserve
University 229
Cassillis, Earl of 6
Cat-Stane, Linlithgow 191
Catholic Emancipation Act, 1829 50
Cauliflower Tumours 77
Central Board of Health 91, 92
cervix, amputation of 76, 77
Chalmers, Thomas 86, 128, 221
Chambers, Robert 66, 82, 85, 86,
88, 173, 176
Chambers, William 86
Charenton Asylum 42
Chegoin, Hervez de 77
Chemistry Society 36
Chenry, Thomas 177
chloric ether (also called
Dutch Liquid and Sweet
Whiskey) 118, 119
chloroform 1, 116, 117–37, 150,
152, 167, 168, 193, 218, 232,
241
banned in the USA 125
causing sexual arousal 127, 128
experiments by JYS 118–22
first use in dentistry 122
first use in obstetrics 121
means of administering 135–7
pamphlet on by JYS 123, 124
producing hydrochloric acid 126
religious objections to 129, 130
unexplained deaths from 133,
134
use by Queen Victoria 167

cholera 89–104, 177
  in the Crimean War 177
  pandemics, 1831–54 89, 90, 96
Cholera Board 92
Christison, David 178
Christison, Sir Robert 22, 25, 54,
  117, 227, 228
Church of England 128
Church of Scotland 128, 131, 221
Churchill, Dr Fleetwood 76, 77, 132
Churchill, John 87
'Cinderella' *see* Girdwood, Miss
Clarendon, Lord 178
Clarke, Samuel 41
Clay, Charles 74, 75
Cleland, Mary (grandmother of
  JYS) 10
Clerk, Sir James 167
Clerke, Sir Charles 77
Clift, William 40
Cobden, Richard 226
Cockburn, John of Ormiston 4
Cockburn, Lord Henry 15, 19
Coghill, Mr 243
Coldstream, John 154
Cole, Lord 231
Collins, Robert 154
Coombe, Dr 132
Coote, Holmes 178
Cormack, John Rose 69
Corn Laws 139
Cowan, William 163
Cowper, William 184, 185
Cox, Robert 88
Craig, Sir William Gibson 227
Crimean War 124, 125, 177–9, 211
Crowe, Catherine 111
Cullen, Professor William 18, 64
Culzean Castle 6

Dalzel, Alexander 19
Darwin, Charles 40, 87, 88, 109,
  154, 171
Darwin, Erasmus 80, 81

Davis, David 77
Davy, Humphry 107
Dawson, Mr (surgeon in
  Bathgate) 30–2, 45
De Beers Mining Company 141
De Quincey, Thomas 222
Dickson, Professor 99
diphtheria 190
Dodsley, Robert 14
Douglas, Andrew 171, 174
Douglas, Marquis of 66
Drummond, Mr 243
Drysdale, Lady 132
Drysdale, Sir William 54
Dunbar, Professor George 18
Duncan, Professor Andrew 18
Duncan, James Matthews 67, 117,
  119, 120, 122, 215
Duncan, Flockhart & Co 117, 119,
  125, 126
Dundas, Henry 16–18, 35, 37
  Dundas Despotism 16, 50
Dundas, Lady 65
Duns, Rev John 222, 223, 226, 242
Dutch Liquid *see* chloric ether

East India Company 16, 90
Edinburgh Cholera Health
  Board 92, 93
Edinburgh Daily Review 206
Edinburgh Fever Board 92
Edinburgh Homoeopathic
  Dispensary 155
Edinburgh Lying-In Hospital 45,
  58–60, 62, 202, 203
*Edinburgh Medical and Surgical
  Journal* 23, 44, 69, 77, 84, 97,
  98, 100, 135, 204, 213, 215, 216
Edinburgh Medical Missionary
  Society 224
Edinburgh Medico-Chirurgical
  Society 74, 76, 84, 88, 115,
  120, 122, 148, 149, 188, 198,
  199

Edinburgh Monthly Journal of Medical Science 162
Edinburgh Obstetrics Society 159
Edinburgh Philosophical Institution 226
Edinburgh Philosophical Journal 23
Edinburgh Review 19, 81
Edinburgh Royal Dispensary for the Poor 32, 62
Edinburgh Royal Infirmary 35, 36, 109, 137, 171, 175, 188, 208, 211, 214, 216, 219, 224
Edinburgh Royal Maternity Hospital 59, 60, 70, 142, 148, 210
Edinburgh Town Council 21, 50, 170–2
Edinburgh University 13
Elcho, Lord 182–185
Elliotson, Professor John 158
emigration from Scotland 5
Empress Eugenie 142
Encyclopaedia Britannica 20
Episcopal Church of Scotland 131
Erichsen, Professor 206
Esquirol, Jean-Etienne 42
ether 105–16, 128, 133–5, 151
    first use in an operation 105
    first use in obstetric delivery 112
    social use of 111
    sulphuric ether 128
    use in an amputation 108, 109
Evangelical Movement 86, 88, 104, 128, 221, 222, 224
evolution, theories of 78–82
    opposition to 86–88
Ewart, Colonel 142

Fairbairn, Mr 147
Falkirk Public Dispensary 30
famines in the late seventeenth century 2
Ferguson, Professor Adam 18, 79

Fergusson, Professor Sir William 25, 27, 206
Fettes, Sir William 18
Fife, Sir John 133, 134
Fleming, J.B. 110
Flourens, Marie Jean Pierre 134
Fohmann, Professor 41
Forbes, Professor Edward 170
Fox, Charles James 37
Free Church of Scotland 86, 88, 128, 131, 156, 164, 171, 221
    formation in 1843 86, 221
French Academy of Sciences 168
French Revolution 17, 22, 35
Friends of the People 17
Frost, Eban 108
Fyfe, Baillie 227

Gairdner, Dr William T. 32, 171, 174
Galen 106
galvanism 70–3
Gaskell, Elizabeth 235
Gavarret, Jules 72
General Medical Council, establishment of 185
Geological Society 81
Gilchrist, W. 95
Gillon, Andrew of Wallhouse 11
Girdwood, Miss ('Cinderella') 47, 48
Glasgow Arms Bank 4, 9
Glasgow Royal Infirmary 214, 216, 225
Glenmavis distillery 8
Glover, Dr 152
Gold Fields of South Africa Ltd 141
gold mining 141
Gooch, Richard 77
Gordon, Alexander 194, 195, 201
Graham, James 180
Graham, Professor Robert 56–8
Grangemouth 10
Grant, Sir Alexander 227–9

graverobbers 24–9
Gream, Dr George 127, 128
Great Exhibition, 1851 126, 150, 167, 211
Great Pyramid of Giza 191, 192
Greener, Hannah 132–4
Greenhow, Dr Edward 98
Gregory, Professor James 37
Gregory, Professor John 18
Gregory, Professor William 117, 119, 158
Greig, Dr 205
Grenville, Charles 90–2
Grey, Earl 68
Grey, Sir George 183
Grieve, Baillie 54
Grindlay, Elisabeth (wife of Walter) 140
Grindlay, Isabella (grandmother of JYS) 5
Grindlay, Jessie (later wife of JYS) 48, 52, 53
  proposal from JYS 53
Grindlay, Richard (son of Walter) 139, 140
Grindlay, Walter (father-in-law of JYS) 31, 52–4, 61, 62, 65, 138–40
  death of 140
  loans to JYS 61, 138
Grindlay, Williamina (daughter of Walter) 119, 120, 232, 245
Guislain, Dr 42
Gull, Dr 232
Guthrie, Samuel 118, 119
Guthrie, Rev Thomas 164, 165, 221, 238
Guy's Hospital, London 40, 153, 214
gynaecology 73, 187

Hall, Dr John 124, 125
Hambro, C. J. 111
Hamilton, Alexander 58, 59

Hamilton, Professor Alexander 194
Hamilton, Duke of 49, 66
Hamilton, Professor James 32, 45, 49–51, 58, 59, 63, 73, 160, 196
Hamilton, Professor Sir William 222
Hammond, William 213
Handyside, Peter 205
Hanna, Dr 238, 245
Hahnemann, Samuel 155, 156
Hare, Margaret 25
Hare, William 25, 26
  Burke and Hare trial 22, 25, 26
hashish (as an anaesthetic) 106
Hastings, Sir Charles 169, 184–6
Headlam, Thomas 182–5
Hebra, Ferdiand von 197
henbane (as an anaesthetic) 106
Henderson, William 155, 157
Herbert, Sydney 178, 179
Herder, Gottfried 70
Herodotus 191, 192
Hippocrates 94
Hogg, Mr (bank manager) 34, 35
Holmes, Oliver Wendell 105
Holmes, Thomas 212–15
Home, David Milne 227
homoeopathy 155–9, 162
Honourable Society of Improvers 4, 5
Hooper, Robert 77
Hope, Professor John 18
Hope, Thomas of Rankeillour 4
Hopetoun, Earl of 3–5
Horner, Francis 19, 36
hospitalism 210–17, 238
hospitals 210–17, 236
  design 210, 211
  diseases in 211
  overcrowding 210
Huguenots 10
Hugo of Lucca 106
Hunter, John 35

Hutton, James 78–81
hydrochloric acid 126

Imperial Academy of Medicine,
     Paris 168
inflammation 33
     JYS thesis on 33
Inglis, John 227
Inveraray Castle 6, 168
Inverkip 30
Ireland, Alexander 87, 88
Irons, Isaac (pen-name of Robert
     Lee) 157–9, 161

Jackson, Charles 107, 116
Jacobite Rebellions 15
Jameson, Professor Robert 170
Jardine, Mr 11
Jarvey, George (great-uncle of
     JYS) 12, 30
Jarvey, Mary (mother of JYS) *see*
     Simpson, Mary
Jarvis (manservant to JYS) 65, 142,
     144, 240, 242
Jeffrey, Francis 19
Jenkinson, Mr 243
Jervais, George (uncle of JYS) 190
Jex-Blake, Sophia 229, 230
Johnson, Dr Samuel 5
Johnstone, Mrs 151, 152
Johnstone, Sir Frederic 231
Jones, Professor Thomas
     Wharton 25

Kaffir Wars 23
Karolinska Instituet, Sweden 114
Kay, William (uncle of JYS) 7
Keate, Robert 36
Keiller, Alexander 189
Keith, Dr George 67, 112, 119, 120
Keith, William 206
Kennedy, Professor Evory 54, 132,
     216
Kilian, Hermann 70

King Henry III of England 85
King Henry VIII 182
King Louis IX of France 85
King Robert Bruce 10
King Robert II of Scotland 85
King's College Hospital,
     London 214
Kirk, John 178
Kirkliston 7, 8
Klein, Professor Johannes 199
Knights Hospitallers 82
Knox, Robert 22–8, 33, 234, 235
     accused of graverobbing 26–8
     support from Simpson family 27,
     28
Kolletschka, Professor 197

L'Isere, Marc Colombat de 73, 77
Laennec 65
Lair, Samuel 65
Lambeth Water Company 104
Lancet, The 91, 97, 123, 127, 133,
     153, 157, 158, 161, 162, 167,
     206, 215, 216, 223, 225–8
Larrey, Baron Dominique 41
Latta, Dr Thomas 93
Lauderdale, Earl of 35, 37
'laughing gas' (nitrous oxide) 107
Lavoisier, Antoine 35
Lawson, Thomas 109, 124
Laycock, Dr Thomas 172–6
Lee, Robert 54, 77, 159, 160
     opposition to JYS use of
          forceps 160
Lemaire 225
leper hospitals 82–5
leprosy 82–5
Letheon (patent anaesthetic) 108,
     116
Lewins, Dr 76
Liebeg, Justus 197
Lincoln, Countess of 66
Lister, Professor Joseph 178, 208,
     209, 216, 225

Liston, Professor Robert 21, 25, 27, 41, 50, 64, 108, 109, 111, 115, 150
Livingstone, David 235
Lizars, John 22, 24, 27, 152, 168
Locock, Charles 114
London Gazette 219
London Hospital 214
Londonderry, Marquess of 19
Long, Crawford 107
Lorne, Marquis and Marchioness of 67
Loudon, J.C. 210, 211
Louis, Pierre 41
Lowe, Robert 226
lycanthropia 82
Lyell, Charles 81

mandragora (as an anaesthetic) 106
Marjoribanks, Alexander of Balbardie 8, 11
Massachusetts General Hospital, Boston 105, 107, 108, 116, 125
  ban on use of chloroform 125
  first operation using ether 105
Maxwell, Robert of Arkland 4
MacArthur, Dr Alexander 14, 15, 19, 27
McDougal, Helen 25
McDowell, Ephraim 74, 75
McGrigor, Sir James 41
Mackenzie, Richard 125, 178
McKie, Thomas 228, 240
Mackintosh, John 45–47
Maclagan, Douglas 39
McLaren, Duncan 54
McLeod, Dr 216
measles 82, 203
Medical Gazette 160, 225
Medical Times 168, 169
Medical Society of Ghent 47
Meigs, Professor Charles 113, 114, 132, 195, 196

Melbourne, Lord 38, 160
Mesmer, Franz Anton 158
mesmerism 158, 222
Mid Calder Oil Company 141
Middlesex Hospital 40, 214
midwifery 55, 152, 187
Miller, Alexander 25
Miller, Professor James 117, 122, 150–2, 206
Milton, John 13
Moir, Dr John 59, 111, 112, 243, 244
Moncrieffe, Sir Thomas 230, 231, 238
Monro, Alexander I 21, 234
Monro, Alexander II 18, 21, 234
Monro, Alexander III 14, 21–25, 234
Monthly Journal of Medical Science 69, 112, 113, 123, 169
  co-founded by JYS 69
Monthyon Prize 168
'moral treatment' of the insane 42
Mordaunt, Sir Charles and Lady Harriet 230–2, 237, 238
Morgan, Dr 243, 245
Morrison, T. D. 122
Morton, William T. G. 107, 108, 116
Munro, Dr 240, 241, 243
Mylne, Robert 6

Napoleon Bonaparte 41
Napoleon III 176
Neudorfer, Professor 206
Newbridge 95
Newhaven Free Church, Edinburgh 147
Newland, John and Elizabeth 10,11
Newnham, Dr 109
Newton, Sir Isaac 192, 193
Nichol, John Pringle 82
Nightingale, Florence 178, 235
nitrous oxide (as an anaesthetic) 107
Noble, Dr 175

North, Christopher *see* Wilson, John

North London Hospital 40

Norton, Caroline 235

O'Neil, Mr 140

O'Shaughnessy, Dr W.B. 93

Oakbank Oil Company 141

opium (as an anaesthetic) 106, 242

Order of St Olaf 218

Orford, Dr 230, 231

ovarian cysts 74

ovariotomy 74, 75

Owen, Sir Richard 40

Paisley Bank 34

Paley, William 13, 222

Palmerston, Lord 178–80

Panmure, Lord 179

Paris, Matthew 82

Pasteur, Louis 208, 211

Paterson, David 25

Paxton, Joseph 210

Pearson, John (brother-in-law of JYS) 45, 55, 68

Peel, Sir Robert 138, 139

Pender, John 228, 239, 240, 242

Peninsular Wars 39

Peters Field slaughter 17

Petrie, Agnes 119, 120

Petrie, Captain 119, 220

Philip, Mr 243

phosgene 126

phrenology 158

Pickford, Dr James 114

Pillans, Professor James 19, 20

Pinel, Philippe 41, 42

Pirrie, Professor William 205, 225

Pitt, William 16, 17, 35, 37

placenta, diseases of 43, 44, 47

Playfair, John 81

Pliny 191

Pneumatic Medical Institute 106, 107

Pope Alexander III 82

Porter, John 124

Positions held by James Y. Simpson
  assistant to Dr Gairdner 32
  assistant to Professor Thomson 33, 38
  consultant at Edinburgh Lying-In Hospital 58
  consultant obstetrician, Edinburgh Royal Maternity Hospital 59
  deputy to Professor Thomson 44
  director of Edinburgh Royal Maternity Hospital 60
  Doctor of Civil Law, Oxford University 224
  Fellow of the Royal College of Physicians of Edinburgh 47
  Knight of the Ordfer of St Olaf 218
  partner of John Mackintosh 45
  Physician to Queen Victoria 68
  President of the Medico-Chirurgical Society of Edinburgh 148, 188
  President of the Royal College of Physicians of Edinburgh 148, 154, 188
  President of the Royal Medical Society 38, 43, 44
  Professor of Archaeology, Royal Scottish Academy 190
  Professor of Midwifery 55

press-gangs 7

Priestley, Joseph 106

Priestly, William 173, 176, 185

Prince Albert 67, 150, 167, 168

Prince George, Duke of Cambridge 66

Prince of Wales (later Edward VII) 230–2

Princess Marie Amelia of Baden 65, 66

Pringle, George 178

Privy Council 11

Provincial Medical and Surgical Association (later the British Medical Association) 169, 182, 183

Provincial Medical and Surgical Journal (later the *British Medical Journal*) 70, 123, 154

puerperal fever 193–201, 202, 203

Queen Charlotte's Lying-In Hospital, London 127

Queen Victoria 1, 67, 68, 127, 167, 232

use of chloroform in childbirth 167

Quinton, James and Mary 163–6

Quinton, Rochester 163–6

Radford, Thomas 70

Ramsbotham, Francis 198

Reform Act, 1832 50

Reid, John 14, 15, 22, 25, 40, 46, 47, 52, 53, 77, 222

Renton, Robert 54, 154

resurrectionists *see* graverobbers

Retzius, Professor Magnus 114

Ritchie, John 54

Robertson, Argyll 145

Robertson, Professor William 18, 25, 79

Rokitansky, Carl 197, 199

Roux, Professor 23

Royal Bank of Scotland 13

Royal Burghs Act, 1833 50

Royal College of Physicians of Edinburgh 2, 21, 47, 89, 148, 152, 155, 156, 158, 171, 188, 219

Royal College of Physicians of London 78, 89, 181–6, 232

Royal College of Surgeons of Edinburgh 21, 23, 26–8, 30, 35–7, 64, 118, 202, 219

Royal College of Surgeons of England 40

Royal Faculty of Physicians and Surgeons of Glasgow 181

Royal Free Hospital, London 214

Royal Medical Society 35, 38, 43, 44, 219

Royal Naval Dockyard, Chatham 10

Royal Naval Dockyard, Port Royal, Jamaica 10

Royal Physical Society 38

Royal Scottish Academy 190

Royal Society 67, 123, 160, 171

Royal Society of Arts 150

Royal Society of Edinburgh 23, 78, 79, 192, 204, 227

Royal Society of Scotland 191

Ruskin, John 235

Russell, Baillie 227

Russell, James 16, 27

Russell, Lord John 68, 218, 235

Russell, William 177

Sacred Cubit 193

St Bartholomew's Hospital, London 23, 40, 214, 215

St Columba 191

St George's Hospital, London 40, 212, 214, 215

St Mary's Hospital, London 214

St Matthew 235

St Thomas's Hospital, London 40, 212

scarlet fever 203

Scotsman newspaper 123, 211

Scott, Sir Walter 14, 48, 66, 191

Scottish Enlightenment 79

Second Sikh War, 1848–49 124

Secretary of State for Scotland 15, 168

Semmelweiss, Ignaz 196–201, 202

thesis on puerperal fever 200

shale oil production 141

Sharpey, Professor William 171, 172, 174–6
Ship Bank 4
Sibbald, Sir Robert 2
Siddons, Sarah 235
Silliman, Professor Benjamin 118
Simmons, Mrs 133, 134
Simpson, Alexander or Sandy (brother of JYS) 10, 13, 30, 43, 45, 47, 59, 61, 65, 67, 68, 138, 232, 240, 245
Simpson, Alexander (grandfather of JYS) 1, 3–8
Simpson, Alexander (nephew of JYS) 234, 240, 242, 243, 245
Simpson, Alexander (uncle of JYS) 5, 7
Simpson, David (brother of JYS) 10, 31, 42, 45, 68
Simpson, David (father of JYS) 7–9, 28
    death of 28
Simpson, David (son of JYS) 147, 148, 219, 234
    death of 219
Simpson, Eve (daughter of JYS) 147, 148, 220, 221, 237–239, 241–245
Simpson, George (brother of JYS) 10
Simpson, George (uncle of JYS) 7, 8
Simpson, James (son of JYS) 147, 223
    death of 223
Simpson, Sir James Young
    admitted as a Freemason 30
    appearance as a child 12
    appearance as an adult 63
    appointed assistant to Dr Gairdner 32
    appointed assistant to Professor Thomson 33, 38
    appointed deputy to Professor Thomson 44
    appointed Physician to Queen Victoria 68
    arrival at Edinburgh University 13
    attacked over use of chloroform 153, 154
    award of Baronetcy 218, 219
    award of Stewart Bursary 20
    birth and early childhood 9, 10
    candidature for Principal of Edinburgh University 227–9
    character of as a child 12
    co-founding *The Monthly Journal of Medical Science* 69
    consultant at Edinburgh Lying-In Hospital 58
    daily routine as a GP 143, 144
    death of 232, 233, 245
    debts to Walter Grindlay 60, 61, 138
    development of acupressure 204–9
    drafting bill to regulate medicine in the UK 183–6
    early use of stethoscope 65
    enrolment as medical student 20
    experiments with chloroform 117–22, 126, 151
    experiments with galvanism 70–3
    Fellow of the Royal College of Physicians of Edinburgh 47
    first obstetric delivery using ether 112
    Freeman of the City of Edinburgh 229
    funeral of 233
    GP at 2 Teviot Row 60, 61
    graduation as MD 33
    honours received 148, 168, 218, 229
Simpson, Sir James Young (*contd*)
    interest in archaeology 190–3
    investments in business 140, 141

joining Free Church of Scotland 88, 221
leprosy, study of 82–5
Licentiate of the Royal College of Surgeons 30
marriage to Jessie Grindlay 53
obstetrics, study of 32
onset of angina 220, 230, 232
opposition to homoeopathy 157, 158, 162
pamphlet on chloroform 123, 124
partner of John Mackintosh 45
performing first cervical amputation 76
pioneer in gynaecology 73
poetry of 48, 49
positions at Edinburgh Royal Maternity Hospital 59, 60
President of the Medico-Chirurgical Society of Edinburgh 148
President of the Royal College of Physicians of Edinburgh 148
President of the Royal Medical Society 38, 43, 44
Professor of Midwifery, campaign for 50–5
Professor of Midwifery, election as 55
puerperal fever, views on 196–201
purchase of Viewbank, Trinity 146
research into cholera 94–104
research into anaesthesia in surgery 110, 188
start of education 12
studies in Greek and Latin 18–20
suffering from depression 30, 145
support for John Knox 27, 28

support for women doctors 229, 230
thesis on inflammation 33
tour of France and Belgium, 1835 39–42
treatment of aristocracy 65–7
use of Air Tractor forceps 159
use of vaginal speculum 65
visit to London, 1835 39–41
working in Bathgate 30, 31
Simpson, Jessie (daughtet of JYS) 147, 219, 220
death of 220
Simpson, Jessie (*nee* Grindlay, wife of JYS) 53–5, 61–3, 119, 120, 139, 140, 147, 150, 164, 168, 187, 232, 239, 245
death of 232
taking chloroform 119, 120
Simpson, John (brother of JYS) 10, 13, 31, 46, 47, 68
Simpson, John (uncle of JYS) 5, 7
Simpson, Maggie (daughter of JYS) 147
death of, aged 4 147
Simpson, Magnus (son of JYS) 147, 148, 221, 239, 240, 242
Simpson, Margaret (aunt of JYS) 7
Simpson, Mary (daughter of JYS) 147
death of, aged 2 147
Simpson, Mary *nee* Jarvey (mother of JYS) 8–10, 12
death of 12
Simpson, Mary (sister of JYS, later Mrs Pearson) 10, 12, 47, 55, 61, 68
Simpson, Thomas (brother of JYS) 10, 31, 68
Simpson, Thomas (uncle of JYS) 7, 8
Simpson, Walter (son of JYS) 147, 148, 219, 221, 224, 225, 232, 233, 236, 239, 240, 242–5

Simpson, William (son of JYS) 147, 148, 221, 239, 243–245
Sims, Marion 73
Sinclair, Sir John 6
Sisters of Charity 178
Skoda , Joseph 65, 197, 199
Slackend Farm 5, 7, 8
smallpox 82, 203
Smith, Adam 79
Smith, Dr Andrew 178
Smith, Protheroe 131
Smyth, Professor Piazzi 191–3
Snow, John 102–4, 134, 135, 137, 232
Society for Relieving Indigent Pregnant Women 58
Society for the Promotion of Christian Knowledge 223
Society of Antiquaries of Scotland 191
Society of the Friends of the People 17, 22, 26, 35
Southwark and Vauxhall Water Company 104
Spence, Professor James 206, 225
Spurgeon, Mr 240
Standard Life Assurance Company 13, 68
Statistical Account of Scotland 6
stethoscope, use of 65
Stewart, Rev Alexander 232
Stewart, Professor Dugald 18
Stewart, Rev James 20
Stewart Bursary 20
Storer, Dr 240
Storrer, John 183, 184
Struthers, Alexander 178
surgical fever 202–4
Sutherland, Duke and Duchess of 67, 235
sweating sickness 82
'Sweet Whiskey' (chloric ether) 118
Syme, Professor James 27–9, 54, 120, 124, 125, 150, 151, 155, 163, 165, 168, 171, 172, 176, 178, 206, 207, 226
syphilis 191

Tait, Lawson 215
Thackeray, William Makepeace 63, 235
Thatcher, John 54
Theodoric 106
Thistle Bank 4
Thomson, Professor John 27, 32, 33–40, 44–6, 89, 154
Thomson, William 44, 45
Todd, Dr 125
Tootal, Mrs 175, 176
Torphichen 7
Torrisdale Castle 168
Treaty of Fontainebleau 9
Treaty of Union, 1707 16
Trollope, Anthony 66
Tsar Nicholas I of Russia 176
Tuke, John 232
Turner, John 38
Tyler, Dr 132

uniformitarianism 80
United States Dispensatory 118
University College Hospital, London 108, 109, 158, 171, 212

vaginal speculum, use of 65
Ventouse Vacuum Extractor 159
Vienna Lying-In Hospital 196, 198, 199, 201

Wakley, Thomas 223
Waldie, David 117, 119
Walker, Dr 97
Wallace, Alfred Russell 88
Wallace, Professor William 20
Waller, John 77
Walpole, Robert 185
Wardell, Dr 126
Warren, John Collins 105, 108

Watson, Heron 178
Watson, Sir Thomas 89, 104
Weir, Dr Graham 112
Wells, Horace 107, 116
Wells, Spenser 178
Westminster Confession of
      Faith 221, 222
Westminster Hospital, London
      214
Westminster Medical Society 128,
      135
whisky distilling 7, 8
White, Dr 34
whooping-cough 82
Wilde, Sir William 192

Wilson, Professor John
      ('Christopher North') 20
Winchburgh 3, 5
Wollstonecraft, Mary 141
Wood, Alexander 228
Wood, Dr Andrew 171, 172, 174–6,
      242–4

York County Hospital 173
York Medical School 173
Young, Rev Robert 238
Young's Paraffin Light and Mineral
      Oil Company 141

Zeigler, Dr 76, 112